HANDBOOK OF
SKELETAL RADIOLOGY

HANDBOOKS IN RADIOLOGY SERIES

Other Volumes in Series

Handbook of Chest Radiology
STUART A. GROSKIN, M.D.

Handbook of Gastrointestinal and Genitourinary Radiology
STEPHEN R. ELL, M.D., Ph.D.

Handbook of Head and Neck Imaging, Second Edition
H. RIC HARNSBERGER, M.D.

Handbook of Interventional Radiology and Angiography
Second Edition
MYRON WOJTOWYCZ, M.D.

Handbook of Neuroradiology: Brain and Skull, Second Edition
ANNE G. OSBORN, M.D. AND KAREN A. TONG, M.D.

Handbook of Nuclear Medicine, Second Edition
FREDERICK L. DATZ, M.D.

Handbook of Pediatric Radiology
VESNA MARTICH KRISS, M.D.

HANDBOOK OF
SKELETAL RADIOLOGY

B. J. MANASTER, M.D., Ph.D.
Professor of Radiology
Vice Chair, Department of Radiology
University of Utah School of Medicine
Salt Lake City, Utah

SECOND EDITION

with 123 *illustrations*

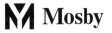 Mosby

St. Louis Baltimore Boston
Carlsbad Chicago Naples New York Philadelphia Portland
London Madrid Mexico City Singapore Sydney Tokyo Toronto Wiesbaden

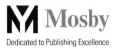

Dedicated to Publishing Excellence

A Times Mirror
Company

Vice President and Publisher: Anne S. Patterson
Editor: Elizabeth Corra
Associate Developmental Editor: Christine Pluta
Project Manager: Chris Baumle
Production Editor: Anthony Trioli
Designer: Nancy McDonald
Manufacturing Manager: William A. Winneberger, Jr.

SECOND EDITION
Copyright © 1997 by Mosby-Year Book, Inc.

Previous editions copyrighted 1989, by Year Book Medical Publishers, Inc.

Printed in the United States of America
Composition by Maryland Composition Company, Inc.
Printing/binding by Maple-Vail Book Manufacturing Group

Mosby–Year Book, Inc.
11830 Westline Industrial Drive
St. Louis, Missouri 63146

Library of Congress Cataloging in Publication Data
Manaster, B.J.
    Handbook of skeletal radiology / B.J. Manaster. — 2nd ed.
      p.   cm. — (Handbooks in radiology series)
    Includes bibliographical references and index.
    ISBN 0-8151-7032-7 (pbk.)
    1. Skeleton—Radiography—Handbooks, manuals, etc. 2. Skeleton—
Diseases—Diagnosis—Handbooks, manuals, etc. I. Manaster, B. J.
Skeletal radiology. II. Title. III. Series.
    [DNLM: 1. Bone and Bones—radiography—handbooks. WE 39 M267h
1997]
RC930.5.M36   1997
616.7'107572—dc20
DNLM/DLC
for Library of Congress   96-9383
                                               CIP

97 98 99 00 / 9 8 7 6 5 4 3 2

To Steve, Tracy Joy, and Katy Rose

Preface

This book is designed primarily for use by diagnostic radiology residents, who will find it a handy source in day-to-day film interpretation, as well as a complete source for board review. Orthopedic residents and clinicians in rheumatology and rehabilitative medicine will find pertinent information relating to their interests.

The book is divided into major sections covering tumor, arthritis, trauma, metabolic bone disease, congenital abnormalities, and a few miscellaneous items. Outline form has been used to allow a quick review. The tumor and arthritis sections begin with an introductory chapter outlining the author's approach to the work-up and diagnosis of these disease processes. The introduction is followed by discussions of the individual diseases, each of which is outlined using the same format; with repeated use, the reader will find that this organization allows easy reference.

The second edition updates many facts, most of which relate to MR anatomy and pathology. Also, this edition features 50% more illustrations, and a trauma section that is double the size of that in the previous handbook. It may be of interest to the reader to know that the ACR Learning File (Musculoskeletal Section), produced on videodisk as well as CD-ROM, was produced by the same author, and is organized to mirror this handbook. Together, the two act as a completely illustrated orthopaedic radiology text.

A "key concepts" box is found at the beginning of each section. This, by its nature, cannot be all-inclusive, but does give quick reference to the most common features of each disease process.

B. J. Manaster, M.D., Ph.D.

Contents

1

Tumors

GENERALIZATIONS

Individual tumors are discussed according to a slightly modified World Health Organization (WHO) classification in this chapter. The reader is strongly urged to read this introductory chapter first.

A. The purpose of learning the characteristics of musculoskeletal tumors is to be an effective consultant to the clinician in terms of:
   1. Work-up of a new lesion: Identify a lesion or arrive at a reasonable differential diagnosis. Determine whether work-up beyond plain radiograph is necessary. If so, provide a cost-effective work-up that leads neither to over-treatment of a benign lesion or under-treatment of an aggressive lesion.
   2. Guidance of biopsy and/or surgical resection: The radiologist must understand the natural history of the lesion and must be conversant with the surgeon's treatment options in order to give a complete assessment of tumor involvement. The radiologist must also be aware of which diagnostic modality is most suitable for this purpose for each tumor.
   3. Knowledgeable post-treatment follow-up: Given the natural history of the lesion and the treatment in the individual case, the radiologist should know which diagnostic modalities can most effectively monitor for recurrence and complications.
B. The work-up of any musculoskeletal tumor must begin with a plain radiograph. This usually does not add much information regarding soft tissue tumors, but may reveal fat density or dystrophic calcification in these tumors. On the other hand, with osseous tumors, the plain film is the most useful imaging tool in determining biologic activity and, often, histology. The plain film will often provide the definitive diagnosis. If it does not, it should be used to place the lesion in one of the following categories:
   1. A benign "leave-me-alone" lesion that is best totally ignored. The most notable example is benign fibrous cortical defect.
   2. A lesion that is almost certainly benign and can be safely watched

for confirmation of the diagnosis. Examples of this type of lesion are nonossifying fibroma, fibrous dysplasia, or myositis ossificans.

3. A benign symptomatic lesion which needs no further work-up prior to surgery.
4. A lesion with uncertain diagnosis regarding benign or malignant status, requiring work-up and biopsy.
5. A malignant lesion requiring preoperative work-up and biopsy.

In order to categorize an osseous tumor properly, radiologists have developed *ten determinants* which must be assessed in each case. If they are accurately assessed, the diagnosis, or the two or three most likely diagnoses, usually becomes obvious. Generalizations applicable to each determinant are discussed below:

1. Age of patient: This is more important in some lesions than in others and may occasionally lead to the correct diagnosis when the tumor is otherwise atypical. Common tumors in various age groups are as follows:

Age (yr)	Lesion
1	Metastatic neuroblastoma
1–10	Ewing's sarcoma (tubular bones)
10–20	Aneurysmal bone cyst
10–30	Osteosarcoma, Ewing's sarcoma (flat bones)
Skeletally immature	Chondroblastoma
Skeletally mature—50	Giant cell tumor (GCT)
30–60	Chondrosarcoma, primary lymphoma, Malignant fibrous histiocytoma, Fibrosarcoma
50–80	Metastasis, multiple myeloma

2. Soft tissue involvement.
   a. Cortical breakthrough of a bone lesion to create a soft tissue mass generally suggests an aggressive lesion.
   b. Such a soft tissue mass generally distorts muscle planes but otherwise leaves them intact; infection, on the other hand, often obliterates these planes.
   c. Soft tissue sarcomas (such as liposarcoma, malignant fibrous histiocytoma [MFH], synovial sarcoma) often appear radiographically and at surgery to be very distinct and even encapsulated, leading to the mistaken assumption that they can be "shelled out" successfully; benign soft tissue tumors (especially desmoids) may, on the other hand, appear very infiltrative and locally aggressive.
3. Pattern of bone destruction.
   a. Geographic: least aggressive, well-defined margin.

   b. Moth-eaten: more aggressive; margin less well-defined.
   c. Permeative: highly aggressive, poorly demarcated, and often even very difficult to visualize.
4. Size of lesion.
5. Location of lesion.
   a. The *particular bone* may be important. For example, certain tumors—adamantinoma, ossifying fibroma, chondromyxoid fibroma—occur much more commonly in the tibia than elsewhere. Another example might be thin tubular bones, such as the ulna and fibula, where lesions such as nonossifying fibroma [NOF] and aneurysmal bone cyst [ABC], which are usually eccentrically placed, appear centrally placed owing to the small diameter of the bone.
   b. Flat vs. tubular bones: Many lesions are found more commonly in one than the other.
   c. Appendicular vs. axial skeleton: Again, many lesions are found more commonly in one than the other.
   d. Epiphysis, metaphysis, or diaphysis: Some lesions are dependably found in one region or another; for example, chondroblastoma is the only lesion frequently found in the epiphysis, osteosarcoma is most commonly metaphyseal, and Ewing's sarcoma is usually diaphyseal.
   e. Central, eccentric, or cortical epicenter of the lesion: For example, an expanded nonaggressive lytic lesion in the metaphysis of a tubular bone is more likely a solitary bone cyst, ABC, or NOF if the epicenter is located centrally, eccentrically, or cortically, respectively.
6. Zone of transition from abnormal to normal bone.
   a. Wide: Aggressive.
   b. Narrow: Nonaggressive.
7. Margin of lesion: Sclerotic or nonsclerotic.
   a. Note that ''margin'' is a different entity than ''zone of transition.'' Logically, most nonaggressive lesions have a sclerotic margin and narrow zone of transition, and most aggressive lesions do not have a sclerotic margin and have a wide zone of transition; there are, however, some lesions that typically have a narrow zone of transition but no sclerotic margin (GCT and occasionally, plasmacytoma).
   b. These characteristics are important determinants in these lesions.
8. Presence of visible tumor matrix.
   a. Aggressive bone-forming tumors produce amorphous osteoid, which may be less dense than or as dense as normal bone.

      b. Less aggressive bone-forming tumors produce better organized dense bone.

      c. Cartilage-forming tumors produce a stippled matrix with C and J shapes; the matrix is denser than normal bone.

  9. Host response.

      a. Cortical thickening, expansion, or penetration.

      b. Periosteal reaction.

  10. Polyostotic vs. monostotic lesion: Polyostotic lesions automatically restrict the disease process to:

      a. Benign: Fibrous dysplasia, Paget's, histiocytosis, multiple exostoses, multiple enchondromatosis.

      b. Malignant: Metastases, myeloma, or primary bone tumors with bony metastases (Ewing's sarcoma, osteosarcoma, MFH).

  11. After the ten major determinants are identified, a *conclusion* should be drawn that states whether the lesion is *aggressive or nonaggressive*. Note that the conclusion should *not* be whether the lesion is malignant or benign; several aggressive lesions are, in fact, benign (e.g., histiocytosis, ABC, infection).

C. Surgical staging of solitary bone tumors and soft tissue sarcomas, Enneking methodology,[1] utilized when the lesion is felt to be aggressive.

  1. Accepted in the orthopaedic community as a guideline to both prognosis and treatment; uses both histologic and radiographic information.

  2. This staging system does not apply to metastatic lesions or round cell lesions, but does include Ewing's sarcoma.

      a. G: grade (histologic). Appropriate grading requires representative tissue sampling at biopsy, often guided by imaging.

        (1) G_0—benign.

        (2) G_1—low-grade, malignant.

        (3) G_2—high-grade, malignant.

      b. S: site (radiographic and clinical features). This is determined by cross-sectional imaging (usually magnetic resonance [MR]).

        (1) T_0—true capsule surrounds lesion (reactive rim of tissue).

        (2) T_1—extracapsular, intracompartmental; compartments are defined as follows:

          a Skin—subcutaneous.

          b Parosseous—a potential compartment is seen when a lesion pushes muscle away from bone without invading either muscle or cortex.

          c Bone—intracortical; also a lesion in ray of the hand or foot is considered intracompartmental.

          d Muscle compartments—may contain more than one muscle if the muscle group is limited by a fascial plane:

        i Posterior compartment calf.
      ii Anterior compartment calf.
    iii Anterolateral compartment calf.
    iv Anterior thigh.
     v Medial thigh.
    vi Posterior thigh.
   vii Buttocks.
 viii Volar forearm.
    ix Dorsal forearm.
     x Anterior arm.
    xi Posterior arm.
   xii Deltoid.
 xiii Periscapula.

(3) T_2—extracapsular, extracompartmental extension from any of the above-named compartments or abutment of major neurovascular structures; in addition, some sites are extracompartmental by origin:

a Midhand, dorsal or palmar.
b Mid- or hindfoot.
c Popliteal fossa.
d Femoral triangle.
e Obturator foramen.
f Sciatic notch.
g Antecubital fossa.
h Axilla.
i Periclavicular.
j Paraspinal.
k Periarticular, elbow or knee.

c. M: metastases, usually bone or lung.
(1) M_0—no metastases.
(2) M_1—metastases present.
d. Staging. Uses grade, site, and metastases as follows:
(1) *Benign:*

1 (Inactive)	2 (Active)	3 (Aggressive)
G_0	G_0	G_0
T_0	T_0	T_{1-2}
M_0	M_0	M_{0-1}

(2) *Malignant:*

Ia: Low-grade without metastases, intracompartmental.
Ib: Low-grade without metastases, extracompartmental.
IIa: High-grade without metastases, intracompartmental.

IIb: High-grade without metastases, extracompartmental.

III: Low- or high-grade with metastases.

Ia	Ib	IIa	IIb	III
G_1	G_1	G_2	G_2	G_2
T_1	T_2	T_1	T_2	T_2
M_0	M_0	M_0	M_0	M_1

D. Surgical treatment options. Be ready to discuss these with your surgeon, and be certain your cross-sectional imaging answers all potential questions required to plan the surgery.

1. Intralesional excision (curettage): Tumor is found at the margin.

2. Marginal excision (excisional biopsy): Plane of dissection passes through the reactive tissue or pseudocapsule of the lesion; satellites of residual lesion may be found; inadequate for malignant or recurrent benign lesions.

3. Wide excision: Removal of lesion surrounded by an intact cuff of normal tissue. The plane of dissection is well beyond the reactive tissue surrounding the lesion, but the entire muscle or bone is not removed. Because the plane of resection passes through the compartment, skip lesions may remain. Adequate for recurrent, aggressive benign tumors, low-grade sarcomas, and some high-grade sarcomas that have been reduced in bulk by chemotherapy.

4. Radical resection: Removal of the lesion along with the entire muscle, bone, or other involved tissues in the compartment (bones removed joint to joint and muscles removed origin to insertion).

5. Any of these margins can be achieved by either amputation or limb salvage procedures. Limb salvage *en bloc* procedures most commonly fall in the category of wide excisions, offering tumor control without sacrifice of limb. Consideration of limb salvage is based on the staging of the lesion, anatomical location, age (and expected growth) of the patient, extent of local disease, expected function after the procedure, and the efficacy of adjuvant therapy. Studies have shown that the significant factor in tumor surgery is the margin achieved rather than the method of achieving that margin (limb salvage vs. amputation).

E. Philosophy of tumor work-up.

Once a lesion is deemed aggressive and biopsy is planned, the diagnostic work-up should be tailored to the individual lesion to (1) stage the lesion and (2) assist in treatment planning. Preoperative staging should have the following goals: (1) avoid overly extensive (and overly expensive) staging; (2) avoid overly aggressive surgery on low-grade lesions; (3) avoid irreversible undertreatment of aggressive lesions; and (4) if the aggressiveness of the lesion cannot be determined by plain film, it should be completely worked up to determine stage, assuming aggressiveness. Staging is done radiographically by discovering the presence or absence of metastatic disease and by determining whether the lesion is encapsulated, intracompartmental, or extracompartmental. For treatment planning, communication with the surgeon is essential to ensure that the correct questions are addressed and answered by the diagnostic procedures. For example, if amputation is the only surgical option, the work-up need be directed only toward defining the proximal end of the lesion. If, on the other hand, limb salvage is considered, both the proximal and distal extent of bone and muscle involvement must be determined, as well as involvement of vital neurovascular structures. Soft tissues involved by the tumor must be specifically identified. If the lesion is adjacent to a joint, involvement of that joint must be assessed. Bear in mind that it is extremely helpful to the surgeon to have an external landmark on the images, so that measurements of tumor extent can be made with reference to that palpable landmark. Certain surgical options have mechanical requirements. For example, approximately 2 cm of tumor-free superior acetabulum is required for an ideal internal hemipelvectomy. Discuss any such requirements in advance with your surgeon so you can be certain the necessary information is provided with your imaging.

Choice of biopsy site should also be guided by the radiographic work-up. Biopsy must be made of the most aggressive viable portion of the lesion. Typically, the central portion of an aggressive lesion is necrotic, so more information is gained from a peripheral biopsy. Biopsy should be made through an approach that can be resected at the definitive surgical procedure and that, therefore, does not (through possible tumor spill) compromise vital tissue planes or skin that may be needed to close over a resected area. The biopsy site should be within a single compartment and should not approach neurovascular structures. The two most common sites of biopsy error are found with knee and pelvic lesions. When a knee lesion is biopsied, it is often forgetten how large the suprapatellar bursa can be and it may be violated. In the pelvis, it is tempting to pass the needle across the glutei muscles to approach lesions of the iliac wing or sacrum. However, this tissue may be needed as a flap should the patient require a hindquarter amputation; do not violate this tissue without prior discussion with the surgeon.

Percutaneous biopsy by the radiologist has become quite popular since it may reduce both cost and morbidity. The site must be chosen carefully, as described above, and at least three needle passes made. It should be remembered that histologic diagnosis of metastatic disease and myeloma can be made with very little tissue, often with cytology alone, but that diagnosis of primary malignant bone tumors requires a larger amount of tissue. Primary benign bone tumors often require tissue obtained by open biopsy, as even larger specimens are needed for histologic diagnosis.

Keeping in mind the need to arrive at a logical differential diagnosis, the need to stage the lesion correctly, and the need to assist in biopsy and treatment planning, the radiographic work-up may utilize the following imaging studies:

1. Plain film.
    a. The best method for assessing bone detail, aggressiveness of the lesion, and certain diagnostic features, as detailed in Section B of this chapter.
    b. Extent of lesion often can be determined.
    c. Used to assess whether further work-up is required.
2. Radionuclide studies.
    a. Technetium ^{99m}Tc MDP scans are used primarily to determine whether a lesion is monostotic or polyostotic. Such a study is often useful in staging a bone tumor. Although the degree of abnormal uptake may be related to the aggressiveness of the lesion, this does not correlate with histologic grade, and, in fact, some benign lesions, such as osteoid osteoma, show very significant uptake owing to hypervascularity and host bone reaction. A bone scan may not accurately demonstrate extent of lesion: some lesions show an "extended uptake" pattern beyond the margin of tumor, perhaps secondary to hyperemia.
    b. Gallium ^{67}Ga may show uptake in a soft tissue sarcoma and may help differentiate a sarcoma from a benign soft tissue lesion (sensitivity 85%, specificity 92%).[2] This is generally not utilized.
3. Computed tomography (CT). Generally MR is preferred. However, there are a few specific reasons to chose CT:
    a. May add diagnostic features to the lesion. For example, matrix calcification may be better seen.
    b. Thin rim calcification or detail of cortical involvement is seen well.
    c. If CT is chosen for the above reasons, osseous extent can be defined very clearly by measuring Hounsfield units within the marrow. Accuracy is much better in diaphysis than metaphysis or epiphysis.
    d. Extraosseous relations are much better defined than by plain film; most radiologists and clinicians prefer MR for evaluation of extraosseous tissues.

e. Remember always to image the contralateral extremity so that intra- and extraosseous extent can better be identified.

f. Disadvantages: Restricted to axial views or reconstructions in other planes; soft tissue contrast may be limited, especially in a forearm or leg of a thin person; large dose of intravenous (IV) contrast medium may be required.

4. Magnetic resonance imaging (MRI).

a. Tumor work-ups usually require either CT or MRI but should rarely require both because of high cost relative to benefit. Therefore, the more appropriate modality should be chosen at the outset; the choice will depend on the questions that need to be answered. An entirely intraosseous lesion may be examined best by CT, while an entirely extraosseous lesion is far more clearly delineated by MRI. Intraosseous lesions that extend into the soft tissues may be examined by either modality, but many authors feel that MRI more easily answers the pertinent staging and surgical treatment questions of this type of lesion.[3]

b. MR is superior to CT in defining extraosseous relations since soft tissue contrast is superb; T1-weighted images enhance contrast with fat, while T2-weighted images enhance contrast with muscle. Neurovascular structures are seen well without the use of contrast medium.

c. According to the recent Radiologic Diagnostic Oncology Group (RDOG) study, MR is thought to be as accurate as CT in defining marrow extent of the lesion. T1-weighted or inversion recovery images are required for this, as it enhances the contrast between fatty marrow and the lesion. Do not be misled into describing a lesion on MR as "geographic" or having a "narrow zone of transition." Even the most aggressive osteosarcomas often appear on MR as well-defined lesions even though they are highly permeative on plain film. Plain film is more reliable in judging biologic activity.

d. Direct coronal, sagittal, and axial planes are all available.

e. Disadvantage: Neither calcification nor disturbance in cortex is seen as well on MR as on CT.

f. Two sequences are usually obtained in order to best contrast the lesion with surrounding tissue, whether they are fat or muscle. A lesion may appear isointense with surrounding soft tissues on any single sequence. The most commonly used sequences are T1 and T2 spin echo (fast spin echo is acceptable for T2). Other specialized sequences may be used for specific reasons. For example, inversion recovery (STIR) imaging may make a subtle osseous lesion more conspicuous. Although some radiologists feel that gadolinium adds conspicicity to the lesion, it has not been shown to significantly alter diagnostic or site considerations. Remember that axial images are mandatory as specific soft tissue site involvement and neurovascular bundle involvement are not accurately assessed with coronal or sagittal imaging.

g. Different pulse sequences have not, at this writing, achieved the ability to make specific histologic diagnoses based on tumor signal intensity. There are a few exceptions to this statement, including lipomas, hemangiomas, fibromatosis, and pigmented villonodular synovitis. These will be further discussed in later sections of this chapter, but remember that up to 20% of the latter three above-mentioned diagnoses may not follow their MR signal intensity ''rules.'' Thus, when the MR findings are typical, specific diagnoses may be made in a few instances, but this is not the general rule. Most tumors have low T1 osseous signal, T1 soft tissue signal that is isointense with muscle, and high T2 signal. There are a few exceptions to the ''isointense with muscle on T1'' and ''high signal intensity (SI) on T2'' nonspecificity of tumors:

(1) Differential diagnosis for mass with short T1 (high SI):
a lipoma
b hematoma (subacute)
c intralesional hemorrhage
d gadolinium enhancement

(2) Differential diagnosis for mass with low SI on T2:
a hypocellular fibrous tumor
b scar tissue
c dense mineralization
d melanin
e acute hematoma
f vascular flow void
g air
h foreign body
i hemosiderin or iron-containing tissue

h. Avoid using MR for nonaggressive osseous lesions. The results may be confusing, especially if there is a pathologic fracture with hematoma appearing as an inhomogeneous ''mass.''

i. Not only does MR generally not provide a histologic diagnosis, but it also does not reliably differentiate between benign and malignant lesions.[4,5] Generally, benign lesions are smaller, homogeneous, and circumscribed, while malignant lesions are larger, inhomogeneous, and infiltrative. There are many exceptions to this however. Malignant soft tissue lesions frequently develop a ''pseudocapsule'' that appears on MR and at surgery as an encapsulation of a benign lesion. However, nests of tumor cells may be found outside the pseudocapsule. Such lesions need to be treated with wide excision. Conversely, some benign lesions are locally aggressive and may appear on MR as inhomogeneous, large, and infiltrative. These lesions include histiocytoses, fibromatoses, and infection. It is therefore very difficult to reliably diagnose a benign versus malignant musculoskeletal lesion using MR.

j. Hematoma seen on MR may have a complex and variable appearance. Acutely, hematoma may be isointense with muscle on T1 and hypointense on T2 due to the paramagnetic effect of deoxyhemoglobin in red blood cells. With progression, the hematoma becomes bright on T2 and eventually bright on T1 due to conversion to methemoglobin (the hyperintensity begins peripherally and progresses to fill in the lesion). The hematoma may eventually become a seroma (fluid collection with low SI on T1, high SI on T2). Occasionally, one sees fluid-cellular layers, usually in patients who are anticoagulated or have intratumoral bleeding. Large subacute hematomas with rebleeding may have marked signal inhomogeneity and may elicit surrounding tissue edema.

k. Two conditions may overestimate lesion size. Reactive edema around a tumor may appear somewhat ''veil-like'' and be diagnosed correctly as edema, or may simply make the lesion itself seem larger, being similarly low SI on T1 and high on T2 sequences. Chronic hematoma may be even more confusing, appearing very inhomogeneous, mass-like, and involving several compartments in a very infiltrative-appearing pattern. These are often misdiagnosed as tumors, or hematomas arising from a necrotic tumor, which may make the mass seem much larger than it truly is. If biopsy indicates a sarcoma, the optimal treatment is wide excision, which should include this abnormal tissue, whether it is tumor, reactive edema, or hematoma.

5. Tomography: Used only occasionally, when more detailed views of bony architecture are required.

6. Angiography: Rarely used to diagnose or define a tumor, but may be used if embolization of a highly vascular lesion is required prior

to surgery. The study should be tailored to the individual patient. For example, a popliteal fossa angiogram should be performed in the lateral position, once with the knee flexed and once with the knee extended and using vasodilators in each injection to determine vascular involvement by the tumor.

7. Chest film and CT for evaluation of metastatic disease.

8. Ultrasound is often the most effective modality for guidance of soft tissue biopsy, after full-site evaluation is provided by MR and the approach is agreed upon with the surgeon. Spring-loaded biopsy guns are highly effective soft tissue samplers, as they create little artifact but can produce excellent tissue cores with an 18-gauge needle.

9. Suggested algorithm for osseous lesion work-up:

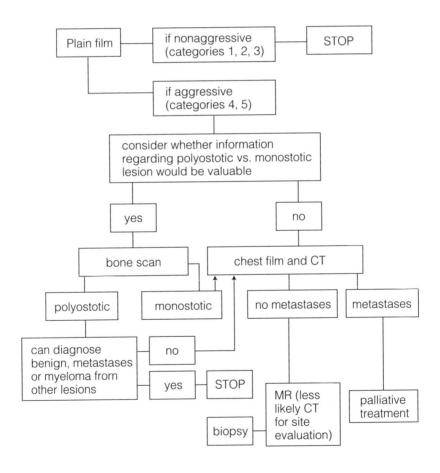

10. Suggested algorithm for soft tissue musculoskeletal lesion work-up:

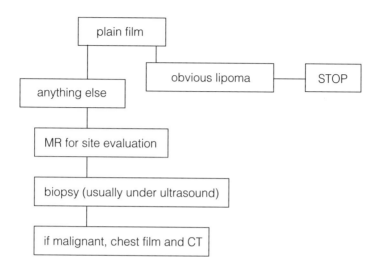

Notice that examination of the chest for metastases is delayed until after the biopsy, since MR is unreliable in predicting malignant vs. benign lesions.

F. Complications of tumor therapy:
   1. Radiation therapy:
      a. Tumor recurrence.
      b. Growth cessation and/or deformities if epiphyses or apophyses are included in the field of radiation; epiphyseal plate widening and metaphyseal fraying may resemble rickets.
      c. Radiation-induced osteochondroma.
      d. Increased susceptibility to infection.
      e. Radiation osteonecrosis: A permeative change seen in bones restricted to the radiation port, often appearing aggressive and producing pathologic fracture. This may be difficult to differentiate from tumor recurrence radiographically, but tends to occur 7 to 10 years after therapy.
      f. Radiation-induced sarcoma: A sarcoma (osteosarcoma, MFH, fibrosarcoma, or chondrosarcoma) arising in a previously irradiated bone, usually 4 to 20 years after therapy. These sarcomas may be difficult to differentiate initially from radiation osteonecrosis, but a soft tissue mass and their aggressive nature is soon demonstrated, and prognosis is very poor (20% 5-year survival).

g. During chemotherapy, reconversion to hematopoietic marrow in nonirradiated bones is often seen, especially if growth-stimulating hormone is given concurrently. This may be potentially confusing, since regions of previously normal-appearing fatty marrow develop low SI on T1 type sequences.

2. Chemotherapy:
   a. Tumor recurrence.
   b. Increased incidence of infection.
   c. Tumor response to chemotherapy: The radiologist's role falls between art and science. The most important indicator is the percentage of viable tumor, with 90% necrosis representing a good response; histologic evaluation is best, but it is subject to sampling and judgement errors; imaging predictors:
      (1) Size: A 50% decrease in the product of the two largest diameters suggests a good response; a pathologic fracture may falsely suggest increased size due to hemorrhage; osteosarcoma often shows little change in size, since the soft tissue mass may develop a more mature, denser osteoid matrix.
      (2) Blood flow: Fast dynamic contrast enhanced MR often differentiates between hypervascular viable tumor and an inflammatory necrotic tissue response to therapy; not completely reliable since not all sarcomas are hypervascular; also subject to sampling error.
      (3) Matrix: Increasing reactive calcification weakly correlates with tumor response.
      (4) Margins: Poor correlation, since a non-tumor-containing "pseudocapsule" may form.
      (5) Metabolic: P-31 MR spectroscopy may show decline in intralesional ATP; PET may show a decrease in glycolosis; not yet completely proven.

3. Limb salvage with allograft:
   a. Tumor recurrence.
   b. Increased incidence of infection (in a large nidus of dead bone, in hardware, or in an immunocompromised patient).
   c. Hardware failure.
   d. Graft resorption.
   e. Late fracture: 15% to 20% of large allografts will fracture; these insufficiency fractures may be best seen by CT with reconstruction.
   f. Delayed union: May take up to 2 years for union with the graft to be demonstrated. The limb must be protected from weightbearing during this process; union with vascularized fibular grafts may progress considerably faster.

   g. Large osteoarticular allografts show a pattern of early cortical graft resorption, followed by slow thickening (over several months); resorptive "cysts" may be prominent for the first two years; late remodeling is manifest as a subcortical sclerotic rim (a "neocortex"): Initially the cancellous graft bone is more sclerotic (higher attenuation by CT) than the host bone—this equalizes over 3 years if there is successful graft incorporation[6]; late articular collapse may occur.

4. Follow-up for recurrence:

   a. CT lungs at intervals appropriate for hazard rate of metastases. For example, osteosarcoma patients should have lung CTs far more often than a patient with grade II chondrosarcoma.

   b. Local osseous recurrence should be monitored by plain film, supplemented if necessary by MR or CT. The presence of hardware complicates the latter option. If plain film is the only option for examination due to hardware, watch for soft tissue contour changes or matrix as indicative of tumor recurrence. If cement or cryosurgery with bone graft packing has been used as structural treatment, be aware that a "halo" of lucency may develop early at the lesion margin (local cell necrosis from treatment) and need not represent recurrence and may fill with lucent fibrous tissue.

   c. Sites of soft tissue resection are generally monitored with MR, with timing as suggested by hazard rate for recurrence. Soft tissue alteration due to surgery or radiation therapy may initially be indistinguishable from recurrent tumor since all may show high T2 signal. Eventually, generally over 6 months to 2 years, the therapy-related high signal decreases so it is isointense with muscle or low signal on T2. Therefore a "baseline" follow-up MR should be obtained approximately 6 months following surgery or therapy and should be available for comparison with later follow-up exams. Early in this follow-up period, you will not be able to distinguish between recurrence and therapy-related T2 high signal regions in the tumor bed except perhaps by morphology. Needle biopsy may need to be performed for any of these regions which appear "mass-like." After 2 years of follow-up exams, tumor bed signal characteristics are usually more reliably that of low-signal fibrosis and this, combined with morphology of the region and comparison studies, should reduce the necessity for biopsy. There are ongoing studies suggesting fast dynamic contrast-enhanced MR studies for tumor viability or recurrence, but those examinations relying on perfusion alone to differentiate tumor from non-tumor are not yet sufficiently reliable for all individual cases.[7,8] Metabolic-based imaging may prove more reliable but is not yet proven or generally available.

The musculoskeletal tumors and tumorlike conditions will be discussed in the text in the following order. Categories are indicated by roman numerals in the text as they are listed in the outline below, which represents a modification of the WHO classification.

 I. Bone-forming tumors.
   A. Benign.
      1. Osteoma.
      2. Enostosis.
      3. Osteoid osteoma.
      4. Osteoblastoma.
      5. Ossifying fibroma.
   B. Malignant.
      1. Conventional osteosarcoma.
      2. Telangiectatic osteosarcoma.
      3. Parosteal osteosarcoma.
      4. Periosteal osteosarcoma.
      5. Low-grade intraosseous osteosarcoma.
      6. Osteosarcoma of the jaw.
      7. Osteosarcoma in the older age group.
      8. Multicentric osteosarcoma.
      9. Soft tissue osteosarcoma.
 II. Cartilage-forming tumors.
   A. Benign.
      1. Chondroma.
      2. Osteochondroma.
      3. Chondroblastoma.
      4. Chondromyxoid fibroma.
      5. Juxtacortical chondroma.
   B. Malignant.
      1. Chondrosarcoma.
III. GCT.
IV. Marrow tumors.
      1. Ewing's sarcoma.
      2. Primary lymphoma.
      3. Hodgkin's disease.
      4. Multiple myeloma/plasmacytoma.
 V. Vascular tumors.
   A. Benign.
      1. Hemangioma.
      2. Lymphangioma.
      3. Cystic angiomatosis.
      4. Massive osteolysis.
      5. Glomus tumor.

B. Indeterminate for malignancy.
　　1. Hemangiopericytoma.
　　2. Hemangioendothelioma.
C. Malignant.
　　1. Angiosarcoma.
VI. Other connective tissue tumors.
　A. Benign.
　　1. Fibromatoses (soft tissue, intraosseous, and cortical desmoid).
　　2. Lipoma (intraosseous, extraosseous, and parosteal).
　　3. Peripheral nerve sheath tumors.
　　4. GCT of tendon sheath.
　B. Malignant.
　　1. Fibrosarcoma, MFH.
　　2. Liposarcoma.
　　3. Synovial cell sarcoma.
VII. Other tumors.
　　1. Chordoma.
　　2. Adamantinoma.
VIII. Tumorlike lesions.
　　1. Solitary bone cyst (SBC).
　　2. ABC.
　　3. NOF/benign fibrous cortical defect.
　　4. Eosinophilic granuloma.
　　5. Fibrous dysplasia.
　　6. Brown tumor of hyperparathyroidism (HPTH).
　　7. Myositis ossificans.
IX. Metastases.

The organization in each section is as follows:
　A. Eleven determinants.
　　1. Age.
　　2. Soft tissue involvement.
　　3. Pattern of bone destruction.
　　4. Size of lesion.
　　5. Location of lesion.
　　6. Zone of transition.
　　7. Margin of lesion.
　　8. Tumor matrix.
　　9. Host response.
　　10. Polyostotic vs. monostotic.
　　11. Other features.
　B. MR appearance.
　C. Aggressiveness of lesion.
　D. Major differential diagnoses.

      E. Metastatic potential.
      F. Radiographic work-up.
      G. Treatment.

BONE-FORMING TUMORS
A. Bone-Forming Tumors: Benign

Osteoma
A hamartomatous process, with abnormal proliferation of bone and no stromal abnormalities.

Key Concepts

    Sclerotic; calvarium or sinuses; may be associated with Gardner's syndrome.

A. Determinants:
    1. Age: Tends to be seen in adults.
    2. Soft tissue involvement: None.
    3. Pattern: Geographic; may expand adjacent bony margins.
    4. Size: Usually greater than 2 cm.
    5. Location: Membranous bone—calvarium, usually arising from the external table, or paranasal sinuses.
    6. Zone of transition: Narrow.
    7. Margin: Entire lesion is sclerotic.
    8. Tumor matrix: Dense homogeneous bone.
    9. Host response: None.
    10. May be polyostotic.
    11. Other features: May be part of the autosomal-dominant Gardner syndrome, occurring with multiple adenomatous colonic polyps.
B. MR appearance: Low signal on all sequences, without other features.
C. Nonaggressive.
D. Major differential diagnoses:
    1. Blastic metastasis.
    2. Hyperostosis from meningioma in calvarium (however, the latter usually involves the inner table).
E. Metastatic potential: None.
F. Radiographic work-up: Plain film diagnosis.
G. Treatment: None.

Enostosis (Bone Island)
A hamartomatous proliferation of bone.

Key Concepts

Small round sclerotic lesion; may be polyostotic and be mistaken for sclerotic metastasis; peripheral spiculation.

A. Determinants:
    1. Age: Any, but most seen after puberty.
    2. Soft tissue involvement: None.
    3. Pattern: Geographic, generally round, but with spicules at the margin which blend with surrounding trabeculae.
    4. Size: 2 mm to 2 cm, but occasionally they are larger.
    5. Location: Medullary canal of any bone.
    6. Zone of transition: Narrow, blending over a very short distance peripherally into normal bone, with spiculation at the margins.
    7. Margin: Entire lesion is sclerotic.
    8. Tumor matrix: Dense homogeneous bone.
    9. Host response: None.
    10. May be polyostotic, at one end of the spectrum of sclerosing dysplasias, including osteopoikilosis (multiple epiphyseal enostoses).
    11. Other features: Very common lesion, usually discovered fortuitously; occasionally will increase or decrease in size due to osteoblastic or osteoclastic activity, not related to patient age.
B. MR appearance: Low signal on all sequences (similar to cortical bone).
C. Nonaggressive.
D. Major differential diagnoses:
    1. Blastic metastasis.
    2. Dense osteoid osteoma.
    3. Osteoblastoma.
    4. Sclerosing intramedullary osteosarcoma.
E. Metastatic potential: None.
F. Radiographic work-up: None, unless painful; with pain, either of the differentials listed might be considered. Bone scan might differentiate enostosis, which shows little or no increased uptake; larger lesions may show more prominent bone scan activity, as will those with increased osteoblastic activity.
G. Treatment: None.

Osteoid Osteoma
A benign entity with distinctive radiographic and clinical findings.

Key Concepts

Painful; lytic lesion with or without sclerotic nidus; sclerotic host reaction which may be distant if the lesion is intracapsular; may cause a painful scoliosis; "hot" on bone scan.

A. Determinants:
1. Age: Second and third decades.
2. Soft tissue involvement: Only in the rare subperiosteal form (see below).
3. Pattern: Geographic—a circumscribed nidus, with or without central calcification, surrounded by a lucent, highly vascular stroma, surrounded by dense reactive bone.
4. Size: Nidus less than 2 cm.
5. Location: (Fig. 1-1) The most common variety is cortically based in the tubular bones. These elicit such a densely sclerotic reaction that the nidus may actually be masked on plain film.

   Another variety is intramedullary and often intracapsular. These are most commonly found in the proximal femur at the medial aspect of the femoral neck. These lesions elicit a sclerotic host reaction, which may be located at a considerable distance from the nidus; calcar buttressing is also a common feature. In a child, osteoid osteomas of the femoral neck may cause irreversible growth deformities (valgus, with a thick neck and overgrowth leading to limb length discrepancy), muscle atrophy, and associated early osteoarthritis.

   Subperiosteal osteoid osteomas, the third and least common variety, demonstrate a round soft tissue mass immediately adjacent to bone with underlying scalloping and irregular bone resorption. The talus is one of the most common sites of the subperiosteal osteoid osteoma.

   The spine is a relatively common site for osteoid osteoma. The posterior elements rather than the vertebral body are involved, and there is a painful scoliosis with the apex at the lesion, concave on the side of the lesion and without a rotatory component.
6. Zone of transition: Narrow.
7. Margin: Sclerotic host reaction.
8. Tumor matrix: Nidus may or may not be calcified.

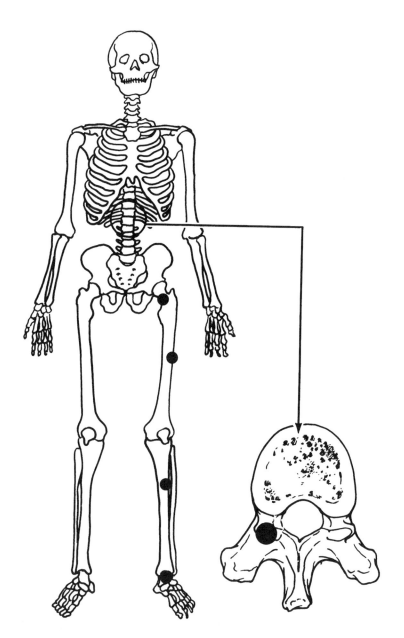

Fig. 1-1   Most common locations of osteoid osteoma.

9. Host response: Varying amounts of sclerosis, depending on location (see Section A-5).
10. Rarely may be polyostotic with a nidus in adjacent bones; may also have double or multiple nidi.
11. The clinical features of aching pain, worse at night, relieved with aspirin, and dramatically relieved by excision are typical; however, the intramedullary intracapsular variety may present as a less painful synovitis. Muscle atrophy of the involved limb is common. The subperiosteal osteoid osteoma not uncommonly presents clinically as arthritis. Overall incidence: 1.6% of excised primary bone tumors.

B. MR appearance: While CT of osteoid osteoma is diagnostic, MR may be inaccurate and confusing. If MR slices are not small, the lesion may be missed altogether (though seen retrospectively once located with CT). The nidus shows low SI on T1, but variably low to high SI on T2, enhancing inconsistently if contrast is given. These are nonspecific findings. However, adjacent marrow sclerosis or edema as well as adjacent soft tissue inflammatory changes seen in many cases may mislead the reader toward diagnosis of a larger, more aggressive lesion.[9] MR should be avoided if osteoid osteoma is clinically suspected, or at the very least interpreted with reference to plain films or CT.

C. Nonaggressive, but recurs if nidus is excised incompletely.

D. Major differential diagnoses:
1. Dense cortical osteoid osteoma:
   a. Brodie's abscess.
   b. Enostosis.
   c. Subacute stress fracture.
2. Intramedullary intracapsular: If the nidus is not obvious and it is confusing radiographically, may consider a synovitis or dysplasia.
3. Subperiosteal:
   a. Arthritis.
   b. Juxtacortical chondroma.
4. Posterior elements of spine:
   a. Metastasis.
   b. Spondylolysis with sclerosis of contralateral posterior elements.

E. Metastatic potential: None.

F. Radiographic work-up: If the lesion is radiographically confusing, a bone scan is very useful. The lesion almost invariably shows significantly increased uptake, occasionally with a double density. With localization guided by the bone scan, the nidus may then be demonstrated by CT, which provides information on exact location and whether there is more than one nidus. Injection of a small amount (one drop, <0.05 cc) of methylene blue dye mixed with radiographic contrast into the periosteum under CT control immediately prior to surgery will localize the lesion, allowing the surgeon to minimize the amount of cortical bone destroyed in the resection.

G. Treatment: Complete marginal excision of the nidus. Recurrence is due to incomplete excision. If there is any question regarding completeness of excision, filming of the specimen may be useful. Intraoperative bone scanning has also been described but is cumbersome. Recent reports abound of percutaneous resection or ablation under CT control. Spontaneous healing over several years has been reported.

Osteoblastoma

A rare benign tumor (0.5% of bone tumor biopsies) that is difficult to differentiate histologically from osteoid osteoma. Radiographically, it is quite distinct from osteoid osteoma. Historically, the two entities have been arbitrarily distinguished by size, with osteoid osteoma measuring less than 2 cm and osteoblastoma measuring greater than 2 cm.

Key Concepts

Expansile, usually nonaggressive; lucent or sclerotic; posterior elements of spine.

A. Determinants:
1. Age: Second and third decade with wide range.
2. Soft tissue involvement: Usually none; occasional epidural extension in spine.
3. Pattern: Geographic—expands bone in a fusiform shape.
4. Size: Greater than 2 cm.
5. Location: Most common in the posterior elements of the spine (42%; Fig 1-2); in the long bones, either metaphyseal or diaphyseal and central to eccentric.
6. Zone of transition: Narrow.
7. Margin of lesion: Thin rim of sclerosis.
8. Tumor matrix: May be lucent, mixed, or completely blastic.
9. Host response: Expansion without large amount of sclerosis; periosteal reaction mild.
10. Monostotic.
11. Other features: Patient presents with a dull, aching pain, less severe than that of osteoid osteoma.
B. MR appearance: Mineralization of the lesions may or may not be visible, affecting the SI on both T1 and T2 imaging; most are indistinguishable from MR of other bone lesions, being low SI on T1 and mixed to high SI on T2; surrounding edema may be prominent.[10]

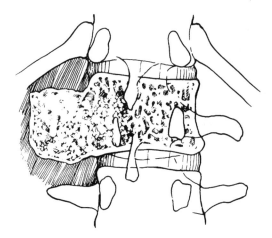

Fig. 1-2 Osteoblastoma, a geographic, expanded lesion most commonly located in the posterior elements of the spine.

C. Generally, as described, appears nonaggressive; occasionally, though, the cortex may be broken through and the lesion may appear to be more aggressive.
D. Major differential diagnoses:
    1. Osteosarcoma (If the lesion appears aggressive and contains calcified osteoid.)
    2. Osteoid osteoma (If the size is borderline.)
    3. Brown tumor of HPTH: Usually has other findings of HPTH.
    4. ABC: Usually located more eccentrically but may be associated with osteoblastoma, especially in the spine.
    5. GCT: Usually located more eccentrically, subarticular, and less well marginated.
E. Metastatic potential:
    1. Generally not malignant, but there have been a few reports of malignant transformation; some of these may be a true transformation, whereas others were osteosarcomas originally misdiagnosed as osteoblastoma.
    2. There are also cases that appear benign radiographically but are "pseudomalignant" histologically; these patients have a benign course.
F. Radiographic work-up: These usually fall into the "radiographically benign, symptomatic" category, which can undergo biopsy and elective surgery without further work-up. If there is a question of aggressiveness, bone scan followed by CT or MR is useful to differentiate osteoblastoma from osteosarcoma.

G. Treatment: Curettage (marginal or intracapsular excision) with bone graft; recurrence is rare; if surgically inaccessible, radiation has been used.

Ossifying Fibroma

An extremely rare benign lesion found almost exclusively in the proximal femur, tibia, and facial bones.

Key Concepts

Rare, looks like NOF since it is cortically based and expansile; location in tibia is an important factor in suggesting the diagnosis.

A. Determinants.
   1. Age: Second and third decades.
   2. Soft tissue involvement: None.
   3. Pattern of bone destruction: Geographic oval lesion.
   4. Size of lesion: Varies widely.
   5. Location: In the proximal third of the tibia, in the anterior cortex, often causing an anterior cortex bowing (Fig. 1-3); also found as an oval geographic femoral neck lesion.
   6. Zone of transition: Narrow.
   7. Margin of lesion: Sclerotic rim.
   8. Tumor matrix: May be lucent or contain osteoid and look like ground glass.
   9. Host response: None except sclerotic margin.
   10. Monostotic.
   11. Other features: This lesion can be similar, both histologically and radiographically, to either fibrous dysplasia or adamantinoma. Since there are no other distinguishing features, the radiologist should consider this lesion whenever the *location* is appropriate (i.e., upper third of tibia in anterior cortex or femoral neck).
B. Initially not aggressive but may become highly aggressive with recurrence.
C. Major differential diagnoses:
   1. Adamantinoma (generally more distal in the tibia).
   2. Cortically based fibrous dysplasia.
   3. NOF.
D. Metastatic potential: None.
E. Radiographic work-up: Diagnosis, biopsy, and treatment are usually based on the plain film alone.
F. Treatment: Wide excision (*en bloc*) of the bony lesion; if the lesion

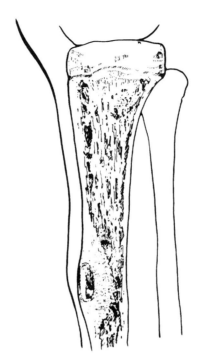

Fig. 1-3 Typical ossifying fibroma, cortically based on the anterior aspect of the proximal one-third of the tibia; the same appearance at a different site would be more suggestive of NOF.

is misdiagnosed as fibrous dysplasia or NOF and treated with curettage (marginal excision) rather than wide excision, the recurrence rate is unacceptably high. With recurrence, the lesion behaves much more aggressively; accurate diagnosis is therefore very important.

B. Bone-Forming Tumors: Malignant

Osteosarcoma
Common (20% of primary bone tumor biopsies, second only to myeloma in primary bone tumor frequency), primary bone tumor that produces malignant osteoid in either large or small foci. Several variants are described.

Key Concepts

Conventional osteosarcoma is extremely aggressive, with tumor matrix in soft tissue mass; childhood and adolescent tumor; metaphyseal.

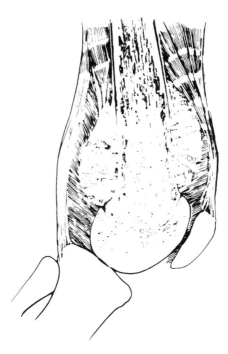

Fig. 1-4   Conventional osteosarcoma, with permeative change, large soft tissue mass, amorphous calcification, and periosteal reaction. Metaphyseal site around the knee is typical.

Conventional Osteosarcoma.—The most common osteosarcoma (75%) (Fig. 1-4).
A. Determinants:
    1. Age: 10 to 25 years is most common; a smaller peak is seen in older adults (see below).
    2. Soft tissue involvement: Cortical breakthrough with large mass, often containing tumor bone.
    3. Pattern: Permeative.
    4. Size: Rarely discovered before it is large.
    5. Location: (Fig. 1-5) Metaphysis, 90%, diaphysis, 10%; even though the lesion arises in the metaphysis, involvement of the growth plate occurs often (75%); 66% around knee, with involvement of the distal femur more common than involvement of the proximal tibia, which is, in turn, more common than involvement of the proximal humerus. Flat bones are less commonly involved than long bones, but osteosarcoma in the iliac wing is not uncom-

mon (more likely in the second than first decade). The extremely rare intracortical osteosarcoma may give the appearance of a metadiaphyseal fibrous cortical defect and is felt to be a very early manifestation of the conventional osteosarcoma.

6. Zone of transition: Wide.
7. Margin: No sclerotic margin.
8. Tumor matrix: 90% produce tumor bone matrix visible on plain films or CT, but the amount varies, producing an appearance ranging from densely blastic to nearly completely lytic. Histologically, 50% produce enough osteoid to be termed ''osteoblastic''; 25% produce predominantly cartilage, and 25% produce predominantly spindle cells. The radiographic appearance often corresponds to these histologic findings, with the matrix calcification in the cartilage and spindle cell varieties either very subtle or entirely lacking.

   It should also be noted that many lesions excite reactive host bone formation, which can appear quite blastic; thus, it may be difficult to differentiate a Ewing's sarcoma with extensive reactive bone formation roentgenographically from an osteosarcoma unless amorphous tumor bone formation is seen within the soft tissue mass (this confirms osteosarcoma).

9. Host response: Periosteal reaction, often in an aggressive sunburst or Codman's triangle pattern.
10. Usually monostotic; however, between 2% and 10% may have skip lesions of medullary involvement within the bone of primary occurrence. Most of these are too small to detect by plain film, bone scan, or MR (as shown by the RDOG study).

B. MR appearance: depends on mineralization of the matrix; if very dense, that portion will appear to have low SI on all sequences; if less dense, T1 weighting will have nonspecific low SI and T2 will have inhomogeneous high SI, often appearing infiltrative; in lesions around the knee, it is crucial to evaluate for tumor extension into the joint via ligaments or tendons—coronal and/or sagittal planes are necessary for full evaluation of the knee joint involvement.

C. Highly aggressive, radiographically as well as clinically (50% to 60% survival).

D. Major differential diagnoses:
   1. Ewing's sarcoma, especially if the osteosarcoma is diaphyseal and has no calcified matrix in the soft tissue mass.
   2. Cortical desmoid: An avulsive irregularity posterior to the adductor tubercle. Location is key to the diagnosis: the cortical desmoid is always on the posterior aspect of the medial femoral condyle; it appears as a scalloped defect in the cortex, sometimes with a small soft tissue mass with periosteal elevation, and occasionally with

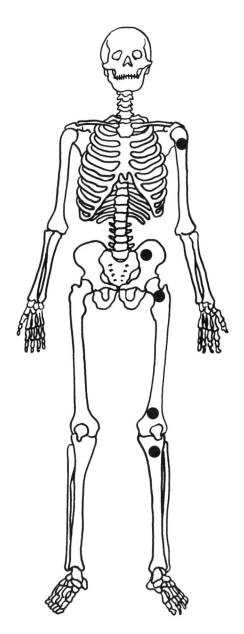

Fig. 1-5   Most common distribution of conventional osteosarcoma.

matrix calcification due to repair. Biopsy material taken during the active repair phase is difficult to distinguish from osteosarcoma, so the lesion is best diagnosed by the radiologist.

3. Early myositis ossicans: In the first 4 to 8 weeks, amorphous calcification may occur in soft tissues overlying bone, and periosteal reaction may be seen, which is highly suggestive of osteosarcoma. Careful evaluation of patient history may mitigate a potentially confusing biopsy (see Chapter 3, Myositis).

4. Aggressive osteoblastoma: Very rare.

E. Metastatic potential: Very significant, with hematogenous spread to lungs or bone and lymphangitic spread more locally; intramedullary skip lesions may also occur. Ten percent to 20% present with metastases to lung or bone; 80% of relapses occur in lung and 20% in bone. Those in bone do very poorly, while those in the lung have a 10% to 20% 5-year survival with resection of metastases and chemotherapy. Relapses usually occur within 2 years of the initial diagnosis.

F. Radiographic work-up:

1. Plain film: Usually diagnostic.
2. Bone scan: To assure it is monostotic.
3. Chest x-ray and CT: To exclude metastatic disease.
4. MRI: To evaluate extent of lesion, plan biopsy, and plan definitive therapy.

G. Treatment (if not metastatic):

1. Induction (neoadjuvant) chemotherapy prior to limb salvage surgery is viewed as very useful.

   a. Helps control the development of micrometastases in the interval needed to order the custom prosthesis or allograft.
   b. May produce regression of the primary tumor, allowing easier excision *en bloc* for limb salvage.
   c. Allows pathologic assessment of the chemotherapy regimen through evaluation of tumor necrosis at the time of limb salvage.
   d. Requires restaging with MR.

2. Radical (amputation) or wide excision *en bloc* (limb salvage). Evaluate carefully for involvement of the epiphysis, even though the lesion originated in the metaphysis. Epyphyseal extension is seen more commonly with MR (up to 80%), especially using coronal or sagittal planes.[11] Depending on lesion staging, a similar protocol may be undertaken in a patient with limited, resectable metastases.

3. Chemotherapy: Adjuvant polydrug chemotherapy has a favorable impact on survival for patients with nonmetastatic high-grade osteosarcoma. It is possible that adjuvant chemotherapy may de-

crease the number of lung metastases and delay their development, thus affecting short-term survival rather than cure rate.[12,13]

Telangiectatic Osteosarcoma.—A rare variant of osteosarcoma that may be difficult to diagnose radiographically, since it is entirely lytic.
A. Determinants:
   1. Age: 10–25 years (same as conventional osteosarcoma).
   2. May or may not have soft tissue involvement.
   3. Pattern: Geographic, though the borders may be somewhat indistinct; definitely has more of a round, blow-out appearance than the permeative, conventional osteosarcomas.
   4. Size: Large (usually greater than 5 cm).
   5. Location: Metaphyses of long bones (as in conventional osteosarcoma); 60% in femur or tibia.
   6. Zone of transition: Somewhat indistinct but much narrower than conventional osteosarcoma.
   7. Margin: Generally no sclerosis.
   8. Tumor matrix: None.
   9. Host response: May or may not have periosteal reaction. If present, should be a "red flag" that this is not a nonaggressive lesion.
  10. Monostotic.
  11. Lesion is highly vascular and may contain grossly visible necrotic tissue with large pools of blood, with tumor at the periphery only.
B. MR appearance: May have prominent fluid-fluid levels, reinforcing the perception that this is a benign lesion; T1 may have high SI due to the presence of methemoglobin.
C. From the description above, this lytic lesion may be confusing radiographically, having some features that appear aggressive and others that appear much less aggressive. The radiologist must keep this lesion in mind when a moderately aggressive lytic metaphyseal lesion occurs in a teenager or young adult, since the lesion itself lacks the cardinal features of osteosarcoma (highly aggressive, with calcified matrix). Telangiectatic osteosarcoma is much more aggressive clinically than the lesions considered in the differential diagnosis and, therefore, must be treated differently.
D. Major differential diagnoses:
   1. Less aggressive looking:
     a. ABC.
     b. GCT.
   2. More aggressive looking:
     a. Fibrosarcoma/MFH.
     b. Ewing's sarcoma.

E. Metastatic potential: Great, in same distribution as conventional osteo-sarcoma (lungs, bones, local lymph nodes) with an equal malignant potential.

F. Radiographic work-up:
   1. Plain film; considering the possibility of this as the diagnosis is the key here, avoiding a misdiagnosis as a less aggressive lesion.
   2. Bone scan.
   3. Chest x-ray and CT.
   4. MRI of lesion.

G. Treatment:
   1. Radical or wide marginal excision *en bloc.*
   2. Chemotherapy.

Parosteal Osteosarcoma.—Well-differentiated osteosarcoma with epicen-ter adjacent to the periosteum and significantly better prognosis than con-ventional osteosarcoma.

A. Determinants:
   1. Age: Wide range, including childhood, but 80% occur between 20 and 50 years of age (therefore usually older than conventional osteosarcoma).
   2. Soft tissue involvement: Although attached to underlying cortex at the site of origin, the lesion is otherwise located nearly entirely in the soft tissues, wrapping around the underlying bone in a lobulated fashion (Fig 1–6). The peripheral zone may consist only of cortical bone and a thin fibrous pseudocapsule, or there may be neoplastic tissue infiltrating the adjacent soft tissues.
   3. Pattern: Geographic.
   4. Size: Often large (greater than 5 cm) at time of discovery.
   5. Location: Juxtacortical, metaphyseal; 60% distal femur; others, proximal tibia, proximal humerus, and other metaphyseal regions (Fig 1–7).
   6. Zone of transition: Usually narrow; with MR evaluation, most demonstrate at least a small amount of tumor extending from the cortex into the adjacent marrow.
   7. Margin: Entire lesion tends to be sclerotic.
   8. Tumor matrix: Densely sclerotic mature osteoid, with lobulated masses centrally; more peripherally, these may be less mature bone or a nonossified soft tissue mass. This zoning pattern distinguishes the lesion from myositis ossificans, in which the more mature bone is found peripherally.
   9. Host response: None.
   10. Monostotic.

B. MR appearance: Variable, depending on degree of maturation of the bone matrix. If it is not cellular and contains little cartilage, there will

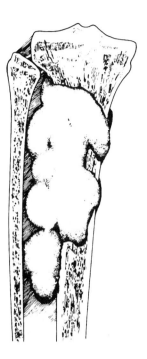

Fig. 1-6   Parosteal osteosarcoma, located typically around the knee and with densely sclerotic mature tumor matrix wrapping around the underlying bone.

be low SI on all sequences. However, there is often more cellularity present, as well as cartilaginous regions, giving an inhomogeneous appearance. Watch particularly for the extent of marrow involvement, as well as central or peripheral areas that are more cellular (yielding low SI on T1, high SI on T2), suggesting a higher grade or dedifferentiation.

C. Aggressiveness: Tends to be very slow growing and low grade, but with inadequate excision, may recur in a more aggressive form; with multiple recurrences, may dedifferentiate. Up to 10% may be dedifferentiated at presentation.

D. Differential diagnosis:

1. Myositis ossificans: Zoning of the mature bone differentiates the two both radiographically and histologically (see Section A–8, above).

2. Osteochondroma: Parosteal osteosarcoma usually has a distinct cleft between the underlying bone and the lesion, except at its origin; in addition, osteochondromas have a matrix of either mature bony trabeculae or the typical cartilaginous snowstorm appearance. In parosteal osteosarcomas, MR shows tumor invading marrow

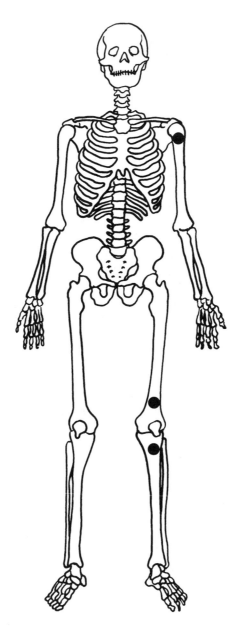

Fig. 1-7   Most common distribution of parosteal osteosarcoma.

rather than marrow extending into the base of the lesion as seen in osteochondroma.

3. Periosteal osteosarcoma.

E. Metastatic potential: Metastases to lung are often late (1 to 10 years) and occur much less frequently than in conventional osteosarcoma; 80% to 90% 5-year survival.

F. Radiographic work-up:
   1. Plain film diagnosis.
   2. MRI for evaluation of marrow involvement and soft tissue extent.
   3. Chest x-ray and CT.
   4. Treatment: Ideal tumor for limb salvage techniques of wide marginal resection *en bloc,* retaining limb function but avoiding the recurrences possible with a marginal excision; no chemotherapy.

Periosteal Osteosarcoma.—Extremely rare surface osteosarcoma without intramedullary involvement and with a better prognosis than conventional osteosarcoma.

A. Determinants:
   1. Age: Second or third decade, usually a little later than conventional osteosarcoma.
   2. Soft tissue involvement: The mass arises juxtacortically, sometimes with perpendicular spicules of bone within the soft tissue mass.
   3. Patterns: Geographic in bone.
   4. Size: Generally 2 to 5 cm.
   5. Location: Diaphysis, most commonly of the tibia or femur.
   6. Zone of transition: Cortex may be involved, with either thickening or "saucerization" but the zone of transition is narrow and the marrow is not involved. The extent of the entire soft tissue mass may be more difficult to determine.
   7. Margin: No sclerotic margin.
   8. Tumor matrix: Amorphous calcific densities or spicules perpendicular to the cortex may be seen in the soft tissue mass.
   9. Host response: Periosteal reaction, often with Codman's triangles.
   10. Monostotic.

B. MR appearance: Since there is such a prominent cartilaginous component to these lesions, contrast-enhanced MR shows cartilaginous lobules with septations and adjacent cortical bone destruction but no marrow invasion. Unenhanced MR shows the typical nonspecific low SI on T1 and high SI on T2-weighted images.

C. Mildly aggressive-looking.

D. Major differential diagnoses:
   1. Conventional osteosarcoma: Any intramedullary involvement should differentiate the two.

2. High-grade surface osteosarcoma: Indistinguishable, though it may have a larger soft-tissue mass; this has the same histologic and survival characteristics of conventional osteosarcoma.
3. Juxtacortical chondroma.
4. Apophyseal avulsion with early repair.
5. Parosteal osteosarcoma.

E. Metastatic potential: May metastasize to lungs, but much less frequently than conventional osteosarcoma; 80% 5-year survival.

F. Radiographic work-up:
1. Plain film suggests diagnosis.
2. MRI defines extent (especially with regard to intramedullary involvement, which would change the diagnosis to conventional osteosarcoma).
3. Chest x-ray and CT.

G. Treatment: Wide marginal resection, limb salvage if possible.

Low-Grade Intraosseous Osteosarcoma.—Very rare (1% of osteosarcomas) variant that is entirely intraosseous and may be so well differentiated as to be mistaken for a benign process; excellent chance for survival if recognized initially.

A. Determinants:
1. Age: 10 to 25 years, but also seen in older patients.
2. Soft tissue involvement: None to minimal.
3. Pattern: Permeative or moth-eaten.
4. Size: Greater than 5 cm.
5. Location: Metadiaphyseal region of long bones.
6. Zone of transition: Wide.
7. Margin: No sclerotic margin.
8. Tumor matrix: Lesions range from lytic permeative to mixed sclerotic and lytic.
9. Host response: Initially contained within bone, so no periosteal reaction or very solid-appearing neocortex; with recurrence, is more aggressive, penetrates cortex, and elicits periosteal reaction.
10. Monostotic.

B. MR appearance: Varies with degree of matrix formation, but showing abnormal SI confined to bone; CT is sometimes more helpful, suggesting aggressive cortical lysis.

C. Appearance ranges from mildly aggressive to more markedly aggressive.

D. Differential diagnosis:
1. Fibrous dysplasia (if only slightly aggressive-looking).
2. Infection.
3. Ewing's sarcoma (if more aggressive-looking).

4. Lymphoma (if more aggressive-looking).
5. Fibrosarcoma/MFH (if more aggressive-looking).
E. Metastatic potential: If recognized initially and completely resected, 80% to 90% 5-year survival. With recurrence it often is highly malignant and proceeds rapidly to metastatic involvement.
F. Radiographic work-up.
   1. Plain film: May be confusing initially, having a moderately aggressive bony destructive pattern but no soft tissue mass.
   2. MR: To assess extent of marrow involvement and confirm that soft tissues are normal.
   3. Chest x-ray and CT.
G. Treatment: Initially, ideal for limb salvage with wide marginal excision *en bloc*. An aggressive recurrence may require more radical surgery plus chemotherapy.

Osteosarcoma of the Jaw.—A variant that occurs later in life than conventional osteosarcoma, has an appearance of variable destruction, may or may not have a tumor matrix, and is generally a lower grade than conventional osteosarcoma, with much better survival (80%) when treated with wide excision.

Osteosarcoma in the Older Age Group (After Age 60 Years).—Generalizations[14]:
A. Location is often different than conventional osteosarcoma:
   1. Axial skeleton 27%.
   2. Craniofacial 13%.
   3. Soft tissue 11%.
B. Eighty percent present as lytic lesions without matrix; all appear aggressive.
C. Fifty-six percent arise in a preexisting lesion:
   1. Paget's disease: Probably no more than 1% of patients with Paget's disease are at risk for developing osteosarcoma, generally in a severely affected bone.
   2. Postirradiation osteosarcoma: Generally in bone receiving more than 3000 rad; location parallels that of commonly irradiated areas (shoulder for breast carcinoma, pelvis for genitourinary tumors, and the common locations of GCT—knee, shoulder, distal radius); degenerates to osteosarcoma (50%), fibrosarcoma, or chondrosarcoma. Interval between radiation and diagnosis ranges from 3 to 40 years, averaging 14 years.
   3. Dedifferentiated chondrosarcoma: Dedifferentiation occurs in up to 10% of well-differentiated chondrosarcomas. Radiographically, there is often a sharp transition between the well-differentiated chondrosarcoma and the highly destructive dedifferentiated

tumor. The dedifferentiated tumor may contain elements of fibrosarcoma, MFH, high-grade chondrosarcoma, as well as osteosarcoma.

4. Osteosarcoma extremely rarely arises from benign conditions (osteochondroma, chronic osteomyelitis, osteoblastoma, bone infarct, fibrous dysplasia).

D. Survival: 37% in osteosarcoma de novo in an older patient; 7.5% in osteosarcoma that arises in a preexisting lesion.

E. Radiographic work-up:
1. Plain film: usually diagnostic.
2. MRI for extent.
3. Chest film and CT.

F. Treatment: Radical excision; adjunctive chemotherapy has no impact on survival at this time.

Multicentric Osteosarcoma (Osteosarcomatosis).—Synchronous appearance of osteosarcoma at multiple sites, often bilaterally symmetric; always osteoblastic, giving the appearance of bone islands (enostoses) early but rapidly progressive; extremely rare; previously believed to occur exclusively in children of 6 to 9 years; early development of lung metastases and extremely poor prognosis. In an Armed Forces Institute of Pathology (AFIP) review, only 50% of cases followed this classic description, with all the lesions approximately the same size, distinguishing this entity from a primary osteosarcoma with multiple bone metastases. The remaining 50% showed fewer, asymmetric sclerotic lesions. In most patients (28 of 29), a radiographically dominant skeletal tumor was seen.[15] This suggests a metastatic origin from a primary dominant lesion rather than a multifocal origin for osteosarcomatosis.

Soft Tissue Osteosarcoma.—Rare extraosseous osteosarcoma, generally occurring later in life (40 to 70 years). They most commonly are found in the thigh, occasionally after radiation therapy. Zoning is reversed from that of myositis ossificans, being more organized and dense centrally with a soft tissue mass peripherally. Occasionally they have no bone matrix. Prognosis is similar to that of conventional osteosarcoma with metastatic disease to lungs and local lymph nodes.

II. CARTILAGE-FORMING TUMORS
A. Cartilage-Forming Tumors: Benign

Chondroma (Enchondroma)
Common benign cartilaginous neoplasm arising in the medullary canal of bone which is asymptomatic in the absence of pathologic fracture or malignant degeneration.

Key Concepts

Geographic lesion; usually with cartilaginous matrix; hands, feet, or metaphyses of long bones; degeneration to chondrosarcoma extremely difficult to detect radiographically: diagnosis must rely on pain and clinical suspicion.

A. Determinants:
  1. Age: Often discovered incidentally in the third or fourth decade.
  2. Soft tissue involvement: None.
  3. Pattern: Geographic; may expand bony margins and cause cortical thinning. Cortical scalloping may also be a feature.
  4. Size: 3 to 4 cm; smaller in hands or feet.
  5. Location: Central lesion (Fig 1-8).
      a. In tubular bones of the hands or feet (50%), phalanges more commonly than metacarpals or metatarsals.
      b. Distributed among metaphyseal region of long tubular bones (especially the humerus, femur, and tibia), the pelvis, and the shoulder girdle (50%).
  6. Zone of transition: Usually narrow, though the lesion may be lobulated.
  7. Margin: Fine sclerotic margin in hands and feet; often no sclerotic margin at other sites.
  8. Tumor matrix: Ranges from lytic (especially in hands or feet) to typical cartilaginous matrix (stippled, often ringlike and denser than normal bone).
  9. Host response: None unless there is a pathologic fracture.
  10. Usually monostotic: There may be several chondromas in the hands. If more than one chondroma is found elsewhere, the patient may have multiple enchondromatosis (Ollier's disease).
B. MR appearance: Enchondromas are often incidentally discovered when MR of a metaphyseal region of a long bone is performed for another reason, presenting on MR as nonspecific low SI on T1 and high SI on T2. In this case, plain film may reveal an extremely subtle central metaphyseal lesion without sclerotic margins or significant matrix calcification; if more calcification is present, it will appear as low SI on all sequences. In those enchondromas that contain large amounts of hyaline cartilage, T2 imaging shows the expected high SI homogeneous lobulated mass.
C. Not aggressive in the absence of malignant change.
D. Major differential diagnoses:

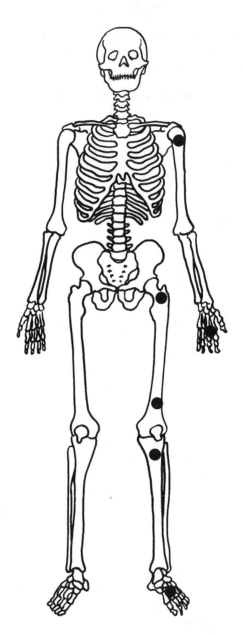

Fig. 1-8   Most common distribution of chondroma.

1. In hands or feet: (Note: Chondromas are much more common than differentials c, d, e, or f, below.)
    a. Inclusion cyst (usually involves the tuft).
    b. GCT of the tendon sheath (usually causes scalloping with the epicenter in the soft tissues).
    c. GCT.
    d. ABC.
    e. Solitary bone cyst.
    f. Fibrous dysplasia.
2. In sites other than hands or feet:
    a. Bone infarct: The pattern of calcification and absence of sclerotic margin may make this indistinguishable from a chondroma.
    b. Chondromyxoid fibroma: A rare lesion in which a calcific matrix is unusual.
    c. Chondrosarcoma: The major diagnostic dilemma, with considerable histologic and radiographic overlap in the low-grade lesions.
E. Metastatic potential:
    1. In hands or feet, the histology may appear ominous but chondroma almost universally behaves in a benign manner.
    2. In sites other than hands or feet, malignant degeneration to chondrosarcoma is not uncommon. Proximal lesions (pelvis or shoulder girdle) have the highest incidence of malignant change. The difficulty lies in the fact that early malignant degeneration may not be detectable radiographically. Even serial plain films, bone scans, and CT or MR scans may show no interval change early in the degeneration. The diagnosis, therefore, often is based solely on local pain, and appropriate treatment should be instituted for a painful chondroma in the absence of pathologic fracture. Histology in early malignant degeneration most commonly shows either low-grade chondrosarcoma or atypical chondroma.
F. Radiographic work-up:
    1. If asymptomatic, plain film diagnosis.
    2. If the lesion is painful and malignant degeneration is clinically suspected, MR is performed to determine extent, aggressiveness, and therapy. Note that MR appearance may be misleading; early sarcomatous change may not be manifest. Serial radionuclide bone scans may, but do not necessarily, show a change with malignant degeneration. A single bone scan is not helpful since chondromas and chondrosarcomas are both highly variable in degree of radionuclide uptake.

G. Treatment:
    1. If asymptomatic (found incidentally), may elect watchful waiting.
    2. If the lesion is painful and suggests early malignant degeneration, the surgeon faces the choice of curettage and bone packing (which usually succeeds without recurrence) or complete excision *en bloc* (limb salvage, a more assuredly curative resection which carries greater morbidity). This decision is made on the basis of the patient's age and condition; thus, an elderly patient might do better with curettage since recurrence or metastatic disease is unlikely to occur during the remainder of his or her life, while a younger patient might benefit more and recover better from the curative limb salvage procedure.
H. Multiple enchondromatosis (Ollier's disease):
    a. A rare developmental abnormality characterized by the presence of enchondromas in the metaphyses and diaphyses of multiple bones.
    b. Not hereditary or familial.
    c. Appears in early childhood.
    d. Tends to be unilateral and localized to an extremity.
    e. The lesions may look like typical enchondromas or may be much larger (even grotesque in a finger).
    f. The metaphyses often have a striated appearance, with vertical lucencies and densities; most have some calcific matrix.
    g. Causes significant limb shortening and growth deformities.
    h. Risk of malignant transformation (usually to chondrosarcoma) 25% to 30%.
I. Maffucci's syndrome:
    a. Enchondromatosis, combined with soft tissue hemangiomas.
    b. Phleboliths may be present, which make the radiographic diagnosis.
    c. Much higher malignant potential than enchondromatosis alone (approaching 100% according to a recent study[16]).

Osteochondroma (Exostosis)

Very common benign neoplasm that results from growth plate cartilage displaced to the metaphyseal region. Underlying bone is completely normal, and normal bone grows as an excrescence from the underlying metaphysis, with continuity of the periosteum, cortices, and marrow of the exostosis and host bone. The exostosis is covered by a cartilaginous cap, the source of growth. Osteochondromas may extend from the host bone on a stalk with a cauliflowerlike head or may be much more broad based and sessile.

Key Concepts

Metaphyseal: may cause growth deformity (especially if multiple and sessile) or mechanical problems (if cauliflowerlike). Growth ceases with skeletal maturity and growth or pain after skeletal maturity is suggestive of degeneration to chondrosarcoma. Multiple exostosis is hereditary (autosomal dominant) and has a 15% incidence of malignant degeneration. MR is useful in diagnosis and differentiating benign from malignant lesions.

A. Determinants:
  1. Age: Mass is usually discovered in first or second decade.
  2. Soft tissue involvement: Soft tissues are displaced by the bony mass, and a bursa may form over the mass if there is mechanical irritation.
  3. Pattern: Geographic.
  4. Size: Range from small to very large (10 cm).
  5. Locations: Metaphyseal, with exostosis pointing away from adjacent joints; 36% are found around the knee; 95%, in the extremities.
  6. Zone of transition: None, since normal bone is found within the exostosis.
  7. Margins; No sclerotic margins, since normal bone extends from host bone to the exostotic bone.
  8. Tumor matrix: Normal bone is within the stalk, but cartilaginous matrix may be seen in the cartilaginous cap.
  9. Host response: None. Remodeling of adjacent normal bone may occur from mechanical erosion.
  10. Ninety percent are solitary (for discussion of multiple exostoses, see Section H).
  11. Other features: Osteochondromas are distinctive in that growth from the cartilage cap normally ceases with fusion of the epiphyses. Growth after maturity suggests malignant degeneration.
B. MR appearance: Normal-appearing bone marrow and cortex extend from the underlying bone into the stalk; the overlying hyaline cartilage is high signal on T2 and is expected to be thin (1–2 cm thickness suggests degeneration to chondrosarcoma); overlying bursal formation is diagnosed by MR.
C. Nonaggressive in the absence of malignant change. Malignant transformation occurs in 1% of solitary exostoses.
D. Major differential diagnoses:
  1. Stalk or cauliflower type:
    a. Parosteal osteosarcoma: Matrix is different and does not have continuity of cortex with host cortex.

  b. Chondrosarcoma: Malignant degeneration of an osteochondroma may be indistinguishable radiographically from benign osteochondroma.
  c. Myositis ossificans: No cortical or marrow continuity.
  2. Broad-based sessile type:
   a. Metaphyseal dysplasia.
   b. Fibrous dysplasia.
E. Metastatic potential: Less than 1% of solitary osteochondromas undergo malignant degeneration to chondrosarcoma. This may be detected radiographically as new mineral deposition beyond previously documented contours or, very rarely, destructive changes at the neck or base of the exostosis. More often, there is no radiographic change, but the patient complains of pain or growth of the exostosis (after closure of epiphyses). In the absence of mechanical reasons for pain or the formation of a bursa simulating growth of the exostosis, such clinical symptoms indicate malignant degeneration until proven otherwise.
F. Radiographic work-up:
  1. Plain film diagnosis of osteochondroma.
  2. If malignant degeneration is suspected, chondrosarcoma work-up is done, which usually requires MRI.
  3. Bone scan shows mildly increased uptake for osteochondroma and variable uptake for chondrosarcoma; a single bone scan, therefore, often is not useful though serial scans may be.
G. Treatment.
  1. Solitary osteochondroma as an incidental finding: None.
  2. Osteochondroma painful for mechanical reasons: Local excision.
  3. Suspected malignant degeneration: See Peripheral Chondrosarcoma, Section IIB.
H. Multiple hereditary exostoses:
  1. Autosomal-dominant disorder but with sporadic cases resulting in development of multiple osteochondromas.
  2. Although some of these exostoses are stalklike, most are broadbased and involve a greater circumference of the metaphysis, simulating dysplasia.
  3. Appears first in childhood as lumps around joints.
  4. Results in shorter limbs and deformities.
  5. Relatively high incidence of sarcomatous degeneration (10% to 20%), especially in more proximal lesions. Degeneration occurs earlier in life than for solitary exostosis.
  6. Treatment: Resect locally as necessary for mechanical problems and observe for sarcomatous degeneration.
I. Dysplasia epiphysealis hemimelica (Trevor-Fairbank disease):

1. Intra-articular osteochondromas arising from the epiphysis.
2. May occur in single or multiple epiphyses, generally on one side of the body.
3. Knee and ankle are most common sites.
4. Histologically identical to exostosis.
5. Radiographically, a lobulated mass arising from an epiphysis, usually well mineralized.
6. Causes joint deformity, pain, and limited range of motion.
7. Treatment: Local resection.

Chondroblastoma

Fairly rare benign cartilaginous lesion found almost exclusively in the epiphysis (one of the few lesions *ever* found in epiphysis).

Key Concepts

Found in epiphysis in skeletally immature patient (most commonly proximal humerus), but may extend into metaphysis with plate closure; cartilage matrix may—but need not—be present; appears benign; but may elicit prominent periosteal reaction.

A. Determinants:
  1. Age: Second decade most common (before epiphyseal closure).
  2. Soft tissue involvement: None.
  3. Pattern: Geographic—oval and sometimes lobulated.
  4. Size: 1.5 to 4 cm.
  5. Location: Eccentric, with epicenter nearly always in the epiphysis; with partial epiphyseal plate closure, the lesion may extend into the metaphysis; very rarely, the epicenter may be in the metaphysis or apophysis; common sites of involvement: proximal humerus, proximal femur, distal femur, proximal tibia (Fig 1-9). The talus and calcaneus may also be involved.
  6. Zone of transition: Narrow.
  7. Margin: Sclerotic.
  8. Tumor matrix: Lytic, with cartilaginous calcifications in 50% (though they may be very subtle).
  9. Host response: 50% show thick periosteal reaction along metaphysis.
  10. Monostotic.
  11. Other features: Mild pain, often referred to the adjacent joint.
B. MR appearance: Low to intermediate heterogeneous SI on T2, in lobulated pattern; less commonly, high SI is seen on T2 imaging; very

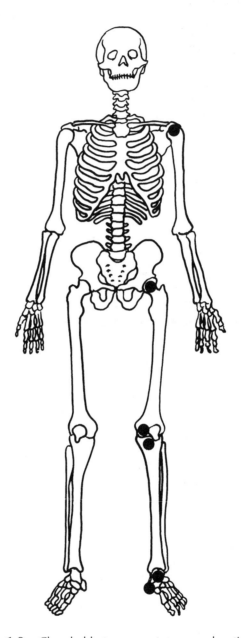

Fig. 1-9 Chondroblastoma: most common locations.

prominent periosteal reaction, bone marrow edema, and adjacent soft tissue reaction is common and may be confusing, simulating a more aggressive lesion.[17]

C. Not aggressive.
D. Major differential diagnoses:
   1. GCT crossing into the epiphysis.
   2. Articular lesions with large cysts such as pigmented villonodular synovitis (PVNS).
   3. Clear cell chondrosarcoma.
E. Metastatic potential: Almost negligible. There are only isolated case reports of malignant chondroblastomas with lung metastases (in the absence of radiation therapy).
F. Radiographic work-up: Plain film diagnosis. CT can be helpful in searching for matrix calcification and in establishing the relationship of the chondroblastoma to the adjacent joint.
G. Treatment: Curettage and bone graft. Recurrence rate is 15%, and recurrence is more likely if the chondroblastoma has an ABC component; recurrent lesions may be more aggressive and may require wider excision.

Chondromyxoid Fibroma
Very rare, benign cartilaginous lesion also containing fibrous and myxoid tissue; found most commonly in the proximal tibial metaphysis.

Key Concepts

Rare bubbly lesion found almost exclusively in proximal tibial metaphysis. That location is the major key to the diagnosis, since typical cartilaginous matrix is rare.

A. Determinants:
   1. Age: Second and third decades.
   2. Soft tissue involvement: None.
   3. Pattern: Geographic; often lobulated, with a pseudoseptate appearance.
   4. Size: Often greater than 5 cm.
   5. Location: Eccentric in metaphysis; one third in proximal tibia; others distributed in the proximal and distal femur, flat bones, and tarsals or other small bones of the hand or foot.
   6. Zone of transition: Narrow.
   7. Margin: Thick sclerotic margin, with endosteal sclerosis at sites of cortical expansion; lobulated.
   8. Tumor matrix: Calcification rare (2%).

9. Host response: Commonly, endosteal sclerosis; periosteal reaction is rare.

10. Monostotic.

B. MR appearance: Nonspecific, with low SI on T1 and high SI on T2, often inhomogeneous.

C. Not aggressive.

D. Major differential diagnoses:
1. GCT (generally does not have a sclerotic margin).
2. NOF.
3. ABC.
4. Chondroblastoma.
5. Enchondroma.

E. Metastatic potential: Malignant transformation (in the absence of radiation therapy) is extremely rare.

F. Radiographic work-up: Diagnosis is suggested by plain film and proven by subsequent biopsy; additional imaging generally is not useful.

G. Treatment:
1. Curettage and bone grafting are commonly the initial therapeutic approach; a high recurrence rate (25% to 30%) may be due to the lobulated nature of the lesion (lobules may be missed on curettage). Interestingly, younger patients tend to have more aggressive lesions and a higher recurrence rate.
2. Wide excision may be attempted after recurrence, or initially for a more aggressive lesion.

Juxtacortical (Periosteal) Chondroma

A benign cartilaginous lesion originating on the periosteal surface of the bone producing a soft tissue mass and cortical erosion that may be difficult to differentiate from more aggressive lesions.

Key Concepts

Rare lesion that appears aggressive, with cortical scalloping, soft tissue mass, and even periosteal reaction; location in hands or feet is suggestive.

A. Determinants:
1. Age: Occurs in both children and adults but generally before 30 years of age.
2. Soft tissue involvement: Soft tissue mass.
3. Pattern: Geographic, with ''saucerization'' or erosion of the cortical surface.
4. Size: Less than 4 cm.
5. Location: Periosteal (juxtacortical) epicenter; most commonly in

the small tubular bones of the hands and feet, though it may be seen in the larger tubular bones.

6. Zone of transition: Narrow.
7. Margin: Sclerotic margin is usually seen at the eroded cortex.
8. Tumor matrix: Calcification in soft tissue in 50% of lesions.
9. Host response: Smooth periosteal reaction is not uncommon.
10. Monostotic.

B. MR appearance: Nonspecific, but soft tissue mass with adjacent bone destruction may appear aggressive.

C. Aggressiveness: Bone involvement does not appear aggressive, but the soft tissue mass makes the lesion appear more ominous and may confuse the diagnosis. The histology may also appear more aggressive than that of central chondromas, but the behavior is benign.

D. Major differential diagnoses: (Note: Lesions 1 through 3 should appear more aggressive than the juxtocortical chondroma and, furthermore, rarely appear in the hands or feet.)

1. Chondrosarcoma.
2. Parosteal osteosarcoma.
3. Periosteal osteosarcoma.
4. GCT of tendon sheath.

E. Metastatic potential: With recurrence, may undergo malignant transformation.

F. Radiographic work-up: With the typical appearance in the hands or feet, it is a plain film diagnosis. A more aggressive appearance in a large tubular bone may require MRI and may present a diagnostic dilemma.

G. Treatment: Excision *en bloc* precludes recurrence and malignant transformation.

B. Cartilage-Forming Tumors: Malignant

Chondrosarcoma
Cartilage-producing sarcoma.

Key Concepts

Third most common primary malignant bone tumor (following osteosarcoma and multiple myeloma); these sarcomas are often asymptomatic, leading to large tumors with late diagnosis; errors in diagnosis are also common, again leading to delay in appropriate treatment; exostotic variety almost always has cartilaginous matrix, but central variety may not; radiographically, the lesion may appear unaggressive or only mildly aggressive. If this is seen in conjunction with pain or growth of an exostosis in an adult sarcoma should be assumed and the appropriate work-up instituted.

Central (Medullary) Chondrosarcoma.—Either primary or secondary (degeneration of enchondromas, usually those lesions located more proximally in the skeleton) chondrosarcoma arising centrally in the bone.
A. Determinants:
   1. Age: Fourth, fifth, sixth decades most common.
   2. Soft tissue involvement: Generally no soft tissue mass, although a high-grade lesion may have soft tissue involvement.
   3. Pattern: Tends to be geographic, but may have portions that appear more permeative. Mild cortical expansion and/or scalloping may occur.
   4. Size: Generally greater than 5 cm.
   5. Location: Central, metaphyseal ends of long bones; also seen in pelvis and shoulder girdle (Fig 1-10).
   6. Zone of transition. Large portions of the tumor may have a narrow zone of transition, but other regions may have a less distinct zone of transition.
   7. Margin: Usually no sclerotic margin.
   8. Tumor matrix: Central chondrosarcomas range from completely lytic to lytic with a few flecks of calcification to dense aggregates of anular calcification.
   9. Host response: Periosteal reaction is variable; the endosteum may be significantly thickened (a feature that may suggest the diagnosis).
   10. Monostotic.
B. MR appearance: A well-differentiated (low grade) lesion may show the lobulated hyaline cartilage; higher grade lesions will appear more nonspecific and have inhomogeneous high SI on T2; mineralized matrix may be seen as low SI on all sequences.
C. Aggressiveness: 90% of central chondrosarcomas are low grade. This corresponds to the determinants listed above, which describe only a moderately aggressive lesion. The take-home lesson is this: Chondrosarcomas are common lesions and are usually not very aggressive-looking radiographically. Therefore, if a central lesion (in the right age group) appears slightly to moderately aggressive (question of permeative pattern or a questionable zone of transition), subtle calcification should be sought and the diagnosis of chondrosarcoma should be offered, whether or not cartilaginous calcification is found. This lesion is very commonly underdiagnosed since it so often appears rather benign; this underdiagnosis results in undertreatment.
D. Major differential diagnoses:
   1. If calcification is present:
      a. Enchondroma, if it looks unaggressive.
      b. Bone infarct degenerating to MFH (if it appears more aggressive).

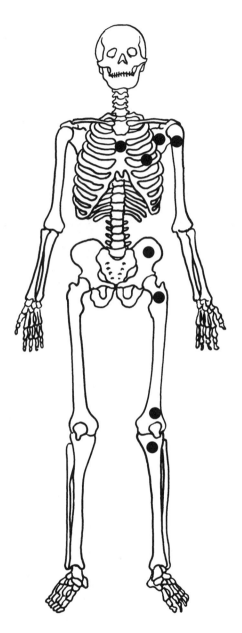

Fig. 1-10 Chondrosarcoma: most common locations.

    2. If no calcific matrix is present:
      a. MFH.
      b. Fibrosarcoma.
      c. Lymphoma.
      d. Osteosarcoma.
      e. GCT (if less aggressive).
E. Metastatic potential:
    1. Ninety percent are low-grade lesions, so local recurrence is more common than metastatic disease. Prognosis is worse for axial than appendicular lesions.
    2. Metastasis involves the lungs, often quite late (even 20 years after diagnosis).
    3. Five-year survival is 75%; this can be improved by:
      a. More prompt radiographic diagnosis.
      b. Meticulous biopsy technique: Chondrosarcoma is very readily implanted in soft tissues since it does not need a blood supply to survive, so recurrences may be due to tumor spill at time of biopsy or resection. Similarly, placement of an intramedullary rod may disseminate tumor cells.
F. Radiographic work-up:
    1. Plain film: Suggests diagnosis.
    2. CT: May detect subtle calcification in a lytic lesion and make the diagnosis; otherwise MRI is useful to determine tumor extent and biopsy and therapy plans.
    3. Bone scan: Variable uptake is not particularly useful.
    4. Chest x-ray and CT.
G. Treatment: Radical excision or limb salvage *en bloc*. Radiation and chemotherapy are effective only as palliative therapy and generally not used initially.

Peripheral (Exostotic) Chondrosarcoma.—Either primary or secondary (degeneration of an exostosis) chondrosarcoma extending peripherally to normal bone.
A. Determinants:
    1. Age: Third, fourth, and fifth decades.
    2. Soft tissue involvement: Unmineralized soft tissue mass may arise from the cartilaginous cap of the exostosis, usually only displacing rather than invading local soft tissue.
    3. Pattern: Geographic.
    4. Size: Greater than 5 cm, usually quite large before detected.
    5. Location: Peripheral, metaphyses of long bones as well as pelvis, shoulder girdle, sternum, and ribs.
    6. Zone of transition: Generally narrow.

   7. Margin: None (see section on osteochondroma).
   8. Tumor matrix: Cartilage cap is often densely calcified. Peripheral streaking or a snowstorm pattern of calcification may help differentiate chondrosarcoma from exostosis. A cartilage cap more than 1 cm thick suggests malignant change to chondrosarcoma, but this may be very difficult to detect and quantify.
   9. Host response: Generally none.
  10. Monostotic.
  11. As described in the section on osteochondroma, degeneration to chondrosarcoma often produces no clear-cut radiographic signs. Therefore clinical signs of pain and growth of exostosis after epiphyseal closure should be considered of primary importance in making the diagnosis of peripheral chondrosarcoma.
B. MR appearance: In an early degeneration of an exostosis to chondrosarcoma, the features of normal marrow and cortex extending into the exostosis will predominate, with an enlarged cartilage cap being the only significantly different feature; higher grade lesions will show more destruction of the stalk, with more high SI on T2 relating to soft tissue mass.
C. Generally not aggressive-looking.
D. Major differential diagnosis: Benign osteochondroma.
E. Metastatic potential: Metastases to the lungs are rather uncommon and generally late, owing to the low-grade nature of most peripheral chondrosarcomas.
F. Radiographic work-up:
   1. Plain film: Watch for change in osteochondroma (growth, change in calcification pattern, destruction of osteochondroma or underlying bone), but pay strict attention to clinical signs in the absence of radiographic changes.
   2. CT or MRI: CT does not reliably show the extent of the cartilaginous cap or soft tissue mass; MRI may show these more reliably.
G. Treatment: Radical or wide excision; generally no radiation or chemotherapy.

Clear Cell Chondrosarcoma.—Very rare lesion most often mistaken for a chondroblastoma because it is low grade and occurs in the ends of long bones.
A. Determinants:
   1. Age: Third decade (older than most chondroblastomas).
   2. Soft tissue involvement: None.
   3. Pattern: Geographic.
   4. Size: Less than 5 cm.
   5. Location: The ends of long bones, most commonly the proximal femur and humerus.

    6. Zone of transition: Narrow.
    7. Margin: Sharp sclerotic margin.
    8. Tumor matrix: Generally absent.
    9. Host response: Periosteal reaction rare.
   10. Monostotic.
   11. The description is identical to that of chondroblastoma, except that it occurs in a slightly older age group, which initially may be the only hint of the true diagnosis. After growing slowly for a number of years, it may become more aggressive.
B. MR appearance: Nonspecific.
C. Generally appears nonaggressive.
D. Major differential diagnosis:
    1. Chondroblastoma.
    2. Later, if more aggressive, MFH, fibrosarcoma, or lymphoma.
E. Metastatic potential: Very low; better prognosis than for conventional chondrosarcoma.
F. Radiographic work-up: Plain film.
G. Treatment: Wide excision; this is more aggressive treatment than that for chondroblastoma (curettage); curettage alone can result in an aggressive recurrence.

Dedifferentiated Chondrosarcoma.—The following are characteristic of this lesion:
A. Degeneration of a typically indolent chondrosarcoma into a highly aggressive lesion.
B. Degenerates to fibrosarcoma, MFH, high-grade chondrosarcoma, osteosarcoma, or a lesion that has several elements.
C. Ten percent of chondrosarcomas may dedifferentiate. This is, therefore, not a rare lesion, since chondrosarcomas are relatively common.
D. The original chondrosarcoma and the dedifferentiated elements coexist, so the biopsy site must be chosen to include the more aggressive lesion.
E. Prognosis is poor (20% 5-year survival), and lung metastases are common.
F. Treatment is radical excision and chemotherapy.

Mesenchymal Chondrosarcoma.—The following are characteristic of this lesion[18]:
A. Exceedingly rare, highly malignant sarcoma.
B. Age group is younger than standard chondrosarcoma (10 to 40 years).
C. Site is unusual: One third arise in soft tissues; in the skeleton, rib and jaw lesions are common while long bone lesions are unusual.
D. Calcification is usually present.
E. Radiographically aggressive; it either looks like chondrosarcoma or is nonspecific. MR shows a lobulated mass, high SI on T2.

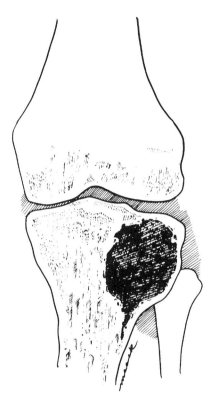

Fig. 1-11   Giant cell tumor demonstrating its typically lytic nature, with a narrow zone of transition but lack of sclerotic margin. The eccentric and subarticular location is also typical.

F. Treatment is radical resection. Hematogenous metastases may be expected to occur commonly and early.

III. GIANT CELL TUMOR (GCT)

A relatively uncommon (5% of primary bone tumors) lesion consisting of multinucleated giant cells in a fibroid stroma; these are distinct from many other lesions that may contain reactive giant cells (Fig 1-11).

Key Concepts

Subarticular, eccentric lytic lesion with a narrow zone of transition but no sclerotic margin; most common around the knee or distal radius; recurrence after curettage is very common.

A. Determinants:
  1. Age: Lesion nearly always occurs after epiphyseal fusion (85% after 20 years of age); 70% fall between 20 and 40 years of age.
  2. Soft tissue involvement: Cortical breakthrough and soft tissue mass may be seen in 24%.
  3. Pattern: Geographic expanding lesion.
  4. Size: Often large (3 to 5 cm) by time of diagnosis.
  5. Location:
      a. In tubular bones: Lesion starts *eccentrically in the metaphysis, it later extends to the subarticular end of the bone.* Because of the eventual subarticular extension of most GCTs it is sometimes mistakenly believed that these are epiphyseal lesions. However, purely metaphyseal early GCTs occur.
      b. About the knee (distal femur and proximal tibia) or wrist (distal radius or ulna): 65% of cases (Fig 1–12).
      c. In thin tubular bones: Appear to be central rather than eccentric.
      d. Metaphyseal equivalents may be sites of involvement in flat bones (especially around the acetabulum).
      e. In the spine: Often involves the sacrum or body of the vertebrae (rarely the posterior elements).
  6. Zone of transition: Narrow.
  7. Margin: No sclerotic margin. (Note: This combination of narrow zone of transition and no sclerotic margin is a highly reliable feature of GCT that is rarely seen in other lesions.)
  8. Matrix: None.
  9. Host response: No periosteal or marginal reaction in the absence of fracture.
  10. Generally monostotic: May be multicentric, especially in the skull and facial bones affected by Paget's disease. In the case of multicentric GCTs, hyperparathyroidism with multiple brown tumors should be excluded. Multicentric GCTs may be difficult to differentiate from metastatic GCT; fortunately both are rare.
B. MR appearance: The lesion is solid, with typical low SI on T1. About 60% of GCTs will have high T2 SI that contain low SI areas that may be nodular, zonal, whorled, or diffuse (the low SI regions occupy 20% to 25% of tumor volume)[19]; these relate to hemosiderin and collagen content. Forty percent of GCTs will simply show high SI on T2.
C. Aggressiveness: Generally appear unaggressive, but occasionally destroy cortex and present with a soft tissue mass.
D. Major differential diagnoses:
  1. In long bones:
      a. Chondroblastoma: Generally skeletally immature with sclerotic margin.

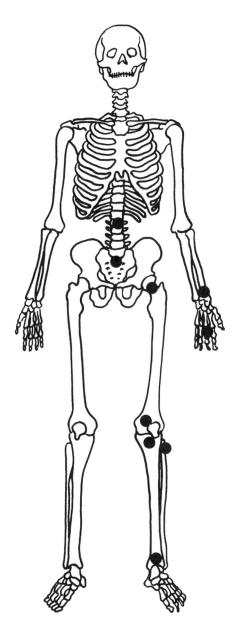

Fig. 1-12   Giant cell tumor: most common locations.

    b. Brown tumor of hyperpara-thyroidism (HPTH): Usually have subperiosteal resorption or other signs of HPTH.

    c. NOF: Metaphyseal with sclerotic border.

    d. Chondrosarcoma: If epiphyseal and only slightly aggressive.

    e. Plasmacytoma.

  2. In flat bones or spine:

    a. Aneurysmal bone cyst.

    b. Osteoblastoma.

    c. Chordoma.

    d. Plasmacytoma.

    e. Metastasis.

E. Metastatic potential:

  1. Majority are benign: grade I or II.

  2. Malignant (often secondary to previous radiation) with metastases to lungs in 5%.

  3. Of those that metastasize, prognosis may be good (25% mortality) with surgical resection of lung metastases.

  4. Problem: One cannot reliably differentiate benign from malignant GCT radiographically; similarly, the histologic features are not predictive of the tumor's ultimate behavior. However, a higher-stage GCT that has recurred does increase the likelihood of developing metastatic disease.[20]

  5. Rarely, a histologically benign GCT will metastasize to the lung, with the lung lesion also showing benign histology; the lung nodules often have a thin calcific rim.

F. Radiographic work-up:

  1. Plain film diagnosis: The radiographic appearance and location are quite characteristic, and the diagnosis is usually easily made.

  2. MRI may be required, depending on the type of surgery anticipated. It may be especially valuable in assessing subchondral breakthrough and intraarticular tumor extension.

G. Treatment:

  1. Curative treatment would be to regard the lesion as a low-grade malignant neoplasm and treat it with a wide resection *en bloc*, after which the rate of recurrence is only 10% to 15%. However, the subarticular nature of the lesion often requires resection of the joint and fusion or the placement of a long-stemmed custom prosthesis; in a young patient, such a prosthesis almost inevitably loosens and requires multiple revisions throughout life, causing considerable morbidity.

  2. To avoid the potential morbidity of wide resection *en bloc*, curettage and bone grafting may be the initial treatment. *A recurrence rate of 55% is expected following curettage.*

3. A compromise seems to be initial treatment with curettage and cryosurgery if resection *en bloc* seems unacceptable initially. Another method is wide resection at the metaphyseal margins and curettage of the subarticular margin; recurrence rates seem to be lower with these methods.

4. Radiation therapy should be avoided: Besides having an unacceptable cure rate of only 50%, 10% to 15% of irradiated GCTs develop radiation sarcomas, with extremely high mortality. In the Mayo Clinic series, nearly 100% of malignant GCTs were secondary to radiation treatment. In rare cases when a GCT is unresectable radiation may be the only treatment option.

H. In 15% of GCTs, a secondary ABC may be found. This combination may make the radiographic picture somewhat confusing.

I. Patients with Paget's disease may develop GCT. The patients are older and location tends to be different (skull, facial bones, axial skeleton) than the usual GCT patient. The lesions may be multicentric, are usually benign, but may be malignant.

IV. MARROW TUMORS

The "round cell" tumors; *round cell lesions include tumors (Ewing's sarcoma, lymphoma, multiple myeloma), metastatic neuroblastoma, histiocytosis, and infection. These lesions often are not easily distinguished radiographically.*

Ewing's Sarcoma

A highly malignant round cell tumor found in children, it is the *second most common primary bone tumor in children,* after osteosarcoma.

Key Concepts

Highly aggressive, usually diaphyseal with large soft tissue mass and periosteal reaction. Dense host bone sclerosis is common, but no matrix is seen in the soft tissues. Most frequently affected are tubular bones in young children and flat bones in adolescents and young adults.

A. Determinants:
1. Age: 4 to 25 years (95%), most commonly 5 to 14 years.
2. Soft tissue involvement: A soft tissue mass is almost invariably present and often very large.
3. Pattern: *Permeative;* rarely expands the bone.
4. Size: Greater than 5 cm.

5. Location: *Central* (based in medullary canal), *most commonly diaphyseal or metadiaphyseal* but metaphyseal epicenter is not uncommon; 75% involve the *pelvis or long tubular bones.* Other sites are shoulder girdle, rib, and vertebral body. Tends to involve the tubular bones in children under age 10 years and the axial skeleton, pelvis, and shoulder girdle in older children (Fig 1–13).
6. Zone of transition. Wide.
7. Margin: No sclerotic margin.
8. Matrix: *No tumor matrix is produced, but sclerotic reactive bone may be seen:* 62% are completely lytic; 23% have minimal reactive bone; 15% have marked sclerotic reactive bone. Reactive bone, however, is not found in the soft tissue mass, helping to differentiate Ewing's from an osteosarcoma with tumor bone formation in the soft tissue mass.
9. Host response:
   a. Aggressive periosteal reaction is a prominent feature.
   b. Sclerotic reactive bone formation in medullary canal.
   c. Rarely, thick reactive endosteal bone is seen.
10. Initially monostotic, but metastases to bone are common, so the lesion may appear to be polyostotic.
11. Other features:
    a. *One third of patients with Ewing's present with fever, leukocytosis, and elevated erythrocyte sedimentation rate (ESR), simulating infection.* The overlying skin may even be warm and red. Clinical findings may, therefore, be misleading.
    b. Ewing's is extremely rare in black persons.
B. MR appearance: Nonspecific low SI on T1 and high SI on T2, with large soft tissue mass; this mass may contain necrotic areas which have lower SI.
C. Highly aggressive appearance.
D. Major differential diagnoses:
   1. Primarily other round cell lesions: osteomyelitis, histiocytosis (may appear highly aggressive), neuroblastoma metastasis, low-grade intramedullary osteosarcoma.
   2. The duration of symptoms may be helpful in differentiating the round cell lesions. Histiocytosis (eosinophilic granuloma) may be one of the most aggressive locally, with the shortest time course (1 to 2 weeks). Osteomyelitis has a relatively short course of destruction (2 to 4 weeks), and Ewing's sarcoma has a slower course (destructive changes seen at 6 to 12 weeks).
E. Metastatic potential:
   1. Five-year survival, 50%.
   2. Fifteen to 30% have metastases at time of diagnosis; *metastases*

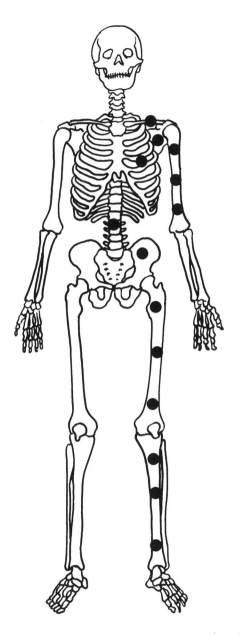

Fig. 1-13   Ewing's sarcoma: most common locations.

affect lung and bone with equal frequency. Central and larger lesions have a worse prognosis than more distal ones.

F. Radiographic work-up:
1. Plain film suggests diagnosis.
2. Bone scan to rule out polyostotic lesion or metastases.
3. Chest x-ray and CT.
4. MRI to determine extent and biopsy site.

G. Treatment is controversial:
1. Combined radiation and chemotherapy: High complication rate, with sarcomatous degeneration and growth disturbance.
2. Some protocols now call for postirradiation resection because local recurrence is found at autopsy following radiation alone in 23% of patients. Local recurrence is difficult to differentiate radiographically from radiation osteonecrosis and tumor necrosis. Since viable tumor cells are found in so many autopsy cases, wide excision following radiation and chemotherapy may be logical in selected cases; it is too early to determine the efficacy of such a protocol.

Primary Lymphoma of Bone (Reticulum Cell Sarcoma)

Uncommon lymphoma that arises initially in bone.

Key Concepts

Permeative and aggressive, as other round cell lesions; soft tissue mass may be enormous.

A. Determinants:
1. Age: Ten to 60 years, but usually 30 to 60 years.
2. Soft tissue involvement: *Soft tissue mass may be huge* since it enlarges very rapidly and is usually asymptomatic until pathologic fracture develops.
3. Pattern: *Permeative lytic.*
4. Size: Very large.
5. Location: *Central appendicular* diaphyseal sites are more common than axial; in descending order of occurrence: femur, pelvis, tibia, humerus, scapula. (Fig. 1-14).
6. Zone of transition: Wide.
7. Margin: No sclerotic margin.
8. Matrix: Usually lytic (77%), but some reactive sclerosis may be seen. Sequestra have been reported in 10%, likely due to rapid bone destruction and soft tissue mass overwhelming residual pieces of bone.[21]

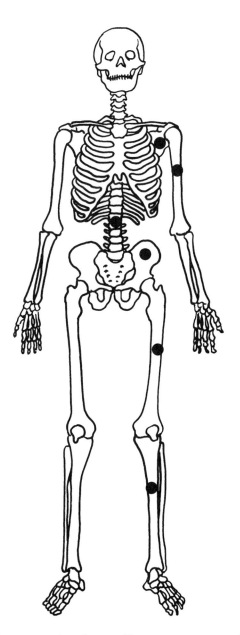

Fig. 1-14   Primary lymphoma of bone: most common locations.

    9. Host response: Often have periosteal reaction.

    10. Monostotic.

B. MR appearance: Nonspecific.

C. Aggressive appearance.

D. Major differential diagnosis:

    1. Fibrosarcoma/MFH.

    2. Osteomyelitis.

    3. Histiocytosis.

    4. Ewing's sarcoma.

E. Metastatic potential:

    1. Five-year survival 55%.

    2. Metastasizes to lymph nodes and bone; lung metastases are unusual, but, when present, may develop and grow extremely fast (much faster than other metastatic lung nodules).

F. Radiographic work-up:

    1. Plain film suggests diagnosis.

    2. Bone scan to determine whether monostotic.

    3. Chest x-ray and CT.

    4. MR to determine local extent and lymphadenopathy.

G. Treatment:

    1. Whole bone radiation.

    2. Chemotherapy for disseminated disease.

Hodgkin's Disease

In bone, is almost always secondary to a primary lymph node lesion; 20% of patients with Hodgkin's disease have radiographic evidence of bone involvement; extremely rare as a primary bone tumor. Metastatic Hodgkin's disease can involve bone by either hematogenous dissemination or contiguous spread from adjacent nodes (the sternum is a common site, with extension from internal mammary nodes).

Key Concepts

Especially common in vertebral bodies, and so sclerotic that it is a cause of "ivory" vertebral body; often polyostotic.

A. Determinants:

    1. Age: Second through fourth decade.

    2. Soft tissue involvement: Mass is common.

    3. Pattern: Often geographic with some permeative areas.

    4. Size: Wide range.

5. Location: *Axial skeleton* (77%) much more common than appendicular; especially common in *vertebral bodies.*
6. Zone of transition: Wide.
7. Margin: May or may not show sclerosis.
8. Matrix: *Sclerotic reactive bone often seen.*
   a. Lytic, 25%.
   b. Blastic, 15%.
   c. Mixed, 60%.
   d. The *ivory vertebra* is a classic manifestation of Hodgkin's disease, though it is seen also in Paget's and other metastatic disease processes.
9. Host response: Minimal periosteal reaction.
10. Sixty-six percent polyostotic.
B. Moderately aggressive in appearance.
C. Major differential diagnosis: Metastatic disease.

Multiple Myeloma

A neoplastic proliferation of plasma cells; the most common primary bone tumor with the most common clinical presentation being back pain and anemia; both multiple myeloma and its solitary form (plasmacytoma) will be discussed.

Key Concepts

Plasmacytoma may be expansile and appear relatively non-aggressive; multiple myeloma may present with punched-out lytic lesions or merely generalized "osteoporosis" with compression fracture. Bone scan and skeletal survey are complementary studies, since each misses a significant number of myeloma lesions.

A. Determinants:
1. Age: Most (95%) over 40 years.
2. Soft tissue involvement: Small soft tissue mass is common.
3. Pattern:
   a. *Seventy percent are multifocal myeloma with focal punched-out lesions*—a moth-eaten pattern.
   b. *Fifteen percent show generalized infiltration without focal lesions:* appears only as a generalized osteopenia.
   c. *Thirty percent are plasmacytomas with an expansile geographic pattern* (which may have permeative components).

4. Size:
   a. Multiple myeloma lesions generally are less than 5 cm.
   b. Plasmacytomas usually are greater than 5 cm.
5. Location:
   a. Multiple myeloma: Originates in the red marrow but progresses to cortex and other areas. *The skull, vertebral bodies, and ribs are most commonly involved, followed by the proximal appendicular skeleton.*
   b. Plasmacytoma: Involves vertebral bodies, pelvis, femur, and humerus most commonly; rib and skull lesions are much less commonly seen.
6. Zone of transition: Relatively narrow in both the punched-out lesions of multiple myeloma and the more cystic lesions of plasmacytoma.
7. Margins: No sclerotic margin except in sclerosing myeloma (see 11, below).
8. Matrix: None except in sclerosing myeloma.
9. Host response: None.
10. Polyostotic if multiple myeloma. Plasmacytoma progresses to multifocal disease.
11. Other features:
    a. Ten to 15% are associated with amyloidosis. When amyloid is in the synovium, it simulates rheumatoid arthritis.
    b. One percent may be sclerosing myeloma, with either a sclerotic margin around the lesion or else entirely sclerotic lesions. Sclerosing myeloma is associated with a syndrome with the acronym POEMS: *p*olyneuropathy, *o*rganomegaly, *e*ndocrinopathy, *m*yeloma, *s*kin changes.

B. MR appearance: Nonspecific pattern of homogeneous diffuse, mottled, or localized decrease in SI on T1 and increased SI on T2; work is currently being done to evaluate MR correlation with disease progression/regression markers.

C. Appearance: Mildly aggressive.

D. Major differential diagnoses:
   1. Multiple myeloma:
      a. Metastatic disease (the latter usually involves the pedicles, not the vertebral body, as does myeloma).
      b. Osteoporosis.
      c. HPTH.
      d. Osteopoikilosis (if sclerotic).
   2. Plasmacytoma:
      a. GCT.
      b. Chondrosarcoma (intramedullary).

E. Metastatic potential:
   1. Multiple myeloma: 5-year survival, 10%.
   2. Plasmacytoma: Most go on to multifocal or generalized disease,
      though a few remain localized; 5-year survival, 30%.
F. Radiographic work-up:
   1. This is controversial, but it seems that skeletal surveys and bone
      scans are complementary studies in multiple myeloma.
      a. ^{99m}Tc bone scanning is positive in 25% to 40% of myeloma
         lesions.
      b. ^{99m}Tc is less reliable than a skeletal survey in a lesion search,
         but is more sensitive than plain film in 18% of lesions.
      c. Plain film is more sensitive than ^{99m}Tc in 38% of lesions.
      d. MRI appears to be quite sensitive and may be helpful when
         one must resolve a discrepancy between scan and plain film
         results.
   2. Other work-up: (Note: *20% of plasmacytoma patients* will have
      neither serum electrophoresis or bone marrow aspirate abnormali-
      ties; in these cases, biopsy of the lesion is diagnostic.)
      a. Serum electrophoresis.
      b. Bone marrow aspiration.
G. Treatment:
   1. Multiple myeloma: Chemotherapy and palliative radiation therapy
      for painful lesions and large lesions likely to develop pathologic
      fracture.
   2. Plasmacytoma: Radiation therapy; occasionally ablative surgery is
      performed.

V. VASCULAR TUMORS
A. Vascular Tumors: Benign

Hemangioma–Osseous
Hamartomatous lesion composed of vascular channels.

Key Concepts

Vertebral bodies and skull are most commonly involved and show dense
vertical striations. High SI on both T1 and T2.

A. Determinants:
   1. Age: Fourth and fifth decades predominate, but wide range.
   2. Soft tissue involvement: May have a soft tissue mass; in the verte-
      bral bodies, this may lead to neurologic symptoms if the mass is
      epidural.

3. Patterns: Geographic cystic lesion.
4. Size: Usually greater than 2 cm.
5. Location: *75% in vertebral bodies (especially thoracic spine), skull (involved outer table, nor inner table), and facial bones.* Vertebral body hemangiomas are found in 10% to 15% of the population in autopsy series.
6. Zone of transition: Narrow.
7. Margin: Sclerotic.
8. Tumor matrix: None.
9. *Host response is characteristic and makes the diagnosis: In the vertebral bodies, there is a coarsened vertical trabecular pattern without collapse; in the skull, there are also coarsened trabeculae, but they radiate in a sunburst pattern to the expanded outer table.*
10. Usually monostotic in the skull; often multiple in the spine.

B. MR appearance: Osseous hemangiomas characteristically have variably high SI on both T1 and T2 imaging, due to the variable fatty stroma of the lesion. The vessels themselves are rarely seen in the osseous lesion. CT shows the coarsened trabeculae as a ''polka dot'' appearance in the axial cuts.

C. Not aggressive.

D. Major differential diagnoses:
   1. Multiple myeloma: Usually no coarsened trabecula.
   2. Paget's disease of bone: Usually enlarged vertebral body.
   3. Metastatic disease.

E. Metastatic potential: None.

F. Radiographic work-up:
   1. Plain film is diagnostic but less sensitive than MR.
   2. If symptomatic spine lesion, may need CT or MRI to define epidural extent.

G. Treatment:
   1. Usually none.
   2. If symptomatic, resection and/or radiation.

Hemangioma–Soft tissue

A. Soft tissue hemangiomas are characterized by a mass and calcified phleboliths on plain film.

B. On contrast-enhanced CT, one sees a characteristic ''can-of-worms'' appearance of tortuous, dilated vessels.

C. MR is usually characteristic, with the lesion containing areas of fatty stroma which yields high SI on both T1 and T2 imaging. Tortuous vessels are seen as either high signal or flow void, depending on rate of flow.

D. Some cases have a more nonspecific appearance, with low SI on T1 and homogeneously high SI on T2.

E. Common (7% of all benign soft tissue tumors).[22] Most frequent tumor of infancy and childhood.
F. Usually intramuscular.
G. Soft tissue hemangiomas may scallop or extend into adjacent bone; may cause bone overgrowth locally due to chronic hyperemia.
H. Synovial hemangioma: May cause repetitive bleeding into the joint and an appearance similar to hemophilia; knee and elbow are favored sites, as in hemophilia; MR similar to intramuscular hemangioma.
I. The patient may observe lesion size variability throughout the day.

Lymphangioma–Osseous
Hamartomatous lesion of dilated lymphatic vessels; extremely rare.
A. Determinants:
  1. Age: Usually adult.
  2. Soft tissue involvement: None.
  3. Pattern: Geographic or moth-eaten.
  4. Size: Greater than 2 cm.
  5. Location: Central, flat, or tubular bones.
  6. Zone of transition: Narrow.
  7. Margins: Sclerotic.
  8. Tumor matrix: None (lytic).
  9. Host response: Generally none.
  10. Monostotic or polyostotic.
  11. Other features: Lymphangiomatosis is the form of lymphangioma with multiple skeletal lesions, lymphedema, and chylous pleural effusion.
B. Nonaggressive to mildly aggressive in appearance, generally nonspecific.
C. Major differential diagnoses:
  1. SBC.
  2. Fibrous dysplasia.
  3. Desmoplastic fibroma.
D. Metastatic potential: None.
E. Radiographic work-up: Plain film appearance often leads to biopsy without further work-up since it is a nonaggressive-looking lesion.

Lymphangioma–Soft Tissue[22]
A. Vast majority of lymphangiomas are soft tissue.
B. Most found at birth, or in first 2 years.
C. Most common type is cystic hygroma (involving head, neck, axilla, thorax).
D. Nonspecific on plain film, multilocular cystic characteristics seen by CT, ultrasound (US), MR; may show serpentine vascular channels as well.

Cystic Angiomatosis

Rare, benign, multicentric hemangiomatosis or lymphangiomatosis, often with severe visceral involvement (60–70%).

Key Concepts

Benign lesion that is extremely aggressive locally; phleboliths help make the diagnosis.

A. Determinants:
1. Age: First through third decades.
2. Soft tissue involvement: Mass with calcified phleboliths may be present.
3. Pattern: Moth-eaten.
4. Size: Usually several centimeters.
5. Location: In any bone, most commonly femur, pelvis, ribs, humerus, skull, and vertebrae.
6. Zone of transition: Generally narrow, but may be indistinct.
7. Margin: Sclerotic rim, but may be incomplete.
8. Tumor matrix: Lytic (rarely dense).
9. Host response: Usually none except cortical expansion.
10. Polyostotic.
B. Aggressive-looking large, very expanded lesions.
C. Major differential diagnoses in the usual case of polyostotic lesions:
1. Metastases.
2. Histiocytosis.
3. Fibrous dysplasia.
4. Enchondromatosis (Maffucci's).
D. Metastatic potential: Does not metastasize, but is locally aggressive: 50%, 5-year survival without visceral involvement; visceral involvement associated with chylous effusions and death.
E. Radiographic work-up: Plain film; otherwise symptomatic.
F. Treatment: Curettage or radiation, depending on extent and site of lesion; recurrence is common, and therapy often is not helpful, especially with visceral involvement.

Massive Osteolysis (Gorham's Disease)

Angiomatosis and regional dissolution of bone with much more extensive destruction than in routine angiomatosis.
A. Most commonly seen in children and young adults.
B. There is usually a *history of trauma.*
C. *Rapid destruction of bone* (not permeative—bone simply disappears) *which spreads contiguously across joints.*

D. No host reaction.

E. Shoulder and hip are most common sites.

F. Radiation may possibly help, but lesions may either stabilize or progress relentlessly.

Glomus Tumor

A rare benign vascular tumor found dorsally in the *terminal phalanx* that shows extrinsic osseous erosion by the soft tissue mass, usually with a sclerotic border. It is usually found in adults, is painful, and is treated by marginal excision or curettage. Its location in the terminal phalanx helps differentiate it from enchondroma and sarcoid lesion of the hand.

B. Vascular Lesions Intermediate or Indeterminate for Malignancy

Hemangiopericytoma

Vascular lesion seen in soft tissues which may erode bone cortex, but is extremely rare as an intraosseous lesion. The soft tissue lesion is nonspecific by plain film and MR. The osseous lesion is described here.

A. Determinants:
   1. Age: Fourth or fifth decade.
   2. Soft tissue involvement: Mass common.
   3. Pattern: Permeative or moth-eaten.
   4. Size: Usually less than 5 cm.
   5. Location: Axial skeleton and proximal tubular bones (metaphyseal).
   6. Zone of transition: Wide.
   7. Margin: No sclerotic margin.
   8. Tumor matrix: Lytic.
   9. Host response: Usually none, rare periosteal reaction.
   10. Monostotic.
   11. May be benign, locally aggressive, or malignant.
B. MR appearance: Nonspecific, though vascular channels are occasionally seen; no fatty elements (as seen in hemangioma).
C. Generally aggressive appearance.
D. Major differential diagnoses: Aggressive lesions.
   1. Fibrosarcoma/MFH.
   2. Intramedullary chondrosarcoma.
   3. Lymphoma.
E. Metastatic potential:
   1. Occasional metastases to lung or bone.
   2. Five-year survival, 90%.
F. Radiographic work-up:
   1. Plain film suggests an aggressive lesion and leads to work-up including bone scan, CT or MRI, and chest films. The lesion is

nonspecific and extremely rare, so it is unlikely that the diagnosis will be made radiographically.

G. Treatment: Wide resection.

Hemangioendothelioma

Benign or low-grade malignant vascular lesion, often difficult to differentiate histologically from angiosarcoma.

Key Concepts

Moderately aggressive lesion, very often polyostotic and involving the hands or feet.

A. Determinants:
   1. Age: Second or third decade.
   2. Soft tissue involvement: May have a soft tissue mass.
   3. Patterns: Moth-eaten to geographic.
   4. Size: 2 to 5 cm.
   5. *Location: The most important radiographic feature* of these tumors. *When multicentric, they tend to involve multiple bones of a single extremity, often the hands or feet;* may be cortically based and either diaphyseal or metaphyseal.
   6. Zone of transition: Narrow to intermediate.
   7. Margin: Little or no sclerosis.
   8. Tumor matrix: Lytic.
   9. Host response: Usually none.
   10. *Polyostotic* more common than monostotic.
   11. Other features: Interestingly, the epithelioid hemangioendothelioma has the same histology as intravascular bronchoalveolar tumor (IVBAT).
B. MR appearance: Nonspecific, though vascular channels are occasionally seen; no fatty elements (as seen in hemangioma).
C. Nonaggressive to mildly aggressive appearance.
D. Major differential diagnoses:
   1. Metastases.
   2. Multiple enchondromas.
E. Metastatic potential: Occasionally metastasizes to lungs; interestingly, the *multicentric lesions have a better prognosis* than monostotic ones.
F. Radiographic work-up: Usually a plain film diagnosis.
G. Treatment: Resection if monostotic.

C. Malignant Vascular Tumors

Angiosarcoma

A rare malignant vascular lesion that may be difficult to differentiate histologically from the more benign hemangioendothelioma.

Key Concepts

Aggressive vascular lesion; not uncommonly multifocal; in a young adult, this multifocal character suggests the diagnosis.

A. Determinants:
   1. Age: Fourth and fifth decades; younger if multifocal.
   2. Soft tissue involvement: Mass is common.
   3. Pattern: Permeative.
   4. Size: Usually greater than 5 cm.
   5. Location: Metaphyseal—femur, tibia, humerus, and pelvis are most common sites. (*If the lesion is multifocal, the angiosarcoma may be regional in distribution.*)
   6. Zone of transition: Moderate to wide.
   7. Margin: Usually no sclerotic margin.
   8. Tumor matrix: Lytic.
   9. Host response: Cortex is thinned, expanded, and disrupted without significant host reaction.
   10. *Thirty-eight percent polyostotic.*
B. MR appearance: Nonspecific, though vascular channels are occasionally seen; no fatty elements (as seen in hemangioma).
C. *Aggressive appearance.*
D. Major differential diagnoses:
   1. If monostotic:
      a. Fibrosarcoma/MFH.
      b. Intramedullary chondrosarcoma.
      c. Lymphoma.
   2. If polyostotic: Metastases.
E. Metastatic potential:
   1. *Highly malignant,* with metastases to lungs or skeleton.
   2. Five-year survival 30% to 50%.
   3. *Prognosis better if the lesions are multifocal.*
F. Radiographic work-up:
   1. Plain film.
   2. Bone scan for metastases or multifocal lesion.
   3. MRI as needed for diagnosis or treatment plan.

    4. Chest x-ray and CT.

G. Treatment: Radical or wide resection.

H. Has been associated as a complication of chronic lymphedema (particularly in mastectomy patients).

VI. OTHER CONNECTIVE TISSUE TUMORS

A. Other Connective Tissue Tumors: Benign

Fibromatoses

A heterogeneous group of lesions that have been described with a variety of terms and classifications; the histology of all of these lesions is similar. In this chapter, they are divided into *soft tissue* and *intraosseous* fibromatoses.

Soft Tissue Fibromatoses—Tend to be grouped according to time and location of occurrence; they all tend to be *locally infiltrative,* a characteristic mirrored by CT or MRI scans on which *no pseudocapsule is seen* and the tumor often infiltrates through compartmental barriers. *This local infiltrating nature, as well as its (often) large size may lead to a misdiagnosis of a malignant lesion. The MR characteristics are helpful in making the diagnosis in approximately 80% of cases: because of the hypocellularity of the lesion, it is usually low SI on both T1 and T2 imaging. The remaining 20% of cases show the low SI on T1 and high SI on T2 that is more typical of other lesions and much more nonspecific.*

A. *Juvenile aponeurotic fibroma.*
    1. Slowly infiltrative lesion arising in the aponeurotic tissue of the *hands* (palms), *wrist,* and *feet* (soles).
    2. Forms a painless soft tissue mass, usually less than 4 cm in length.
    3. May calcify, especially in the *interosseous membranes* of the distal forearm.
    4. Seen in children and adolescents.
    5. *Recurrence* after resection is *common.*

B. *Infantile dermal fibromatosis:*
    1. Infiltrates *extensor surfaces of digits,* presenting as multiple firm nodules attached to skin, tendon, fascia, and periosteum.
    2. Bony erosion rarely occurs.
    3. Appears at 1 to 2 years of age.
    4. *Recurrence* after excision is *frequent.*

C. *Congenital generalized fibromatosis:*
    1. Develops in utero.
    2. Disseminated fibromatosis involves much of the *musculature and viscera.*
    3. *Fatal* within a few months.
    4. Another form (congenital multiple fibromatosis) involves only

muscle and has a better prognosis. Small, well-defined bony erosions are seen occasionally.

D. *Desmoid tumor* (also commonly called *aggressive fibromatosis,* desmoid fibromatosis, or fibrosarcoma grade 1 desmoid type). Relatively common (7% of benign soft tissue tumors).[23]

   1. Painless *infiltrative soft tissue masses* originating in abdominal or extra-abdominal muscle.
   2. Aggressive local infiltration of adjacent muscles, vessels, nerves, and tendons.
   3. *Bone involvement* is rare (6%) and is extrinsic, but *may be spectacular:* huge *frondlike excrescences* may form from a stimulated periosteum, with spicules of bone radiating into a soft tissue mass. Less remarkable *pressure erosion of the cortex* also may be seen.
   4. Often presents in children and may be indolent for long periods.
   5. May be difficult to differentiate histologically from a low-grade fibrosarcoma but rarely, if ever, metastasizes.
   6. The postresection *recurrence rate* is 65% to 75%. Since fibromatosis can microscopically infiltrate beyond the margins indicated by imaging studies or direct palpation at surgery, the surgeon should obtain a wide margin beyond the apparent defined tumor limits.

Desmoplastic Fibroma.—The rare form of fibromatosis that is *intraosseous;* same histology as soft tissue fibromatoses.

A. Determinants:
   1. Age: 50% present in *second decade.*
   2. Soft tissue involvement: Generally none.
   3. Pattern: Geographic to moth-eaten, with *cortical expansion* and endosteal erosion.
   4. Size: Variable, but usually greater than 5 cm.
   5. Location: *Central, metaphyseal;* long bones most frequent (around knee); also pelvis and mandible.
   6. Zone of transition: Usually narrow, but may be wider, simulating a very aggressive lesion.
   7. Margin: Sclerotic margin not common.
   8. Tumor matrix: None (lysis).
   9. Host response: Generally none.
   10. Monostotic.

B. *Mildly to moderately aggressive, sometimes difficult to differentiate radiographically or pathologically from a well-differentiated fibrosarcoma.*

C. Major differential diagnoses:
   1. Fibrosarcoma (if aggressive).

   2. ABC.
   3. GCT.
 D. Metastatic potential: Not malignant but *recurrences are very common,*
    though slow (1 to 2 years).
       1. Ten to 50% behave as low-grade aggressive but nonmetastasizing
          neoplasms, but it is impossible to predict which on the basis of
          radiographic appearance.
 E. Radiographic work-up:
       1. Plain film.
       2. CT or MRI.
 F. Treatment:
       1. Extensive cryosurgery and curettage.
       2. With recurrence, wide excision.

Cortical Desmoid (Periosteal Desmoid).—The following are characteristic of cortical desmoids:

A. *Not a true desmoid,* but fibroblastic proliferation, *probably secondary to trauma* at the insertion of the adductor magnus muscle or medial head of gastrocnemius. Essentially a normal variant that is better termed "avulsive cortical irregularity" or "medial supracondylar defect."
B. Causes *erosion of the cortex,* a small soft tissue mass, and *exuberant periostitis* that may simulate tumor bone formation.
C. *May be misdiagnosed* both radiographically and histologically as an *osteosarcoma.*
D. Occurs in the right age group for osteosarcoma (*15 to 20 years*).
E. *Location* is the hallmark of this lesion and leads to the correct diagnosis: it is always found on the *posteromedial cortex of the distal end of the femur,* adjacent to the medial femoral condyle.
F. If the diagnosis is not correctly made on plain film and MR is obtained, it may further confuse the issue. MR is nonspecific, with low SI on T1 and high SI on T2. A low signal rim has been described but is not always present.

Lipoma

Tumor arising from fatty tissue, commonly found in soft tissues and rarely intraosseous. Lipomas and lipoma variants constitute 16% of benign soft tissue tumors.[23]

Soft Tissue Lipoma.—Common lesion:

A. Eighty percent are in subcutaneous tissue; others are inter- or intramuscular. The latter may appear highly infiltrative.
B. Ninety-five percent are solitary.
C. Present as an asymptomatic soft, compressible, and moveable mass.
D. On plain film or CT, they are *radiolucent* (fat tissue density) and *well defined.*

E. Rarely, lipomas contain metaplastic cartilage and bone calcification.

F. MR shows a sharply bordered lesion *with high signal intensity on both T1 and T2 weighting,* corresponding to subcutaneous fat SI. Does not enhance.

Lipomatosis.—The following are characteristic of lipomatosis:

A. Congenital abnormality with multiple lipomas distributed either randomly or symmetrically over body.

B. Macrodystrophia lipomatosa is a more localized form, with overgrowth of soft tissues and bone, usually of a hand or foot. This entity belongs in the differential for localized giantism (neurofibromatosis and soft tissue vascular lesions are the other common causes). It is very difficult to handle surgically.

Lipoblastoma.—An embryonal fatty tumor seen in young children:

A. It is benign, but simulates liposarcoma histologically. CT or MR show nonadipose tissue, characteristically in the periphery (corresponding to fibrous and myxomatous tissue); in this age group, this must not be mistaken for liposarcoma!

B. Recurrence after surgery is common.

C. Age at onset is the major differentiating factor from liposarcoma, which occurs in adults.

Hibernoma.—Tumor of brown (embryologic) fat:

A. May be within a lipoma.

B. Usually in the scapular or axillary region.

C. More cellular than lipoma, which may affect the MR or CT appearance.

Atypical Lipoma.—Well-differentiated lipomatous tumor that recurs locally but does not metastasize. MR should be carefully scrutinized to detect any portion of the lipoma that does not contain typical fat signal in order to rule out a very low-grade, well-differentiated liposarcoma.

Lipoma Arborescens.—Monarticular, usually involving the knee:

A. May be reactive to chronic synovitis.

B. Hypertrophic synovial villi distended with fat.

C. MR: Synovial mass with frondlike architecture; fat SI on all sequences that suppresses with fat-selective presaturation; joint effusion; no significant erosions; lack of hemosiderin differentiates it from PVNS.

Osseous Lipoma.—Rare fatty lesion of bone:

A. Generally asymptomatic.

B. *Lytic lesion* with a distinct, fine *sclerotic margin* and no destructive change or periosteal reaction.

C. Usually of *fat density on CT* (not completely reliable). Fat SI on MR.

D. *May have a central calcified nidus.*

E. Found in the metaphyses of long bones, especially the *proximal femur,* fibula, and *calcaneus,* where the osseous lipoma occurs in the triangular region between the major trabecular arcs (same site as SBC).

F. Occasionally the epicenter is *parosteal,* in which case radiographic studies demonstrate the *soft tissue lucent mass adjacent to cortex* plus occasional periosteal reaction that may take the form of hyperostosis or may produce large bony spicules radiating from the periosteum into the lesion.

Peripheral Nerve Sheath Tumors (PNST).—*Neurofibromas and schwannomas together represent 10% of benign soft tissue tumors.*[23] Nomenclature is confusing; schwannomas are also known as neurilemoma, neurinoma, perineural fibroblastoma, and peripheral glioma.

A. Both types are *associated with peripheral nerves;* they may clinically present as an *exquisitely painful mass;* there are a few features which may help distinguish neurofibromas from schwannomas, but specificity is not complete.

B. Neurofibromas: Most arise in small cutaneous nerves; the lesions involving the deeper major nerves cause *fusiform enlargement; with the nerve fascicles separated and intimately involved with tumor;* on MR, the margins are smooth and, most distinctively, the T2 image may show a *"target" pattern of increased peripheral signal and decreased central signal.*

C. Schwannomas: Most involve the larger deeper nerves (often ulnar or peroneal); the *tumor lies on the surface of the nerve;* MR appearance is not distinctive, appearing isointense with muscle on T1 and high SI on T2, often with inhomogeneity; the distinct target sign of neurofibroma is not usually present.

Giant Cell Tumor of the Tendon Sheath (Pigmented Villonodular Synovitis [PVNS]).—The following are characteristic of this lesion:

A. Painless, slow-growing lesion in the tendon sheath, usually of the finger.

B. Patients are usually 30 to 50 years old.

C. Uncertain whether etiology is neoplastic or reactive.

D. Radiographically, a localized soft tissue mass is seen, not centered around a joint, with bony erosion (pressure type) in 10%.

E. MR appearance: Hypointense to muscle on T1, variably hypo/iso/hyperintense to muscle on T2; similar in this respect to its pathologic counterpart, PVNS.

F. Postsurgical recurrence 30%.

G. Intra-articular PVNS, histologically the same lesion but with different radiographic and clinical manifestations, is discussed in Chapter 2.

Morton Neuroma.—Benign tumor consisting of perineural fibrosis and nerve degeneration occurring in the interdigital space.

A. Etiology likely to be trauma, with abnormal force distributed to the metatarsal heads; the association with high-heeled shoes is suggested by the gender frequency (7.5–18:1, F:M)
B. Most commonly between 3rd and 4th or 2nd and 3rd metatarsal heads.
C. Painful, relieved by rest; usually a clinical diagnosis.
D. MR used if necessary; conventional T1 and T2 imaging demonstrates the lesions poorly since they are isointense with surrounding tissue; contrast-enhanced imaging with fat suppression is recommended.

Elastofibroma.—Slow growing fibroelastic pseudotumors.
A. Considered reactive, resulting from mechanical friction between the chest wall and scapula.
B. Common lesion; often bilateral.
C. Major significance is the possibility of confusion with a more aggressive lesion; the location, bilaterality, and the fact that MR signal intensity is that of muscle (with minor interspersed high- or low-signal regions) should help correctly identify the lesion.

B. Other Connective Tissue Tumors: Malignant

Malignant Fibrous Histiocytoma (MFH)/Fibrosarcoma

Key Concepts

Relatively common bone or soft tissue sarcoma in adults; the bony lesion appears permeative and aggressive; the soft tissue lesion may appear misleadingly "encapsulated" and benign.

Malignant fibrous histiocytoma (MFH) is a recently described lesion that encompasses many tumors previously felt to be distinct entities; many lesions previously diagnosed as fibrosarcomas would now be designated MFH.

Because fibrosarcoma and MFH usually can be distinguished histologically, but not radiographically, the two are described together in this chapter.

Either MFH or fibrosarcoma *may originate in the skeleton,* where it is usually an aggressive sarcoma, or *in the soft tissues* (the most common soft tissue sarcoma in adults), where it may be either low-grade or highly aggressive. In large series, *MFH is found to be the most common malignant sarcoma of soft tissues* (24%).[24] It is worked-up with MR for site evaluation. *MR is nonspecific,* with T1 generally isointense with muscle and high signal intensity T2 (unlike the benign hypocellular fibromatoses), with variable inhomogeneity.

The *soft tissue MFH/fibrosarcomas,* like many soft tissue sarcomas, may have a reactive pseudocapsule that makes it *appear encapsulated* on CT, MRI, and at surgery, when the lesion may "shell out" easily. It is important not to be misled by this pseudocapsule into treating it as a nonaggressive lesion: tumor cells invariably are found outside the margin of the reactive pseudocapsule.

Osseous fibrosarcomas and MFH *may be primary bone tumors or may arise secondarily*. Either may be found secondary to previous irradiation, Paget's disease degeneration, or dedifferentiation of a chondrosarcoma. MFH may, in addition, arise in a previous bone infarct, possibly secondary to chronic repair processes. Infarct-associated sarcomas are rare. Seventy-five percent of patients have multiple infarcts and most have no known cause. Most of the sarcomas are MFH (75%), with a few being osteosarcoma. Survival rate of infarct-associated sarcomas is poor at only 30% to 40%.[25]

Osseous MFH and fibrosarcoma are described below:

A. Determinants:
  1. Age: Second through seventh decades, but fifth or sixth decades is most common.
  2. Soft tissue involvement: Large soft tissue mass is common.
  3. Pattern: Permeative or moth-eaten.
  4. Size: Greater than 5 cm.
  5. Location: *Central* (but may be eccentric); diametaphyseal; 75% in *long tubular bones,* especially around the knee, humerus, and pelvis (Fig. 1–15).
  6. Zone of transition: Wide.
  7. Margin: No sclerotic margin.
  8. Tumor matrix: Lytic lesion, though dystrophic calcification may be seen in 15%; serpiginous calcification may also be seen in residual portions of bone infarcts that have degenerated to MFH.
  9. Host response: Periosteal reaction is variable but often present.
  10. Usually monostotic; multicentric lesions are extremely rare and more likely represent bone metastases.
B. MR appearance: Nonspecific low T1 SI and high T2 SI, with occasional low SI regions relating to dystrophic calcification.
C. *Highly aggressive* lesions.
D. Major differential diagnoses:
  1. Lymphoma.
  2. Intramedullary chondrosarcoma (especially if calcification is present).
E. Metastatic potential:
  1. Very few are low-grade lesions (5-year survival, 85% to 95%).
  2. Most are high-grade, with a 5-year survival of 25% and metastases involving lung, bone, lymph nodes, and viscera.

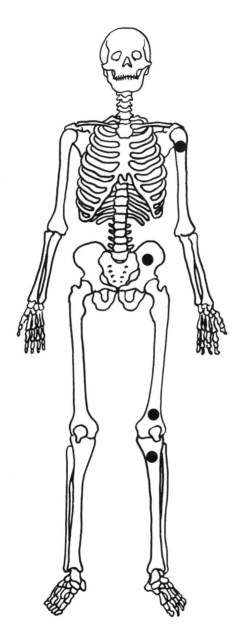

Fig. 1-15 Osseous malignant fibrous histiocytoma: most common distribution.

F. Radiographic work-up:
  1. Plain film: Suggests diagnosis and limited differential of aggressive lesion.
  2. Bone scan for metastases.
  3. Chest film and CT for metastases.
  4. MRI for determination of tumor extent and surgical planning.
G. Treatment:
  1. Low-grade: Wide excision; value of chemotherapy is debated.
  2. High-grade: Wide to radical excision and chemotherapy.

Liposarcoma

A. Liposarcoma of bone is extremely rare. It is aggressive in appearance as well as clinically and is nonspecific radiographically.
B. Soft tissue liposarcoma is the *second most common soft tissue sarcoma* (14% of malignant soft tissue tumors, second only to MFH).[24]
C. It may be well-differentiated or a high-grade lesion.
D. Third, fourth, fifth, or sixth decade.
E. Insidious growth, often asymptomatic, so may be large at diagnosis.
F. Most commonly located in the buttocks, thigh, lower leg, and retroperitoneum.
G. On plain film or CT, *may have fat density if the lesion is well-differentiated. A higher grade lesion is more cellular and more often of nonspecific soft tissue density.*
H. Occasionally may contain dystrophic calcification, bone, or cartilage.
I. MRI shows a high signal intensity T2 (as in nearly all soft tissue lesions) and a variable signal intensity T1 (most other soft tissue lesions except lipoma have a low signal intensity T1). This variability relates to the cellularity of the lesion (the more well-differentiated the tumor, the more closely it appears "fat-like"). Frequently, fat is not detectable at all in a higher-grade liposarcoma! Well-differentiated liposarcomas may occasionally dedifferentiate to a high-grade nonlipogenic sarcoma. Juxtaposition of a predominantly fatty tumor with a nonlipomatous mass suggests this rare occurrence. This happens more often in the retroperitoneum than the extremities. Myxoid liposarcoma can also be potentially confusing in appearance as it often shows amorphous fatty areas within an otherwise nonspecific soft tissue mass, but occasionally appears cystlike on MR.
J. The lesion often elicits formation of a *reactive pseudocapsule;* this is *easily misinterpreted on CT, MRI, and at surgery as true encapsulation* and the lesion is "shelled out," invariably leaving *residual tumor at the margins* since the lesion is never truly encapsulated; thus, recurrence with this type of excision is common and prognosis is poor, with metastatic disease to lungs and viscera.

K. Adequate therapy is wide excision, often with chemotherapy, and often combined with radiation pre- or postoperatively.

Synovial Cell Sarcoma

A. Soft tissue sarcoma of synovial origin. Five percent of malignant soft tissue tumors.
B. Presents with painful swelling but relatively slow growth.
C. Age: 15 to 35 years.
D. Associated with tendon, tendon sheath, and bursa, and therefore may be *remote from joint;* fewer than 10% occur in the joint capsule.
E. Most common in the *lower extremity,* especially about the knee.
F. *Calcification is seen in 20% to 30%.*
G. Adjacent bone erosion or periosteal reaction is rare (15%).
H. MR appearance: Nonspecific, and even misleadingly nonaggressive; usually inhomogeneous on T2, often with areas of hemorrhage and occasional fluid-fluid levels; most appear ''encapsulated'' or clearly delineated from surrounding tissues.[26]
I. Radiographic appearance is, therefore, nonspecific; as in other soft tissue sarcomas, a misleading *pseudocapsule* may be seen, but islands of tumor are found peripheral to it.
J. Recurrence is common unless the lesion is treated initially with wide excision.
K. Metastasizes to lung.

Other Connective Tissue Sarcomas

Radiographically, these are all nonspecific; they tend to be masses of soft tissue density, sometimes containing calcification and often with an apparent pseudocapsule.

Malignant Mesenchymoma.—Contains elements of two or more differentiated sarcomas; may include osteosarcoma, liposarcoma, chondrosarcoma, rhabdomyosarcoma, malignant neurogenic sarcoma, or angiosarcoma. May contain fatty areas or calcification/ossification.

Rhabdomyosarcoma.—Common soft tissue tumor of muscle origin; poor prognosis, with metastases to lung and lymph nodes. Embryonic type occurs in children, primarily in the head and neck and genitourinary tract. The alveolar, or pleomorphic, types occur in adults, usually in the extremities.

Malignant Peripheral Nerve Sheath Tumor.—Arise along major nerve trunks (location is the prime indicator of lesion type), often extremely painful or with neurologic symptoms; 5% to 10% of malignant soft tissue sarcomas; MR appearance is nonspecific, not clearly distinguishing malignant from benign peripheral nerve sheath tumors; signal intensity, margination, and inhomogeneity are not distinctive.

Dermatofibrosarcoma Protruberans.—A distinct fibrous tissue sarcoma accounting for 6% of soft tissue sarcomas[24] (similar in number to malignant schwannoma or synovial sarcoma). Not commonly discussed in radiologic literature since it is so superficial that the diagnosis is usually made clinically; large lesions can penetrate into deeper soft tissue and can be confused with higher-grade sarcomas. Imaging studies show a nonspecific soft tissue mass, usually confined to the skin and subcutaneous tissue.

Clear Cell Sarcoma.—Rare (1%) soft tissue sarcoma. Melanoma of soft tissues, usually foot/ankle.

A. Location may be distinctive, being intimately bound to ligaments, tendons, or musculotendinous junctions.
B. May have associated extrinsic osseous destruction.
C. May be nonspecific on MR, but if melanin is produced, may have hypointense SI.
D. Differential diagnoses include synovial sarcoma, fibromatosis, and giant cell tumor of tendon sheath.

VII. OTHER TUMORS

Chordoma

A low-grade malignant neoplasm that arises from notocord remnants.

Key Concepts

Locally aggressive; because of its origin, it is found only in the *sacrum, clivus, and spine;* recurrence is common.

A. Determinants:
    1. Age: In sacrum, sixth and seventh decades; in clivus or spine, fourth and fifth decades.
    2. Soft tissue involvement: *Local soft tissue mass.* In the sacrum, the soft tissue mass enlarges anteriorly into the pelvis and may be very large by time of discovery; in the spine, there may be a posterior mass with epidural compression.
    3. Pattern of bone destruction: Usually geographic.
    4. Size of lesion: Usually larger than 5 cm in sacrum but smaller in spine.
    5. Location:
        a. *Fifty percent in sacrum (conversely, 40% of sacral tumors are chordomas).*
        b. Thirty-five percent in clivus.

c. Fifteen percent in spine: Body rather than posterior elements; usually lumbar.
6. Zone of transition: Narrow.
7. Margin of lesion: Usually sclerotic.
8. Tumor matrix: No matrix produced, but calcific debris may be present.
9. Host response: No periosteal reaction.
10. Monostotic.

B. Aggressiveness of lesion: *Although extensive local bone destruction and soft tissue mass are seen, the time course is often so slow that the lesion acquires a sclerotic rim and has a narrow zone of transition, making it appear less aggressive.*

C. Major differential diagnoses:
1. In sacrum:
   a. GCT.
   b. Chondrosarcoma.
   c. Plasmacytoma.
2. In vertebral body:
   a. Metastatic disease.
   b. Myeloma.
3. In clivus:
   a. Chondrosarcoma.
   b. Metastatic.

D. Metastatic potential.
1. *Twenty-five percent have distant metastases* (to lung), but these are often very late.
2. *More commonly, patients have significant morbidity and mortality from local recurrence and associated complications.*
3. Five-year survival, 50%.
4. Ten-year survival, 28%.

E. Radiographic work-up:
1. Plain film suggests diagnosis.
2. CT or MRI ideal to diagnose local extent.

F. Treatment:
1. Early wide resection, if possible.
2. *Local recurrence 80% if only marginal resection is accomplished.*
3. Radiation seems to be palliative for recurrence but does not affect survival.
4. Chemotherapy is not helpful.

Adamantinoma (angioblastoma)

Rare lesion of unknown pathogenesis (contains elements of squamous, alveolar, and vascular tissue) and generally low-grade malignancy.

Key Concepts

Location in the tibial diaphysis may be its most distinctive feature; appearance ranges from unaggressive to moderately aggressive; may have satellite foci and may be malignant.

A. Determinants:
   1. Age: Most commonly fourth or fifth decade but may occur in adolescence.
   2. Soft tissue involvement: Rare early, but a soft tissue mass may develop as the lesion becomes more aggressive locally.
   3. Pattern of bone destruction: Geographic.
   4. Size of lesion: Depending on the stage, may be greater than 5 cm.
   5. Location:
      a. *This is the most characteristic aspect of adamantinoma: 90% are found in the tibia.* Other long bones are affected rarely.
      b. It is usually *diaphyseal* (*middle one third*) and *eccentric* (often cortically based initially).
   6. Zone of transition: Geographic (though the more aggressive lesions may be moth-eaten).
   7. Margin of lesion: Usually has reactive sclerosis.
   8. Tumor matrix: None.
   9. Host response: No periosteal reaction unless lesion is very aggressive.
   10. Monostotic, but *may have satellite foci adjacent to the parent lesion or even in the adjacent fibula.*
   11. This lesion is distinct from adamantinoma (ameloblastoma) of the jaw.
B. Aggressiveness of lesion: *Appearance ranges from unaggressive to moderately aggressive.*
C. Major differential diagnoses:
   1. Fibrous dysplasia, osteofibrous dysplasias; there is histologic overlap between fibrous dysplasia, osteofibrous dysplasia (ossifying fibroma), and adamantinoma. All may be cortically based and favor the tibia. Reports show that many patients with diagnosis of fibrous dysplasia or osteofibrous dysplasia of the tibia actually have an adamantinoma. The latter two diseases may possibly be related, and osteofibrous dysplasia may be a precursor of the more aggressive adamantinoma.[27]
   2. NOF.
   3. Vascular lesion (especially when satellite lesions are present).

D. Metastatic potential:
  1. Malignant (20% metastasize to lung, lymph nodes, or skeleton) but generally low-grade, so the lesion may be present for several years prior to metastasis.
  2. Five-year survival, 60%.
  3. Ten-year survival, 40%.
E. Radiographic work-up:
  1. Plain film: Adamantinoma should be suggested by a moderately aggressive midtibial lesion.
  2. CT or MRI: To evaluate local extent and fibular involvement. This is important since the lesion is usually low-grade, and the poor survival statistics are likely to relate to underestimated local extension and inadequate initial treatment.
  3. Chest film.
F. Treatment:
  1. Ideally, wide excision should be performed initially.
  2. Frequently, the initial treatment is an inadequate curettage or cryo-surgery.

VIII. TUMORLIKE LESIONS
Solitary Bone Cyst (SBC)

Also called simple or unicameral bone cyst; common fluid-filled bone lesion of childhood. It is asymptomatic unless fractured.

Key Concepts

Central geographic lesion, common in young children; metaphyseal but may migrate to diaphysis as it matures; proximal humerus is most common site; very high recurrence rate after simple curettage.

A. Determinants:
  1. Age: *First or second decade;* may uncommonly be seen in adults.
  2. Soft tissue involvement: None.
  3. Pattern of bone destruction: Geographic oval lesion with its long axis parallel to the long axis of the bone; may appear multilocular.
  4. Size of lesion: May be 5 cm or larger.
  5. Location: *Proximal humerus (50%) and proximal femur (20%) most common; SBC is metaphyseal, abutting the epiphyseal plate, but migrates into the diaphysis* (normal bone grows away from it). An SBC that has migrated from the growth plate may be less active and, thus, less prone to recurrence than those that remain at the

growth plate; however, activity seems to correlate better with patient age (recurrence is twice as likely in a patient under age 10 than in an older patient). An SBC in an older patient is rare and is found in unusual locations, such as the iliac wing or calcaneus (Fig. 1–16).

   6. Zone of transition: Narrow.
   7. Margin of lesion: *SBCs are mildly expansile and thin the cortex, but have a fine sclerotic rim.*
   8. Tumor matrix: None, but rarely one may see a *fallen fragment sign:* after pathologic fracture of the cyst, a fracture fragment may be displaced inferiorly in the fluid-filled cyst.
   9. Host response: No periosteal reaction unless there is a pathologic fracture.
   10. Monostotic.
B. MR appearance: Low T1 and high T2 SI, typical of cyst; fluid levels occasionally seen.
C. Unaggressive in appearance.
D. Major differential diagnoses:
   1. Fibrous dysplasia.
   2. Eosinophilic granuloma.
   3. Aneurysmal bone cyst (more eccentrically located).
   4. In calcaneus, differential diagnosis is intraosseus lipoma versus pseudocyst.
E. Metastatic potential: None.
F. Radiographic work-up: Plain film diagnosis.
G. Treatment:
   1. *Curettage and bone graft has a recurrence rate of 35% to 50%.*
   2. *Steroid injection* (after proving diagnosis by aspiration of fluid and pressure measurements) or cryosurgery show lower recurrence rates.
   3. Occasionally may heal spontaneously following multiple fractures.
   4. Surgery performed on a lesion adjacent to the epiphysis it may cause acceleration or arrest of growth.

Aneurysmal Bone Cyst (ABC)

An expansile, highly vascular lesion with blood-filled cystic cavities. It is associated with a preexisting osseous lesion (chondroblastoma, fibrous dysplasia, *GCT,* osteoblastoma, NOF) *in 30% to 50% of cases. Trauma* is also a common feature; one theory of the pathogenesis of ABC is that it is a vascular anomaly induced by either trauma or the precursor lesion. It is hypothesized that rapid expansion of the ABC obliterates the precursor lesion in some cases.

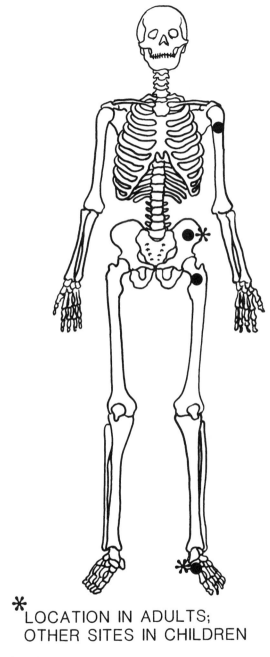

*LOCATION IN ADULTS;
OTHER SITES IN CHILDREN

Fig. 1-16　Solitary bone cyst (SBC): common locations. The femoral and humeral lesions are seen in children; when SBC occurs in adults, it tends to involve the pelvis or calcaneus.

Key Concepts

Very expansile, eccentric, lytic metaphyseal lesion with narrow zone of transition; usually under 25 years of age; may be very rapidly progressive and simulate neoplasm. CT and MR often demonstrate fluid-fluid levels.

A. Determinants:
1. Age: First through third decades; *70% between 5 and 20 years.*
2. Soft tissue involvement: Soft tissues are displaced by the rapidly expanding lesion.
3. Pattern of bone destruction: Geographic.
4. Size of lesion: Often greater than 5 cm.
5. Location: *Metaphyses of long bones, spine (posterior elements), pelvis;* it is *eccentrically* located.
6. Zone of transition: Narrow.
7. Margin of lesion: Fine sclerotic rim; the margin outside the bone may not be seen by plain film, but more commonly can be seen with CT.
8. Tumor matrix: None.
9. Host response: Aggressive recurrence may elicit periosteal reaction, but usually there is no host response.
10. Monostotic.
11. Other features: *May be very rapidly progressive* and elicit periosteal reaction, which may be mistaken for a malignant tumor.
B. Usually the appearance is nonaggressive; rapidly progressive or recurrent lesions may appear more aggressive.
C. Major differential diagnoses:
1. NOF.
2. Fibrous dysplasia.
3. Osteoblastoma (in posterior elements of spine).
D. Metastatic potential: None, but the underlying lesion may occasionally be a sarcoma; therefore, extensive sampling of solid areas should be performed to determine the precursor lesion.
E. Radiographic work-up: Plain film diagnosis usually. If more aggressive, CT or MRI will help further define the lesion; a fluid level may be present. Fluid levels are not specific for this disease process; although much more commonly seen in ABC, they have been described in fibrous dysplasia, SBC, osteosarcoma (especially, but not exclusively, the telangiectatic variety), soft tissue hemangioma, and synovial sarcoma. Note also that a "solid" variety of ABC may occasionally occur (5%).
F. Treatment: Curettage and possibly cryosurgery (there is a 20% to 50%

recurrence rate following curettage). Low-dose radiation may be used only for surgically inaccessible lesions.

Nonossifying Fibroma (NOF)/Benign Fibrous Cortical Defect (BFCD)

Histologically identical, cortically based lesions that are not neoplasms but may be secondary to epiphyseal plate defects that migrate away from the plate with growth. It is estimated that BFCD occurs in *30% to 40% of children* over 2 years of age; they are seen in adults infrequently, indicating that they must heal *spontaneously.* Occasionally BFCD may enlarge, forming an NOF. The lesions are asymptomatic and are so radiographically specific that they are among the "leave-me-alone" lesions that should be ignored unless symptomatic.

Key Concepts

Cortically based metaphyseal lytic lesions with sclerotic border; usually lower extremity long bones; both lesions may ossify during healing phase.

A. Determinants:
1. Age: First or second decade (95% under 20 years).
2. Soft tissue involvement: None.
3. Pattern: Geographic oval lesion, parallel to the long axis of the bone. NOF is expansile and may have pseudotrabeculations.
4. Size:
   a. BFCD less than 2 cm.
   b. NOF greater than 2 cm, occasionally huge.
5. Location: *80% in the long bones of the lower extremity; metaphyseal and cortically based* (an oblique film may be necessary to demonstrate this). *NOF starts in cortex but may enlarge to involve the intramedullary region and even appear central in thin bones (fibula, ulna).*
6. Zone of transition: Narrow.
7. Margin: Sclerotic border.
8. Tumor matrix: None, but *when healing spontaneously one may see dense sclerotic bone formation.*
9. Host response: No periosteal reaction.
10. *Usually monostotic (75%),* but the lesion is so common that polyostotic lesions are seen not infrequently.
11. Other features: NOF may be associated with neurofibromatosis.

B. *Unaggressive appearance.*
C. Major differential diagnoses:
    1. BFCD should be recognized without having to formulate a differential diagnosis.
    2. NOF differential includes chondromyxoid fibroma and ABC, and occasionally Brown tumor of HPTH.
D. Metastatic potential: None.
E. Radiographic work-up: Plain film should be sufficient.
F. Treatment:
    1. *BFCD: "Leave me alone";* natural history is to heal in.
    2. NOF: If treatment is indicated secondary to pain or pathologic fracture, curettage with bone chip packing is performed. Otherwise, NOF gradually migrates away from the metaphysis and is remodeled or ossifies in.

Histiocytosis X (Langerhans' Cell Histiocytosis)

Spectrum of diseases, all with histiocytic infiltration of tissues and *aggressive bone lesions. Eosinophilic granuloma (EG), the most common (60% to 80%) and mildest form, is described below.*

Key Concepts

Consider this lesion when considering round cell tumors. EG may appear as permeative and aggressive as Ewing's (though a soft tissue mass is usually not as large); may develop and enlarge extremely rapidly; often polyostotic, skull, spine, pelvis, and femur are the most common sites.

A. Determinants:
    1. Age: First through third decade, but peaks from *5 to 10 years.*
    2. Soft tissue involvement: Soft tissue mass is common, especially in skull lesions.
    3. Pattern: *Moth-eaten or permeative;* as lesion resolves, becomes more geographic.
    4. Size of lesion: 1 to 5 cm.
    5. Location: (Fig 1–17)
        a. *Skull (calvarium) 50%.*
        b. *Axial skeleton 30%;* pelvis; also involves vertebral body and occasionally an adjacent vertebral body in compression fracture (*vertebra plana*) pattern. Posterior elements and discs are intact.
        c. *Long bones 20%; femur* most common. The lesions are usually central and metadiaphyseal.

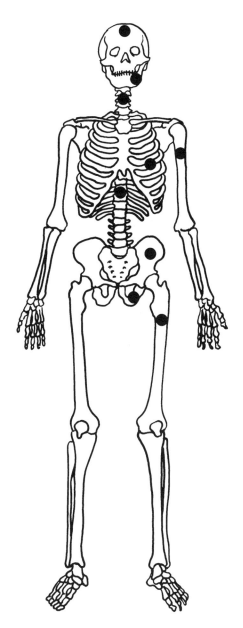

Fig. 1-17   Eosinophilic granuloma: common locations.

6. *Zone of transition: Wide,* especially *in appendicular lesions; skull lesions* have a *narrower* zone of transition, that of a *punched-out* appearance. In addition, the skull lesions often have nonuniform involvement of the inner and outer skull tables, giving a *beveled edge* appearance.
7. Margin of lesion: No sclerotic margin unless in reparative phase.
8. Tumor matrix: No matrix, but occasionally a fragment of bone is left centrally in the lesion, resembling a *"sequestrum." Sclerosis may be seen during healing phases.*
9. Host response: *Periosteal reaction is common.*
10. Monostotic most commonly; 10% to 20% develop polyostotic disease within 6 months of developing the first lesion. Those who present with a lesion at a young age are more likely to develop polyostotic disease.
11. Other features: EG involves only a *single organ system;* it is a *painful lesion.* Rarely, it presents with fever and elevated sedimentation rate, simulating infection. It is very aggressive: the time course of bone destruction may be even shorter than that is seen with infection or tumor.

B. *Highly aggressive lesion, both in time course and appearance.*
C. Major differential diagnoses:
   1. Ewing's sarcoma.
   2. Lymphoma.
   3. Infection.
   4. Metastatic disease.
D. Metastatic potential: None; may have multifocal EG without extraskeletal involvement.
E. Radiographic work-up:
   1. Plain film: Suggests diagnosis and differential.
   2. Bone scan: To determine whether it is polyostotic; other lesions may be in the skull or vertebral bodies and lead to the diagnosis of EG.
F. Treatment:
   1. Many therapeutic regimens have been used. The healing rate seems to be similar for all treatments:
      a. No therapy.
      b. Curettage.
      c. Wide excision.
      d. Low-dose radiation.
      e. Intralesional steroid injection.
   2. *Each of these methods seems to lead to the same rate of recurrence or reconstitution* (including regaining partial height in vertebra plana lesions).

3. Therefore, therapy is often reserved for specific clinical indications, including the painful lesion.

Hand-Christian-Schuller Disease

1. *Chronic disseminated form* of histiocytosis; 15% to 40% of histiocytoses.
2. Involves skeletal, reticuloendothelial, and other visceral sites.
3. The skeletal lesions have the same appearance as in EG.
4. Manifest by age 5 to 10.
5. Variable prognosis, with high morbidity and 10% mortality.

Letterer-Siwe Disease

1. *Acute fulminant* form of histiocytosis.
2. Ten percent of cases.
3. Involves the skin, liver, spleen, lymph nodes, and skeleton.
4. Skeletal lesions may not be focal but are diffuse and poorly defined (as in myeloma or leukemia).
5. Manifest before age 2.
6. Most cases are fatal, though a few may convert to Hand-Christian-Schuller disease and the patients survive.

Fibrous Dysplasia

A hamartomatous *fibro-osseous metaplasia* (a fibrous stroma with islands of osteoid and woven bone) that is relatively *common*.

Key Concepts

The radiographic manifestations all include expansile lesions but differ, depending on the region of body involved. Rib and long bone lesions are mildly expansile, pelvic lesions are bubbly and may be very large, and base of skull lesions are expansile but densely sclerotic. In the femur, a shepherd's crook deformity is common; when polyostotic, tends to be ipsilateral.

A. Determinants:
1. Age: 10 to 70, but most often recognized in second or third decade; the polyostotic form is usually recognized before age 10 years.
2. Soft tissue involvement: None.
3. Pattern of bone destruction: Geographic, expansion with cortical thinning at all sites but may become extremely expansile and bubbly in the pelvis.
4. Size: Usually greater than 5 cm.
5. Location: Found in any bone, but vertebral localization is uncommon. Most *common areas of involvement include the tubular bones*

(central, metadiaphyseal lesions of femur or tibia), ribs *(the most common benign lesion of ribs)*, pelvis, *and skull* (frontal, sphenoid, maxillary, and ethmoid bones) (Fig 1-18).

6. Zone of transition: Narrow.
7. Margin: Fine *sclerotic rim.*
8. Tumor matrix: *Lesions range from completely lucent to a more opaque (ground glass) density, depending on the amount of osteoid or woven bone present). Base of skull lesions often are densely sclerotic.*
9. Host response: No periosteal reaction in the absence of fracture.
10. Seventy percent are monostotic.
11. Other features:
    a. *Polyostotic lesions tend to be more aggressive; 90% are unilateral* in distribution.
    b. Three percent of patients with fibrous dysplasia have *Albright's syndrome*—polyostotic bone lesions, cafe-au-lait spots, and precocious puberty.
    c. Complications of fibrous dysplasia include *fracture (in 40%)* and physical deformity (*shepherd's crook* varus deformity of the proximal femur, *leg length discrepancy,* bowing of long bones).
    d. *Cherubism,* the typical facial deformity, is caused by expanding lesions of the paranasal sinuses and mandible.
    e. *Osteofibrous dysplasia-pseudoarthrosis* of the tibia: In infants to age 5; is a form of fibrous dysplasia resulting in bowing and fracture through the lesion followed by development of pseudoarthrosis; it usually heals with immobilization.
    f. Pregnancy may increase biologic activity resulting in enlarged lesions and pain.
    g. MR is nonspecific, with low SI on T1 and variable SI on T2.
B. Aggressiveness of lesion: Unaggressive in appearance (although polyostotic lesions may appear more aggressive than monostotic lesions).
C. Major differential diagnoses:
    1. For monostotic tubular bone: SBC.
    2. For polyostotic lesions: Ollier's disease or metastases.
    3. For rib lesion: EG, Ewing's, metastasis.
    4. For base of skull lesion: Hyperostosis may suggest meningioma; Paget's may also be in the differential.
D. Metastatic potential:
    1. *Most lesions remain quiescent throughout life, neither improving or resolving;* only 5% continue to enlarge after skeletal maturity.
    2. Malignant transformation (to fibrosarcoma or osteosarcoma) has

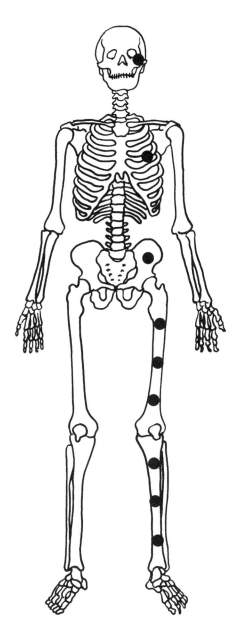

Fig. 1-18   Fibrous dysplasia: common locations.

been reported rarely; one third of the occurrences of malignant transformation are associated with previous radiation.
E. Radiographic work-up:
   1. Plain film diagnosis.
   2. If necessary, bone scan will detect polyostotic lesions.
F. Treatment: Symptomatic only, usually osteotomies to reduce deformities.

Brown Tumor of HPTH

Unaggressive-looking lytic lesion generally occurring in the presence of other manifestations of HPTH, especially subperiosteal resorption. (See Chapter 4, Section III.)

Myositis Ossificans

Posttraumatic bone formation which, in the early stages, may be adjacent to bone and elicit periosteal reaction, simulating osteosarcoma. Time course and zoning within the lesion are characteristic and help make the correct diagnosis; for further details, see Myositis in Chapter 3, Section XIII.

IX. METASTATIC DISEASE OF BONE

A. Frequency of occurrence:
   1. Osseous metastases eventually occur in 20% to 35% of extraskeletal malignancies.
   2. Metastases to bone are significantly more common (25:1) than primary bone tumors.
   3. Eighty percent of bone metastases are from primary breast, prostate, lung, or kidney carcinomas; other common primaries include GI, thyroid, and round cell (lymphoma, neuroblastoma).
B. Imaging modalities:
   1. Plain films and radionuclide bone scan have complementary roles.
   2. Bone scans are highly sensitive compared to plain films: 10% to 40% of metastatic lesions are abnormal on bone scan but normal radiographically. On the other hand, fewer than 5% of metastatic lesions are normal on bone scan but abnormal by plain radiography.
   3. Bone scan specificity is very poor. Abnormalities on radionuclide scan may be due to tumor, trauma, arthritis, or infection; plain film is more specific and differentiates among these possibilities.
   4. In patients with diffuse breast or prostate metastases bone scans may have a ''super scan'' pattern (diffuse excessive bone uptake with no kidney uptake).
   5. While bone scan and plain film remain the major imaging modalities, CT and MRI can demonstrate marrow infiltration and destruc-

tion. MR is more sensitive than bone scan, especially with diffuse metastases. They are, however, nonspecific and are usually not cost-effective diagnostic modalities for metastases unless there is a specific question to be answered that may result in a therapeutic decision.

6. Angiography and embolization may decrease morbidity in highly vascular metastases (particularly kidney).

C. Plain radiographs are used primarily for:
  1. Improving specificity (diagnosis).
  2. Assessment of therapeutic success.
  3. Evaluation for signs of impending pathologic fracture that would indicate prophylactic therapy:
     a. Lesions 2.5 cm or larger.
     b. Fifty percent cortical width destruction.
     c. Pain.

D. Appearance of metastases:
  1. Generally have a moth-eaten pattern with an ill-defined zone of transition, no sclerotic margin, often no periosteal reaction, and a small soft tissue mass. Thus, they appear moderately to highly aggressive.
  2. Occasionally a metastasis may present as a geographic, bubbly, expansile mass. The primary site of lesions in these cases is usually kidney or thyroid.
  3. They are generally polyostotic (only 10% of metastases are solitary, usually from a kidney or thyroid primary site).
  4. The density of metastases is variable.
     a. Purely lytic metastases, in descending order of frequency, include: lung, kidney, breast, thyroid, GI, and neuroblastoma.
     b. Mixed lytic and blastic metastases include: breast, lung, prostate, bladder, and neuroblastoma.
     c. Blastic metastases include: prostate, breast, bladder, GI tract (stomach, carcinoid), lung (small cell), and medulloblastoma.
     d. Changing patterns of density may reflect healing due to therapy, progression of destruction, or radiation osteonecrosis.
  5. The MR appearance of metastases is nonspecific, generally being low SI on T1 and higher SI on T2. Blastic metastases are low signal on all sequences. If a lesion has a ''bull's-eye'' sign (low signal on T1 with central high signal), it usually represents an island of hematopoietic marrow with a central focus of fatty marrow, rather than metastasis.[28] A ''halo sign'' (a rim of high signal intensity around a lesion on T2) and diffuse signal hyperintensity on T2 imaging are strong indicators of metastatic disease.[28]

E. Location:
1. Usually involve marrow spaces centrally (cortex-based metastases are most commonly lung or breast).
2. Eighty percent are located in the axial skeleton (ribs, pelvis, vertebrae, skull, proximal humerus, and femur). Acral lesions, which are distal to the elbows or knees, are usually due to primary lung tumor. Solitary rib lesions in cancer patients are uncommon and 90% of these lesions are due to benign causes. In breast cancer patients, a solitary sternal lesion is rare but has an 80% probability of being due to metastatic disease.
3. Metastases involving the spine are very common (found in 38% of malignancies of autopsy, though fewer are detected radiographically). The spine is the most common site for both solitary and multiple metastases. Vertebral metastases may appear as nonspecific compression fractures, but more commonly have the following features: involvement of a pedicle, focal destruction, focal soft tissue mass, and intact disc. Pedicular involvement is often stated to be the hallmark of metastases. However, vertebral metastases most often originate in the posterior vertebral body, correlating with the sites of entry of vertebral vessels, with secondary pedicular involvement. This has been demonstrated by CT[29]; the plain film appearance of earlier pedicular involvement is due to the fact that early destructive change in the posterior vertebral bodies is extremely difficult to visualize.
4. Lesser trochanter fractures should be considered pathologic until proven otherwise.
5. Breast metastases in the femoral head and neck usually also involve the acetabulum (although not radiographically demonstrable). Total hip arthroplasties rather than bipolar endoprostheses should be strongly considered for these patients if prophylactic or salvage surgery is to be done.
F. Differential diagnosis:
1. In adults:
   a. Multiple myeloma.
   b. Radiation osteonecrosis (may appear highly destructive, tend to involve bones adjacent to one another, and is restricted to a radiation port).
   c. Sclerosing dysplasias.
   d. Posttraumatic osteolysis of the pubis may simulate aggressive metastatic disease. The trauma may be remote and forgotten or may be so minor as to not be noted in a severely osteoporotic patient. The histologic appearance may be aggressive owing to

fracture healing; thus, trauma should be considered as an etiology for a lytic pubic lesion in an elderly patient.
2. In children:
   a. Leukemia.
   b. Disseminated osteomyelitis.
   c. Histiocytosis.
   d. Nonaccidental trauma (e.g., abuse): metaphyseal irregularities and periosteal reaction.
   e. Metabolic stress with deossification: affects rapidly growing parts of bone.
   f. Fibrous dysplasia or Ollier's disease: tends to be unilateral in distribution.
G. In stage I breast carcinoma, baseline and follow-up bone scans have a very low true positive yield and are probably unwarranted. Bone scanning should be done in stages 2, 3, and 4 as well as in patients who have become symptomatic or have positive laboratory studies. With prostate cancer, bone scans are not necessary unless the prostate-specific antigen (PSA) is above 20 ng/ml.
H. Thin-needle biopsy with cytology requires little tissue for diagnosis and is highly accurate.
I. Palliative treatment for pain is usually radiation; if there are structural concerns in a long weightbearing bone, intramedullary rodding may be performed, perhaps supplemented with methylmethacrylate cement. Percutaneous injection of cement can be performed at sites of limited volume (vertebral body, acetabulum).

REFERENCES

1. Enneking WF: Staging of musculoskeletal neoplasms. *Skeletal Radiology* 1985;13:183–194.
2. Kirchner P, Simon M: The clinical value of bone and gallium scintigraphy for soft tissue sarcomas of the extremities. *J Bone and Joint Surg* 1984; 66A:319–327.
3. Pettersson H, Gillespy T, Hamlin D, et al: Primary musculoskeletal tumors: examination with MR imaging compared with conventional modality. *Radiology* 1987;164:237.
4. Ma LD, Frassica FJ, Scott WW, Fishman EK, Zerhouni EA: Differentiation of benign and malignant musculoskeletal tumors: potential pitfalls with MR imaging. *Radiographics* 1995;15:349–366.
5. Moulton JS, Blebea JS, Dunn DM, Braley SE, Bissett GS, Emery KH. MR imaging of soft tissue masses: diagnostic efficacy and value of distinguishing between benign and malignant lesions. *AJR* 1995;164: 1191–1199.
6. Mattila KT, Heikkala JT, Aho AJ, Manner IK, Dean PB. Massive osteoarticu-

lar knee allograft: structural changes evaluated with CT. *Radiology* 1995; 196:657–660.

7. Van der Woude HJ, Bloem JL, Verstraete KL, Taminiau AH, Noog MA, Hagendoorn PC: Osteosarcoma and Ewing's sarcoma after neoadjuvant chemotherapy: value of dynamic MR imaging. *AJR* 1995;165:593–598.

8. Vanel D, Shapeero LG, DeBarre T, Gilles R, Tardivon A, Genin J, Guinesbret-iere JM: MR imaging in the follow-up of malignant and aggressive soft tissue tumors: results of 511 examinations. *Radiology* 1994;190:263–268.

9. Assoum J, Richardi G, Railhac J, Baunin C, Fajadet P, Giron J, Maquin P, Haddad J, Bonnevialle P: Osteoid osteoma: MR imaging versus CT. *Radiology* 1994;191:217–223.

10. Kroon HM, Schurmans J: Osteoblastoma: clinical and radiologic findings in 98 new cases. *Radiology* 1990;175:783–790.

11. Norton KI, Hermann G, Abdelwahab IF, Klein MJ, Gronowetter LF, Rabino-witz JG: Epiphyseal involvement in osteosarcoma. *Radiology* 1991;180: 813–816.

12. Goorin A, Abelson H, Frei E: Osteosarcoma: fifteen years later. *N Engl J Med* 1985;313:1637–1643.

13. Simon M: Causes of increased survival of patients with osteosarcoma: current controversies. *J Bone Joint Surg* 1984;66A:306–310.

14. Huvos A: Osteogenic sarcoma of bones and soft tissues in older persons. *Cancer* 1986;57:1442–1449.

15. Hopper KD, Moser RP, Haseman DB, Sweet DE, Madewell JE, Kransdorf JM: Osteosarcomatosis. *Radiology* 1990;175:233–239.

16. Schwartz H, Zimmerman N, Simon M, et al. The malignant potential of en-chondromatosis. *J Bone Joint Surg* 1987;69:269–274.

17. Weatherall PT, Moole GE, Mendelsohn DB, Sherry CS, Erdman WE, Pascoe HR: Chondroblastoma: classic and confusing appearance at MR imaging. *Radiology* 1994;190:467–474.

18. Shapeero LG, Vanel D, Couanet D, Contesso G, Ackerman CV: Extraskeletal mesenchymal chondrosarcoma. *Radiology* 1993;186:819–826.

19. Aoki J, Tanikawa H, Ishii K, Seo GS, Karakida O, Sone S, Schikawa T, Kashi K: MR findings indicative of hemosiderin in giant cell tumor of bone: frequency, cause, and diagnostic significance. *AJR* 1996;166:145–148.

20. Manaster BJ, Doyle AJ: Giant cell tumor of bone. *Radiologic Clinics of North America* 1993;31:299–323.

21. Mulligan ME, Kransdorf MJ: Sequestrum in primary lymphoma of bone: prevalence and radiologic features. *AJR* 1993;160:1245–1248.

22. Murphey MD, Fairbairn KJ, Parman LM, Baxter KG, Parsa MB, Smith WS: Musculoskeletal angiomatous lesions: radiologic-pathologic correlation. *Radiographics* 1995;15:893–917.

23. Kransdorf M: Benign soft tissue tumors in a large referral population: distribu-tion of specific diagnoses by age, sex, and location. *AJR* 1995;164: 395–402.

24. Kransdorf M: Malignant soft tissue tumors in a large referral population: distribution of diagnoses by age, sex, and location. *AJR* 1995;164: 129–134.

25. Torres FX, Kyriakos M: Bone infarct-associated osteosarcoma. *Cancer* 1992; 70:2418–2430.
26. Jones BC, Sundaram M, Kransdorf MJ: Synovial sarcoma: MR imaging findings in 34 patients. *AJR* 1993;161:827–830.
27. Springfield DS, Rosenberg AE, Mankin HJ: Relationship between osteofibrous dysplasia and adamantinoma. *Clin Orthop* 1994;309:234–244.
28. Schweitzer ME, Levine C, Mitchell DG, Gannon FH, Gomella LG: Bull's-eyes and halos: useful MR discriminators of osseous metastases. *Radiology* 1993;188:249–252.
29. Algra PR, Heinous JJ, Valk J, Nauta JJ, Lachniet M, VanKooten B: Do metastases in vertebrae begin in the body or the pedicle? *AJR* 1992;158: 1275–1279.

BIBLIOGRAPHY

Mirra J: *Bone tumors: diagnosis and treatment.* Philadelphia, 1980, J.B. Lippincott.

Enneking W: *Musculoskeletal tumor staging,* vols I and II. New York, 1983, Churchill Livingstone.

Hudson T: *Radiologic-pathologic correlation of musculoskeletal lesions.* Baltimore, 1987, Williams and Wilkins.

Moser RP, editor: *Imaging of bone and soft tissue tumors.* In The Radiologic Clinics of North America 1993;31:237–452.

2

Arthritis

GENERALIZATIONS

The classic appearance of most arthritides in the chronic stages makes them relatively easy to distinguish radiographically. It is in the early stage of disease that accurate diagnosis may be difficult. A monoarticular arthritis could easily result from trauma, infection, a crystal-induced arthropathy, early rheumatoid arthritis (RA), seronegative arthritis, or osteoarthritis (OA).

Several parameters, when used in combination, usually lead to accurate diagnosis of an early arthropathy. These parameters include clinical evaluation, epidemiologic factors such as age and sex of the patient, distribution of the arthropathy (involved joints), general appearance (erosive versus productive bony changes), and, occasionally, laboratory tests. Because these parameters are usually quite reliable for the various arthropathies, the arthritis section of this handbook is organized to highlight them.

A. Definition.
B. Epidemiology: Age, sex.
C. Clinical signs: Pain, stiffness, swelling, altered range of motion (ROM), deformity.
D. Pertinent laboratory tests (often not necessary but may be confirmatory).
E. Extra-articular manifestations.
F. General radiographic description.
    1. Soft tissue alterations.
    2. Abnormal calcifications.
    3. Bone density.
    4. Cartilage destruction.
    5. Erosive versus productive bone changes. In general, the erosive arthropathies have an initial inflammatory stage which produces pannus (inflammatory granulation tissue), which destroys cartilage and bone by means of lytic enzymes. The classic example of an erosive arthropathy is RA. At the other end of the spectrum, OA also involves cartilaginous and subchondral bone destruction, but abnormal mechanical forces combined with host reactive pro-

cesses lead to productive changes (osteophyte formation, subchondral sclerosis, and buttressing). Many other arthropathies (seronegative, crystal-induced, and erosive osteoarthritis) generally fall between these two ends of the spectrum, often demonstrating both erosive and productive changes.

6. Subchondral cysts.
7. Periostitis or enthesopathy ("whiskering" periostitis at the site of attachment of a ligament or tendon).
8. Ankylosis of joint.
9. Ligamentous abnormality: Rupture, laxity, or contracture leading to subluxation, dislocation, or instability.
10. Magnetic resonance (MR) appearance (if unique).

G. Joints most commonly affected: This distribution is a major diagnostic guide, with specific comments regarding individual sites of involvement.
H. Bilateral symmetry.
I. Other features.
J. Differential diagnosis.
K. Suggested survey films for diagnosis of early disease.
L. MR considerations in arthritis. As with so many other disease processes, MR has been shown to be exquisitely sensitive to early arthritic changes, but generally nonspecific. Effusion, erosion, osteophytes, and synovial proliferation can be seen. IV and intra-articular contrast can be used to follow synovial activity, helping to judge treatment efficacy in experimental models. With very specialized imaging techniques, different cartilage layers can be visualized (based on proteoglycan content), and chondral defects can be seen (fat-suppressed SPGR and magnetization transfer are two favored techniques). However, MR is not as sensitive as arthroscopy in evaluating chondral defects. Physical properties of cartilage relating to degeneration (such as a decrease in diffusion across cartilage) may also be measurable by MR imaging and spectroscopy.[1] With progress being made in treatment of cartilage defects with autologous chondrocyte transplantation, MR techniques may be further developed to provide noninvasive evaluation of this treatment.

In this handbook, the arthropathies have been organized according to the American Rheumatism Association (ARA) classification, with modifications and deletions (either entities that are rare, do not have radiographic abnormalities, or are discussed elsewhere in the handbook):

I. Polyarthritis of unknown etiology.
   A. Rheumatoid arthritis (RA).
   B. Juvenile rheumatoid arthritis (JRA).

    C. Ankylosing spondylitis (AS)/inflammatory bowel disease (IBD) spondylitis.

    D. Psoriatic arthritis.

    E. Reiter's syndrome.

  II. Connective tissue disorders.

    A. Systemic lupus erythematosus (SLE).

    B. Progressive systemic sclerosis (scleroderma).

    C. Polymyositis/dermatomyositis.

    D. Amyloidosis.

 III. Rheumatic fever.

 IV. Osteoarthritis (OA).

  V. Neuropathic arthropathy.

 VI. Arthropathy secondary to biochemical abnormalities.

    A. Gout.

    B. Calcium pyrophosphate dihydrate (CPPD) crystal deposition disease.

    C. Hemochromatosis.

    D. Wilson's disease.

    E. Calcium hydroxyapatite (HA) deposition disease.

    F. Ochronosis.

 VII. Miscellaneous disorders.

    A. Pigmented villonodular synovitis (PVNS).

    B. Synovial chondromatosis.

    C. Osteochondroses/osteochondritis dessicans/spontaneous osteonecrosis.

    D. Hypertrophic osteoarthropathy.

    E. Avascular necrosis (AVN)/transient regional osteoporosis.

    F. Diffuse idiopathic skeletal hyperostosis.

    G. Miscellaneous disorders.

For a much more detailed review of the pathologic basis of these disease processes, the reader is referred to the impressive compilation of data and bibliographies in Resnick D, Niwayama G: *Diagnosis of Bone and Joint Disorders,* ed 3. Philadelphia, W.B. Saunders, 1994.

I. POLYARTHRITIS OF UNKNOWN ETIOLOGY
Rheumatoid Arthritis (RA)

Key Concepts

Erosive arthropathy; synovitis and osteoporosis, bilaterally symmetric; carpus, metacarpo- and metatarsophalangeal joints (MCPs, MTPs), elbows, shoulders (rotator cuff tear), knees (valgus), hips (protrusio), upper cervical spine pathology (facet erosions, atlantoaxial impaction or subluxation).

A. Definition: A common arthritis of unknown etiology that causes synovial inflammation and articular destruction that is invariably polyarticular.

B. Epidemiology:
1. Age: Young or middle-aged.
2. Sex: *Females* more commonly affected (2 or 3:1).

C. Clinical signs:
1. Symptoms may be chronic or episodic.
2. Early morning stiffness.
3. Pain (due to capsular distension).
4. Periarticular muscle wasting, but boggy synovial swelling.
5. Tendon contractures and rupture result in several characteristic deformities (see Section G, below).

D. Laboratory tests:
1. *Rheumatoid factor* (RF) may be negative early in the disease process but eventually becomes positive in 90% to 95% of cases; elderly patients may be false positive.
2. Erythrocyte sedimentation rate (ESR) is elevated and tends to parallel disease activity.

E. Extra-articular manifestations.
1. Subcutaneous or tendon sheath nodules.
2. Tenosynovitis or bursitis.
3. Erosions at estheses.
4. Irregularities at discovertebral junction (especially in the cervical spine).
5. Pleural effusion.
6. Rheumatoid pulmonary nodules.
7. Diffuse interstitial pneumonitis.

F. General radiographic description.
1. Soft tissue alterations: *Fusiform swelling* around joints secondary to effusions and synovitis; in addition, *large synovial cysts* may form that communicate with the joint. The most common of these include the *popliteal cyst at the knee and decompression of hip synovial fluid into the iliopsoas bursa* (*presenting as a fluctuant mass*).
2. Abnormal calcifications: None.
3. Bone density: *Osteoporotic,* owing to a combination of hyperemia and disuse; in early disease, the osteoporosis may be only juxtaarticular; later, generalized; thinning of the subchondral cortex may be seen early as a *dot-dash* pattern.
4. Cartilage destruction: Joint space initially may appear wide due to joint distension. Subsequently, the cartilage is *destroyed in a uniform pattern,* leading to joint space narrowing.

5. *Erosive changes:* Bone destruction initially *is marginal, at the bare areas* (within the joint capsule but not protected by cartilage). Later, with cartilage destruction, *subchondral erosions occur.* Productive bone changes are rare, but secondary osteoarthritis may occur after subsidence of the inflammatory process (burned-out RA). The exception to this rule of no productive changes seen in RA is found in the distal ulna, where bone formation is frequently termed *"ulnar capping."* This may be seen in 10% of RA patients who have long-term disease (longer than nine years).

6. *Subchondral cysts:* Cysts are *common,* communicate with the synovium, and may be so large (especially in the hips and knees) that they simulate tumor. The cysts generally do not have sclerotic margins.

7. Periostitis and enthesopathy: Do not occur in RA.

8. *Ankylosis: Very rare* in RA, limited to the carpals and tarsals.

9. Ligamentous abnormality: Common, with tendon ruptures, laxity, and contractures leading to deformities and altered function.

Magnetic resonance is rarely used in diagnosing RA, but is extremely sensitive to signs of early RA. It also may be used to detect early tendon rupture. Specific sites to monitor for tendon rupture, retraction, and related muscle atrophy include the supraspinatus and glutei. Identification of large synovial cysts is simplified with MR. Unsuspected avascular necrosis may also be seen.

G. Most common joint distribution:

1. Hand: Some of the earliest findings are in the MCP (especially the radial side of the metacarpal head) and *proximal interphalangeal (PIP)* joints (Fig 2-1); distal interphalangeal joints (DIPs) are spared early in the disease. Characteristic deformities are:

   a. MCP ulnar deviation and volar subluxation, often with pressure erosions.

   b. Swan-neck: PIP hyperextension and DIP hyperflexion.

   c. Boutonnière: PIP hyperflexion and DIP hyperextension.

   d. Hitchhiker's thumb: MCP flexion and interphalangeal (IP) extension.

2. Wrist: Early erosions (see Fig 2-1) are found in the *distal radioulnar joint, ulnar styloid, radial styloid, waist of scaphoid, triquetrum,* and *pisiform* (the latter two seen best on the oblique or ball-catcher view; Fig 2-2). Later changes involve the intercarpal and carpalmetacarpal joints; ulnar "capping" is also seen late in the disease; typical wrist deformities include *ulnar translocation* (more than 50% of the lunate articulates with the ulna; often associated with radial deviation of the hand) (see Fig 2-1), *scapholunate dissociation, dorsi- and palmar flexion carpal instability pat-*

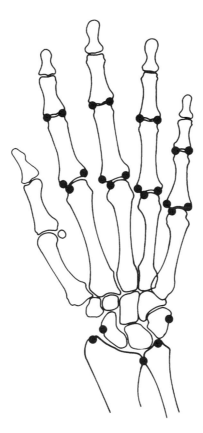

Fig. 2-1   PA view of the hand in RA with characteristic distribution of erosions and ulnar translocation of the carpus.

terns, and *distal radioulnar dissociation.* Adult Still's disease has a different carpal distribution, with pericapitate disease (both erosion and fusion) and DIP disease predominating.
  3. Elbow: The entire articulation is involved with a positive fat-pad sign, indicating effusion and erosions of the distal humerus, radial head, and coronoid.
  4. Shoulder (Fig. 2-3):
    a. Early changes involve *lysis of the distal clavicle,* erosion at the coracoclavicular ligament insertion, and *marginal humeral head erosion* (adjacent to the greater tuberosity, at the insertion of the capsule on the anatomic neck).
    b. Later, secondary signs of *rotator cuff tear* are seen: humeral head elevation and concavity on the under surface of the acro-

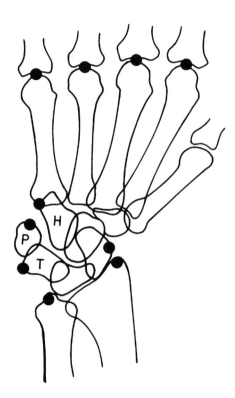

Fig. 2-2   Ball-catcher (oblique) view of hand shows erosions on MC heads, triquetrum, and pisiform to advantage.

mion. With humeral head elevation, *mechanical erosion of the medial surgical neck of the humerus* against the inferior glenoid occurs, occasionally resulting in a pathologic surgical neck fracture.

5. The sternomanubrial and sternoclavicular joints frequently have erosions, but are imaged infrequently.

6. Feet:

   a. *MTPs* very commonly have erosive changes (especially on the medial side of the metatarsal (MT) heads), often before wrist and MCP changes appear.

   b. Associated deformities are lateral deviation at the MTPs, *hammer toes* (flexion of PIPs or DIPs), and *cock-up* deformities (hyperextended MTPs).

   c. Intertarsal erosions occur late in the disease.

   d. *Calcaneal spurs* (plantar and at Achilles tendon insertion) may

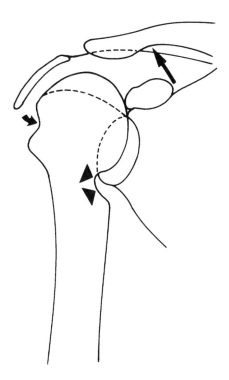

Fig. 2-3 RA of the shoulder with lysis of the distal clavicle, erosion at the coracoclavicular ligament insertion (*long arrow*), marginal humeral head erosion (*short arrow*), elevation of the humeral head secondary to rotator cuff tear, and mechanical erosion of the surgical neck of the humerus (*arrowheads*).

be seen, often with erosions. *Retrocalcaneal bursitis* may obliterate the normal pre-Achilles fat triangle.

7. Ankle: Less commonly involved.
8. Knee (Fig 2-4): Soft tissues demonstrate *suprapatellar effusions* and *popliteal synovial cysts* (Baker's cysts), which may be very large and present as mass lesions. *All three compartments* (medial, lateral, patellofemoral) *demonstrate symmetric cartilage loss, erosion, and subchondral cyst formation.* Deformity most commonly is in *valgus* position. The distal femoral shaft often has an anterior mechanical erosion from patellar pressure.
9. Hip: *Concentric decrease in joint space* and resultant *protrusio* deformity; secondary osteoarthritis is common in the hips, and the two processes may make the diagnosis difficult.
10. Sacroiliac (SI) joints: Involvement by RA is infrequent, mild, and unilateral or asymmetric.

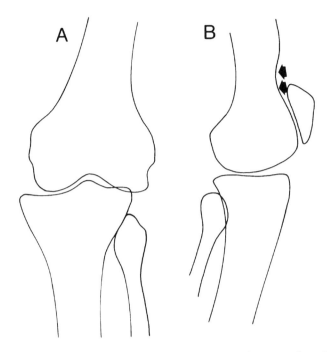

Fig. 2-4 The knee in RA, showing three-compartment disease, valgus deformity, and mechanical erosion on anterior femoral shaft (*arrows*).

11. Spine: Cervical region is much more commonly involved than thoracic or lumbar.
   a. *Atlantoaxial subluxation* (Fig. 2-5, A): Atlantoaxial distance greater than 2.5 mm, secondary to transverse ligament laxity.
   b. *Atlantoaxial impaction* (Fig 2-5, B) due to C_{1-2} facet erosion is perhaps best detected by observation of the relationship of the anterior arch of the atlas with the odontoid process. On the lateral film, the atlas usually articulates with the cranial portion of the odontoid but, with impaction, articulates with the body of C_2; neurologic symptoms more often are associated with atlantoaxial impaction than subluxation.
   c. *Odontoid erosion.*
   d. *Unilateral facet erosion* and collapse at C_{1-2} may result in torticollis and ipsilateral facial pain.
   e. Erosions of the facets and joints of Lushka.
   f. *Discitis* at several levels thought to be due to a combination of osteoporosis and posterior ligament laxity, resulting in de-

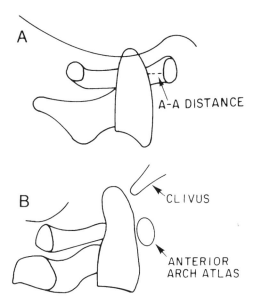

Fig. 2-5 **A,** RA with atlantoaxial subluxation. **B,** RA with atlantoaxial impaction. Note that with impaction, the anterior arch of the atlas articulates with the body of C_2 rather than with the odontoid (as in **A**). Bilateral facet erosion and collapse at C_{1-2} allows this impaction.

creased disk height, irregularity of endplates, and a *"stair-step" deformity* as seen on the lateral film.

    g. *Mechanical spinous process erosion.*

H. Bilateral symmetry: *Symmetry is generally maintained,* especially regarding groups of joints rather than individual ones. *An exception to this is patients with neurologic deficits:* the affected side is protected from rheumatoid changes.

I. Other features:

    1. *"Robust RA":* A type of RA featuring large subchondral cysts and normal bone density, generally seen in patients who maintain normal activity.

    2. *Felty's syndrome: RA, splenomegaly, and leukopenia.*

    3. *Sjögren's syndrome:* Keratoconjunctivitis sicca, xerostomia, connective tissue disease (often RA).

    4. Adult Still's disease: Clinically similar to the systemic form of juvenile chronic arthritis (intermittent fever, skin rash, pleuritis, pericarditis, lymphadenopathy, and hepatosplenomegaly); carpal disease predominates, with pericapitate erosions and fusions distinctly predominating over radiocarpal disease.

J. Differential diagnoses:
   1. Psoriatic arthritis: One form resembles the hand and wrist changes of RA, but DIP distribution tends to predominate.
   2. Reiter's disease: Retrocalcaneal bursitis may appear identical to that of RA, but other distribution is usually characteristic (SI joint, feet more prominent than hand changes).
   3. SLE: Same deformities but rarely erosive.
   4. Septic joint: Monostotic, acute onset.
   5. *Spondyloarthropathy of hemodialysis may have similar discovertebral junction abnormalities,* but C_{1-2} and the facet joints are usually normal, distinguishing this from RA.
K. Survey films for diagnosis of early disease:
   1. Hands: Posteroanterior (PA) and ball-catcher view.
   2. Feet: Anteroposterior (AP) view.
   3. Lateral cervical spine.
   4. Other symptomatic joints.

Juvenile Chronic Arthritis (Including Juvenile Rheumatoid Arthritis—JRA)

Key Concepts

Group of diseases with systemic symptoms and arthropathy; bones are small and gracile, osteoporotic; symmetric distribution; differs from RA in that fusion and periostitis may be present; predilection for large joints, especially hips, elbows; and knees; metaphyseal flaring due to hyperemia.

A–E. Definition: A group of related diseases of unknown etiology arising in childhood with the following symptom complexes[2]:
   1. *Still's disease:* 20% of JRA; *acute systemic disease* occurring in children under 5 years of age. Males and females are affected equally. They present with high fever, anemia, polymorphonuclear leukocytosis, hepatosplenomegaly, lymphadenopathy, and polyarthritis; do not have iridocyclitis. *Radiographic findings are often mild and may not demonstrate erosions;* however, 25% have chronic and destructive arthritis. Another entity, *adult Still's* disease,[3,4] occurs in patients over 18 years of age who present with systemic manifestations and are persistently RF negative; radiographic changes may be identical to adult RA or may be similar to psoriatic arthritis, with predominantly DIP erosion and fusion. Usually, few joints are involved.
   2. *Pauciarticular disease:* Most common type (40%) of JRA; found

predominantly in *young girls*. Involvement of *one to three joints* is rarely severe (usually large joints—knee, ankle, elbow). Chronic *iridocyclitis* occurs in 25%; RF negative and often antinuclear antibody (ANA) positive.

3. *Seronegative polyarticular disease:* 25% of JRA; synovitis with adult type of symmetric and widespread distribution (both large and small joints); female preponderance; occurs at any age; rheumatoid factor negative; no other systemic complaints.

4. *Seropositive polyarticular disease (juvenile-onset adult RA):* 5% of JRA; polyarticular changes typical of RA; multiple joints involved, usually sparing the DIPs; severe erosive changes, generally found in *teenage girls;* most *become RF positive;* like adult RA, may have subcutaneous nodules.

5. *Juvenile ankylosing spondylitis* (AS): Inflammatory arthropathy, male to female ratio is 7:1, strong HLA B27 positivity; *rarely presents with classical signs and symptoms of sacroiliitis and spondylitis* typical of the adult form of AS; *extra-axial arthritis is more common in juvenile than adult AS;* usually affects lower extremities (hips, knees, ankles); may have sacral and lumbar spine tenderness without radiographic changes, but may never develop a clinical back complaint; radiographically, sacroiliac (SI) joint abnormalities may be underdiagnosed because adolescent SI joints are normally wide and have indistinct cortices; symptoms of pain at the symphysis pubis, ischial tuberosities, and costochondral junction are uncommon but strongly support the diagnosis; sternocostal, sternoclavicular, and sternomanubrial joint involvement may result in reduced chest expansion, a finding common in adult AS; enthesitis, especially around the foot, is common; remember that *juvenile AS is often misdiagnosed as JRA because the abnormalities are not typical of those of adult AS and because AS is often simply not considered in an adolescent patient, especially if the SI joints are normal.*[5]

6. *Psoriatic inflammatory bowel disease and Reiter's arthropathies* may also be seen in juvenile patients and should be considered in unusual cases of JRA. The most common type of juvenile psoriatic arthritis is asymmetric pauciarticular, which is not distinguishable from pauciarticular JRA except by the presence of skin or nail changes, or family history of psoriasis. Dactylitis may be seen in either disease process as well. Sacroiliitis may be found in 25%. As in the adult, arthritis may precede the development of psoriatic skin changes, making a misdiagnosis of JRA even more likely.

F. General radiographic description of the arthropathy of JRA (similar in varieties 1–4, above):
   1. Soft tissues: May have muscle wasting with severe disease. Periarticular swelling is fusiform.
   2. Abnormal calcifications: Rarely found in juxta-articular locations.
   3. *Bone density: Osteoporosis* due to hyperemia and disuse; also, metaphyseal lucent lines (similar to those found in leukemia) may be found during disease activity.
   4. *Cartilage destruction: Often a later manifestation than in adult RA.*
   5. Erosive vs. productive changes: *Erosive changes occur, generally as a late manifestation.* Carpal bones often appear highly irregular in outline, or "crenulated."
   6. Subchondral cysts: Rarely present.
   7. Periostitis: *Periosteal reaction may be seen early in JRA* (and is virtually never seen in adult RA). Differential considerations of isolated periosteal reaction in a child include osteomyelitis, psoriatic arthritis, and dactylitis (sickle cell infarcts or tuberculosis); Enthesopathy is not seen.
   8. Ankylosis: *Fusion is much more common in JRA than adult RA.* Carpus and IP joints are most commonly involved.
   9. Ligamentous abnormalities: *Joint contractures are common.*
G. Joints most commonly affected in JRA: Generally, there is a *predilection for large joints* rather than small ones.
   1. Hand and wrist: MCP and PIP involvement similar to adult RA. In the wrist, the *radiocarpal joint may be spared and the midcarpal joint, involved,* especially the pericapitate region,[4] distinguishing JRA from adult RA. Adult Still's disease is similar in this aspect. In JRA, *ankylosis is very common in the hand.*
   2. *Elbow:* Commonly and distinctively involved: there is effusion, often *enlargement of the trochlear notch* due to extensive pannus, as well as *radial head enlargement* due to overgrowth, and uniform cartilage loss and destructive change.
   3. Shoulder: Enlarged glenoid and humeral head with late erosion.
   4. Foot and ankle: Commonly involved with MTPs and tarsal joints.
   5. *Knee:* Distinctive involvement, with *effusion, widened intercondylar notch* from pannus formation, *metaphyseal and epiphyseal flaring and overgrowth, patellar squaring,* and uniform cartilage loss and destructive change.
   6. *Hip: Common* distinctive involvement, with *femoral head enlargement, short neck with coxa valga, and* significant *protrusio acetabuli.* The iliac wings are often hypoplastic and femoral shaft,

very gracile. This constellation of abnormal shapes and sizes makes prosthesis placement difficult.

7. SI joints: Rare asymmetric involvement; if present, should consider juvenile ankylosing spondylitis. Evaluation of SI joints in the adolescent is particularly difficult because of normal widening.

8. Spine: *Cervical spine* may be commonly involved. *Facet joint erosions and ankylosis* are most common in the upper cervical region. The facet ankylosis is thought to protect JRA patients from developing the discovertebral junction abnormalities seen so often in adult RA. With ankylosis there is often *vertebral body hypoplasia* (both in height and AP diameter). *Atlantoaxial subluxation* (greater than 3.5 or 4 mm in children) and *odontoid erosions* are also prominent findings.

9. Temporomandibular joint (TMJ) erosive changes and micrognathia are relatively common.

H. Bilateral symmetry may be present but is not as reliable as in adult RA.

I. Other features: One very distinctive feature of JRA is *growth abnormalities*. With hyperemia, there is *overgrowth of epiphyses* leading to "ballooning" of joints. *Squaring of carpals, tarsals, and patella* is also seen; however, the hyperemia also leads to *advanced skeletal maturation and premature fusion, resulting in limb length discrepancies and overall shortening of limbs.*

J. Differential diagnoses:
1. Psoriatic arthritis can occur in juveniles and may be indistinguishable.

2. AS may also occur in juveniles, usually males; it affects the same regions as adult AS (SI joints, lumbar spine, hips) and is HLA B27 positive.

3. The radiographic appearance of the knee may be indistinguishable from that in hemophilia or tuberculus (TB) arthritis.

4. Eight- to 10-year-olds often have irregularities on the articular surfaces of the knees; this normal variant may be misdiagnosed as early erosion of JRA. As described, the constellation of findings—growth deformities, effusion, erosive changes, large joint involvement, periostitis, and ankylosis—in a child usually make the diagnosis of JRA relatively easy.

K. Survey films for diagnosis of early disease:
1. Hands and wrists PA.
2. Lateral cervical spine.
3. Knees.
4. Hips.
5. Other symptomatic areas, especially elbows or ankles.

Ankylosing Spondylitis (AS) and Inflammatory Bowel Disease (IBD) Spondylitis

Key Concepts
Bilateral, often symmetric sacroiliitis; syndesmophytes and fusion of facet joints of spine, usually without skip areas. Large joints (hips, shoulders) may also be involved.

A. Definition: AS is the most common *seronegative spondyloarthropathy*, of unknown etiology, involving primarily the *axial skeleton and large proximal joints*.
B. Epidemiology:
  1. Gender: Much more common in *males* than females (ratio of 4–10:1, depending on series).
  2. Age: Onset usually *between 15 and 35 years* of age.
  3. *Familial*, but mode of inheritance is unclear.
C. Clinical signs:
  1. *Low back pain*, aggravated by a supine resting position.
  2. *Spine stiffness*, with later postural changes (*increased thoracic kyphosis* and decreased lumbar lordosis).
  3. *Limited chest expansion* (1 inch or less).
D. Laboratory tests:
  1. *HLA B27 positive in greater than* 90% (6% to 8% of the normal population are positive, as are 50% to 80% of patients with Reiter's disease).
  2. RF negative.
  3. ESR increases during disease activity.
E. Extra-articular manifestations:
  1. Iritis.
  2. Heart disease, especially aortic insufficiency.
  3. Pulmonary interstitial disease and fibrosis (especially upper lobes).
F. General radiographic description:
  1. Soft tissues: Generally no change.
  2. Abnormal calcifications: See Section G for discussion of syndesmophytes. Ligamentum flava calcification is frequently noted on computed tomography (CT), but rarely seen on plain film.
  3. *Bone density: Normal* until ankylosis becomes so debilitating that disuse osteoporosis occurs. Later in the disease, osteoporosis can be very significant.
  4. Cartilage destruction: Yes.

5. *Combination of erosive and productive bony changes:* Erosions are smaller and much less prominent than those of RA.
6. Subchondral cysts: Occur, but are not prominent.
7. Periostitis occurs infrequently. *Enthesopathy is common,* especially in the pelvis, calcaneus, and patella.
8. *Ankylosis: Common in SI joints and spine (bodies as well as posterior elements).*
9. Ligamentous abnormalities: Instability not common. Calcification of longitudinal ligaments of the spine may be seen very late in the disease. Ligametum flavum calcification.

G. Joints most commonly affected: *The distribution involving SI joints, spine, and large proximal joints is classic* and crucial in making the diagnosis (Fig 2-6).

1. SI joints: Classically, the *site of initial involvement;* first changes are loss of cortical definition followed by erosions and joint widening (the findings are most prominent on the iliac side of the joint, since the cartilage is normally thinner on the iliac side); later sclerosis and fusion develop. The abnormalities may initially be asymmetric but become *bilaterally symmetric* late in the disease process. While sacroiliitis can usually be diagnosed by plain film, axial imaging is used occasionally. As part of this evaluation, *remember that only part of the "SI joint," the anterior inferior aspect, is a true synovial joint.* The posterior and superior aspects of the sacroiliac apposition have no cartilage, synovium, or capsule. They are joined together by intraosseous ligaments that may ossify in some disorders without representing a true sacroiliitis. MR has been demonstrated to be superior to CT in identifying sacroiliitis via erosion and abnormal cartilage signal.[6] Dynamic gadolinium-enhanced MR imaging appears even more sensitive.[7]

2. Thoracolumbar spine: Involvement classically *follows SI abnormalities* and begins at the *thoracolumbar and lumbosacral junctions* and extends contiguously *without skip areas* (skips and asymmetry may be seen, but not as commonly as in Reiter's or psoriatic arthropathy). Vertebral involvement *begins with osteitis* (erosive changes at the anterior corners of the vertebral bodies). *"Shiny corners"* (reactive sclerosis at the sites of osteitis) may be seen. The osteitis *leads to* loss of the normal concavity of the anterior vertebral body (*squaring*). Syndesmophytes (*thin vertical ossifications*) *form in the annulus fibrosus* at the discovertebral junction (as opposed to bulky horizontal osteophytes that arise from the vertebral body itself, which are seen in Reiter's syndrome and psoriatic arthropathy). Over several segments, *ankylosis* and a *"bamboo"* spine occur, with a change in normal postural align-

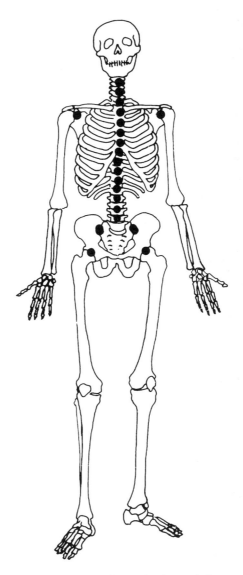

Fig. 2-6   Joints most commonly involved in ankylosing spondylitis.

ment. *Fusion of the apophyseal joints* also occurs: the anterior longitudinal ligament may eventually ossify; *the fused and osteoporotic spine is vulnerable to fracture from minor trauma and "pseudoarthrosis" forms easily.* Pseudoarthroses are most commonly seen at the cervicothoracic and thoracolumbar junctions; the pseudoarthrosis usually goes through the disk space anteriorly and continues through the posterior elements, often appearing extremely subtle. Spine changes are best seen on the lateral film. A traumatically induced fracture of this sort may result in sudden death or severe neurologic sequelae. *MR is often useful in evaluating cord injury* (including contusion, transection, hemisection, central cord syndrome) or compression from disk herniation, fracture fragment encroachment, or epidural hematoma. *If the fracture goes undetected, motion across this segment of osteoporotic bone results in osseous breakdown and appearance similar to a Charcot joint.*

3. Cervical spine: Generally involved late, in an ascending fashion from the thoracic spine. Odontoid erosion and atlantoaxial subluxation are seen, but less commonly than in RA.
4. *Hip: Most common appendicular joint involved* (up to 50% of AS patients); *concentric joint narrowing, mild erosions, protrusio acetabuli, and ring osteophytes give appearance of a combination of RA and OA.* In a young patient, these incongruent findings alone should suggest a diagnosis of AS and lead to careful scrutiny of the SI joints. Involvement is often bilateral but may be asymmetric.
5. *Glenohumeral:* After the hip, the next most commonly involved appendicular joint; again, a combination of erosive and productive findings is manifest. Involvement is often bilateral but may be asymmetric.
6. Symphysis pubis, sternomanubrial, and costovertebral joints commonly are involved, leading to ankylosis.
7. Knees, ankles, hands, and feet are less commonly involved (much less often than in Reiter's disease or psoriatic arthritis). Usually other findings more typical for AS are present, making the diagnosis less difficult, however, when acral sites are involved in AS, the erosive changes may be very prominent.

H. *Bilateral symmetry: An important feature late in the disease* but asymmetry may occur early.
 I. Other features:
1. AS is uncommon, but certainly occurs, in women. The radiographic findings tend to be neither as severe nor as classic in distribution as in male patients.

2. IBD arthritis[8]:

   a. One group of disease processes occurs from *Salmonella, Shigella,* or *Yersinia.* A self-limited polyarthritis may occur, usually without radiographic findings but occasionally with SI joint abnormalities.

   b. Another group of disease processes may occur with ulcerative colitis, Crohn's disease, or Whipple's disease. Ten to 15% of these patients develop an arthropathy; 50% to 60% of these are peripheral arthropathies (predominantly in the lower extremities, in more unusual joints—knees, ankles, elbows—and with milder osseous changes than in AS). The flares of the peripheral arthropathy correlate with disease activity. Twenty to 30% of patients develop a sacroiliitis identical clinically and radiographically to that of AS; the sacroiliitis does not correlate with IBD activity.

J. Differential diagnoses for SI joint disease of AS:

   1. Psoriatic arthritis or Reiter's syndrome: Asymmetry of SI disease is more suggestive of these diseases. The spondylitis pattern is also distinctive, with bulky asymmetric osteophytes and skip regions. Finally, the distribution of peripheral arthritis is helpful. (More acral distribution than hips or shoulders tends to occur in both Reiter's and psoriatic arthritis.)

   2. IBD may not be distinguishable from AS, but tends to be less severe.

   3. RA has less severe and rarely bilaterally symmetric SI disease.

   4. Hyperparathyroidism (HPTH): The subchondral collapse may simulate SI joint arthritis, but generally other findings of HPTH also are present.

K. Suggested survey films for AS/IBD: AP pelvis (looking for SI disease, hip disease, and enthesopathy) and lateral thoracolumbar spine (looking for vertebral body squaring or syndesmophyte formation).

Psoriatic Arthritis

Key Concepts

Predominantly erosive changes involving the carpus, DIP, PIP but less commonly MCP; sacroiliitis, often asymmetric, is common; bulky asymmetric osteophytes at thoracolumbar junction; arthropathy may antedate skin changes.

A. Definition: An arthropathy occurring in 0.5% to 25% of patients with psoriasis. *Five distinct manifestations* are described by Wright and Mall:

1. *Polyarthritis* (predominantly *DIP*).
2. *Arthritis mutilans* (deforming type).
3. *Symmetric type* (*resembling RA*).
4. *Oligoarthritis.*
5. *Spondyloarthropathy* (occurring in 30% to 50% of patients with psoriatic arthritis).

B. Epidemiology:
   1. Age: Generally young adults.
   2. Gender: Affects females and males equally.
   3. Psoriatic skin disease is usually present prior to the arthropathy, but the *arthropathy may antedate skin findings in 20% of cases.*

C. Clinical signs:
   1. Soft tissue swelling, especially in the *small joints of the hands and feet* may involve an entire digit (*sausage digit*). There is pain and reduced range of motion.
   2. Low back pain.
   3. Nail changes (thickening, pitting, or discoloration) are very common and are highly correlated with severity of the arthropathy.

D. Laboratory tests:
   1. Negative RF.
   2. Elevated ESR.
   3. *HLA B27 positive in 25% to 60%.*

E. Extra-articular manifestations: Psoriatic skin and nail changes.

F. General radiographic description of the arthropathy:
   1. Soft tissue: Swelling at involved joints, either fusiform or involving the entire digit (*sausage digit*).
   2. Abnormal calcifications: May develop an *ivory phalanx*—reactive sclerosis of the tuft.
   3. Bone density: Early juxta-articular osteoporosis may be seen, but the *density is generally normal* (an important distinguishing characteristic from RA).
   4. Cartilage destruction: Joint occasionally is widened, but generally narrowing occurs.
   5. Erosive vs. productive change:
      a. *Erosions begin marginally,* as in RA, but progress to severe subchondral erosions, occasionally resulting in a *pencil in cup deformity* (characteristic of, but not pathognomonic for, psoriatic arthritis).
      b. Productive changes are also seen, usually in the form of excrescences at and around the joint.
   6. Subchondral cysts: Not commonly seen.
   7. Periostitis: *Periosteal reaction* is often seen in hand and foot phalanges with the sausage digit pattern of soft tissue swelling. This

periostitis may help differentiate psoriatic arthritis from RA. An *enthesopathy* similar to that seen in AS or Reiter's is also common.
8. *Ankylosis:* Common, especially in the *hands and feet* (again, helping to differentiate this disease from RA).
9. Ligamentous abnormality: Not a prominent finding; however, phalanges with severe pencil in cup deformities may telescope.

G. Joints most commonly affected (Fig. 2-7): *The characteristic distribution is the small joints of the hands and feet, with or without a spondyloarthropathy.*

1. *Hand: Tuft resorption and DIP erosive disease are usually seen earlier and involvement may be more severe than PIP or MCP joints.* This pattern helps differentiate psoriatic arthritis from RA. Also, any compartment of the wrist may be involved, but generally only after DIP abnormalities occur. *Asymmetry is far more common than in RA.*

2. *Foot: IP and MTP erosive disease are common. Ivory tufts* are described. A *retrocalcaneal bursitis* may be seen (as in RA or Reiter's syndrome), along with erosions at the sites of the Achilles tendon and plantar aponeurosis insertions.

3. Larger joint (ankle, knee, hip, shoulder) involvement is *much less common. If large joints are involved, the distal small joints are almost invariably involved as well.*

4. *SI joints: Common* site of involvement (30% to 50%), with erosions, widening, sclerosis, and, eventually, fusion. The disease is usually bilateral, and symmetry is common, though perhaps less common than in AS. The thoracolumbar spine develops bulky asymmetric syndesmophytes (the same pattern as in Reiter's, but differing from the syndesmophytes of AS). Findings in the cervical spine are much less distinctive, including discitis, atlantoaxial subluxation, and apophyseal joint disease. These findings alone do not distinguish psoriatic arthritis from RA, AS, or Reiter's.

H. Symmetry:

1. *Lack of symmetry in the small joints is common, helping to distinguish from RA.*

2. *SI symmetry is common, but less so than in AS.*

I. Differential diagnoses:

1. Reiter's disease: SI joint and spine disease are indistinguishable from psoriatic arthritis. Foot disease is usually more severe in Reiter's, while hand disease is a less prominent feature.

2. RA: Occasionally indistinguishable from one type of psoriatic arthritis, but the predominantly distal distribution in psoriatic arthritis usually leads to the correct diagnosis. Adult Still's disease,

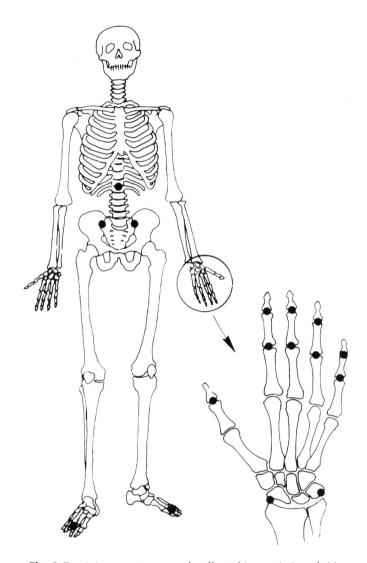

Fig. 2-7 Joints most commonly affected in psoriatic arthritis.

with its DIP distribution, may be distinguishable from psoriatic arthritis.

3. AS/IBD: The SI joint disease may be indistinguishable from that of psoriatic arthritis, but the spine disease is clearly different, as is the small joint distribution.

4. Erosive osteoarthritis (EOA): DIP erosions are potentially confus-

ing, but EOA usually has abnormalities in the first carpometacarpal joint or the scaphoid-trapezium-trapezoid joints. While the carpal distribution is the most reliable distinguishing factor between EOA and psoriatic arthritis, there is also some evidence that DIP erosions are most commonly marginal in psoriatic and directly subchondral in EOA (remember that this is a relative distinction, as both types of erosions can certainly be seen in either disease process).
  5. "Erosions" of hyperparathyroidism: Should also see other findings of HPTH, especially subperiosteal erosion.
 J. Survey films for early diagnosis:
  1. Hands: PA and ball-catcher views.
  2. Feet: AP and lateral views.
  3. AP pelvis: For SI joints and enthesopathy.
  4. AP view of thoracolumbar spine.
 K. SAPHO (synovitis, acne, pustulosis, hyperostosis, osteitis) is likely a form of spondyloarthropathy in which patients can have various osteoarticular manifestations, the most common being *osteitis of the anterior chest wall*. This is seen as hyperostosis and soft tissue ossification between the clavicles, anterior portion of the upper ribs, and manubrium. Many named disease processes likely fit in this spectrum, including the above-named acronym SAPHO, sternoclavicular hyperostosis, palmoplantar pustulosis, hyperostosis syndrome, and pustulotic arthro-osteitis. In addition to the anterior chest wall, the axial skeleton may be involved, and, rarely, extra-axial tumor-simulating bone lesions are seen. Pustulosis, psoriatic lesions, and spondyloarthropathy may be seen. This wide variety of manifestations leaves abundant room for confusion.

Reiter's Disease

Key Concepts

The predominant arthritic pattern includes a spondyloarthropathy and lower extremity erosive disease. The spondyloarthropathy is identical to that of psoriatic arthritis, with asymmetric or symmetric sacroiliitis and bulky thoracolumbar osteophytes. Calcaneal erosive disease and spur formation are particularly prominent.

 A. Definition: A syndrome consisting of the *triad of (1) urethritis (cervicitis in females) in 85% of cases, (2) conjunctivitis in 60% of cases, and (3) arthritis*. The syndrome may be incomplete or may include balanitis or keratoderma blennorrhagicum.

B. Epidemiology:
1. Age: *Young adult.*
2. Gender: Males affected much more commonly than females.
3. The arthropathy only rarely precedes the urethritis or conjunctivitis.
C. Clinical signs: Low back pain, polyarticular arthritis *with heel pain predominating,* urethritis, or conjunctivitis.
D. Laboratory tests:
1. RF negative.
2. Elevated ESR.
3. *HLA B27 positive in 80%.*
E. Extra-articular manifestations: In addition to urethritis and conjunctivitis, pulmonary fibrosis, valvular disease, and diarrhea may rarely be seen.
F. *General radiographic description of the arthropathy: The spondyloarthropathy and mixed erosive-productive acral disease with occasional periostitis, is identical to that of psoriatic arthritis, but the distribution of acral disease is a distinguishing feature.*
1. Soft tissues: Swelling at involved joints may be either fusiform or include the entire digit (*sausage digit,* seen also in psoriatic arthritis).
2. Abnormal calcifications: None.
3. Bone density: May develop osteoporosis around involved joints, but much less consistently than in RA.
4. Cartilage destruction: Decreased joint space.
5. Erosive versus productive change: *Erosions predominate but may be seen in conjunction with mild productive bony changes.*
6. Subchondral cysts: Rare.
7. Periostitis: *Periosteal reaction in phalanges* seen with sausage digits, as in psoriatic arthritis. *Enthesopathy, especially in the pelvis and calcaneus, is common.*
8. *Ankylosis: Occurs in the SI joint but is much less common elsewhere than with psoriatic arthritis.*
9. Ligamentous abnormalities: Uncommon.
G. Joints most commonly affected (Fig 2-8): *The distribution is predominantly distal lower extremity (MTP, calcaneus, ankle, knee), often with a spondyloarthropathy identical to that of psoriatic arthritis.*
1. Foot: Earliest changes:
a. *Small joints of the foot (especially MTPs and first IP) are commonly involved, primarily with erosive changes* (similar to RA, but sausage digit and periostitis, as well as normal hands help to differentiate the two).

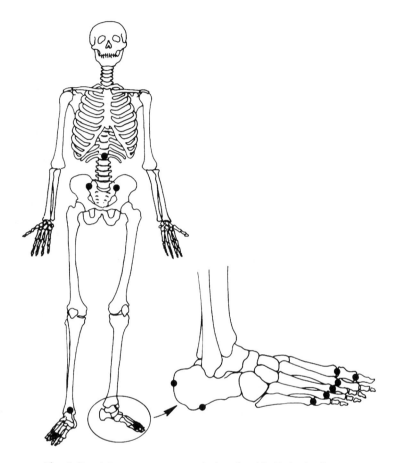

Fig. 2-8 Joints most commonly involved in Reiter's disease.

  b. *Retrocalcaneal bursitis* is common, along with *prominent spur formation* at the Achilles tendon and plantar aponeurosis insertion; erosive changes also are often present.

  c. Erosions are seen in tarsals with more severe disease.

2. Other lower extremity joints (ankle, knee, hip) may have an erosive and productive pattern similar to that of AS or psoriatic arthritis. Hip involvement is less common in Reiter's disease than in the other rheumatoid variants.

3. Upper limb involvement: Rare.

4. *SI joint involvement: Common* (10% to 40%), generally *bilateral* and may be *symmetric or asymmetric* (especially early in the disease process). The appearance of SI joint widening, sclerosis, ero-

sions, followed by fusion is *identical to that seen in psoriatic arthritis.*

5. *Spine: Bulky asymmetric paravertebral osteophytes are often first seen in the thoracolumbar regions, commonly skipping segments.* The appearance is *identical to that of psoriatic arthritis* and is best noted on the AP film, as opposed to AS, where the lateral film best demonstrates the thin vertical syndesmophytes and vertebral body squaring.

H. Symmetry:
   1. *Lack of symmetry* is common in the foot disease, especially early.
   2. *SI joint disease is often symmetric but less dependably than in AS* (especially early).

I. Differential diagnoses:
   1. Psoriatic arthritis: The spondyloarthropathy is identical, the foot disease is identical, but the sites of predominant peripheral involvement usually differs, with hand disease predominating in psoriatic arthritis and foot disease predominating in Reiter's disease. Note that statistically, psoriatic arthritis is significantly more common than Reiter's. This fact alone is helpful in differentiating the two diseases.
   2. AS/IBD: The sacroiliac joint disease is similar, but spine disease is usually quite distinctive. The appendicular distribution is significantly different, with large joint involvement in AS/IBD but primarily foot involvement in Reiter's.
   3. RA: May be confused with Reiter's if there is primarily MTP or calcaneal involvement early in the disease; rheumatoid factor and symmetric hand abnormalities usually distinguish the two.

J. Survey films for early diagnosis:
   1. AP and lateral feet.
   2. AP pelvis looking for SI joint disease.
   3. AP thoracolumbar spine.

II. CONNECTIVE TISSUE DISORDERS
Systemic Lupus Erythematosus (SLE)

Key Concepts

Generally nonerosive deforming arthropathy (but reducible). AVN is very common.

A. Definition: SLE is an immunologic abnormality that produces ANAs that in turn cause severe and widely varied tissue injury. *The musculo-*

skeletal system is most commonly involved with a polyarthritis that is generally nonerosive but may be deforming. There are frequent remissions and exacerbations with severe symptoms, but these are accompanied by remarkably few radiographic abnormalities.

B. Epidemiology:
   1. Gender: *Female* much more common than males (5 to 10:1).
   2. Race: More *blacks* than Caucasians are affected.
   3. Age: *Young adults* (generally under age 40).
C. Clinical signs:
   1. *Polyarthritis in 90% of cases; myositis.*
   2. *Typical skin rash.*
   3. *Constitutional signs:* Malaise, weakness.
   4. Multiple system disease (see Section E, below).
D. Laboratory tests:
   1. Lupus erythematosus (LE) cell prep positive.
   2. ANA positive.
   3. *RF may yield a false positive.*
E. Extra-articular manifestations:
   1. Myositis.
   2. Rash.
   3. Various neurologic abnormalities.
   4. Pulmonary vasculitis, fibrosis, and effusions.
   5. Pericarditis, cardiomyopathy.
   6. Nephritis.
   7. Steroid-induced stress fractures.
F. General radiographic description:
   1. Soft tissue: Symmetric swelling around joints, not chronic.
   2. Calcifications: Subcutaneous calcifications, generally *in the lower extremities, uncommon* (less than 10%).
   3. *Bone density:* Usually *normal,* but periarticular demineralization occasionally is seen.
   4. *Cartilage destruction: Rare.*
   5. *Erosions or productive change:* So *rare* that if erosions are seen, either early RA or a mixed connective tissue disease or overlap disease is considered.
   6. Subchondral cysts. Fairly common in hands and feet, but nonspecific and distinctly not erosive.
   7. Periostitis or enthesopathy: Not present.
   8. Ankylosis: Does not occur.
   9. *Ligamentous abnormality: The classic descriptor of SLE is nonerosive deformity from ligamentous laxity.* This is seen in only approximately *10% of cases.* The deformities are most commonly seen in the *hand,* with *ulnar deviation of the MCPs,* subluxation

of the first carpometacarpal (CMC) joint, and *variable flexion or extension deformities of the IP joints.* The deformities are *reducible,* so they are more prominent on the oblique ball-catcher view of the hand than on the PA view, where the hand and fingers are supported by the film cassette.

G. Joints most commonly affected: *Hand, wrist, knee—all characterized either by nonspecific polyarticular swelling or by a nonerosive ligamentous deformity.*

H. Bilateral symmetry: Generally present.

I. Other features: *Remarkably high incidence of AVN* (up to one third of SLE patients, though only 8% are symptomatic).[9] *Steroid therapy is felt to be the major etiologic factor, but the disease process itself may also predispose to AVN. Femoral head, humeral head, and knee* are common but nonspecific sites. The *dome of the talus and hands or feet are sites that are not uncommon in SLE, but extremely rare sites for AVN of another etiology;* therefore, AVN in these sites suggests SLE.

J. Differential diagnoses:
1. *RA:* The symmetric polyarthritis, deformities, and false-positive RF may be confusing in SLE, but the lack of erosions should make one suspect SLE rather than RA.
2. *Jaccoud's arthropathy:* Identical nonerosive deformities; history of rheumatic fever makes the diagnosis.
3. If the radiographic findings are restricted to AVN, all the other causes of AVN might be considered.

K. Survey films:
1. PA and ball-catcher views of hands.
2. If painful, the hips, shoulders, knees, or ankles may be studied for signs of AVN.

Progressive Systemic Sclerosis: Scleroderma

Key Concepts

Acral soft tissue atrophy, acro-osteolysis, soft tissue calcification; erosions occur, but are not a prominent feature.

A. Definition: A condition of unknown etiology that causes small-vessel disease and fibrosis in several organ systems. Scleroderma is the cutaneous manifestation of the disease.

B. Epidemiology:
1. Gender: Affects *females* more often than males (3:1).
2. Age: Most often diagnosed in the third to fifth decades.

C. Clinical signs:
  1. May present with Raynaud's phenomenon.
  2. Skin changes on the hands, feet, or face.
  3. Distal joint pain and stiffness.
  4. Dysphagia.
  5. Proximal myopathy.
D. Laboratory tests: *Not specific.*
  1. ESR increased in 70%.
  2. ANA increased in up to 95%.
  3. RF positive in up to 40%.
E. Extra-articular manifestations:
  1. Skin changes: Edema, leading to thickening and fibrosis, eventually becoming taut, shiny, and atrophic with progressive distal tapering.
  2. Gastrointestinal (GI): Esophageal atrophy and fibrosis, leading to dysmotility (air-fluid levels may be seen within the esophagus); pseudosacculations seen in the colon.
  3. Pulmonary fibrosis.
  4. Renal fibrosis.
  5. Cardiac: Pericarditis and myocarditis.
F. General radiographic description:
  1. Soft tissue: Extremely common; *acral tapering of digits* (78% in one series).[10]
  2. *Calcification: A prominent feature, with extensive subcutaneous, extra-articular, and occasionally intra-articular calcification;* punctate calcification in the terminal phalanx may also be seen. (Calcification seen in 25% of Bassett's series).[10]
  3. Bone density: Generally normal, but periarticular osteoporosis may be seen.
  4. Cartilage destruction: Joint space narrowing occasionally is seen.
  5. Erosive vs. productive change:
    a. The issues regarding true erosive change in scleroderma are difficult to resolve since, clinically, 25% to 50% of cases of scleroderma look like rheumatoid arthritis as well (often even with a positive RF). Thus, many patients have concurrent RA or overlap syndromes that explain any observed erosive changes.
    b. In addition, some scleroderma patients who are RF negative also have erosions, most commonly in the PIP and DIP joints.
    c. *Overall, joint abnormalities eventually occur in nearly 50% of scleroderma patients, predominantly erosions, but there may also be mild productive changes.*

6. Subchondral cysts: None.
7. Periostitis or enthesopathy: None.
8. Ankylosis: May occur.
9. Ligamentous abnormality: *Flexion contractures are common*, especially in the hands, wrists, and elbows.
G. Joints most commonly affected: PIPs and DIPs, sparing the MCPs and wrists.
H. Bilateral symmetry: Often present.
 I. Other features: *Resorption of bone is extremely common (seen in up to 80%)*:
1. *Tufts: Acro-osteolysis*, initially on the palmar aspect.
2. *Severe resorption at the first CMC joint* (trapezium and base of first metacarpal) *with radial subluxation of the first MC is very distinctive and almost pathognomonic of scleroderma.*
3. Resorption at the angle of the mandible is seen with facial skin changes.
4. Posterior resorption of ribs 3 through 6 (related to intercostal muscle atrophy).
J. Differential diagnoses:
1. *Differential for acro-osteolysis* includes HPTH and thermal injury, among many others; the soft tissue tapering and frequent calcifications help make the diagnosis of scleroderma.
2. *Differential for the erosive changes* includes RA (the sparing of the wrists and MCPs helps differentiate it from RA), and psoriatic arthritis (again, soft tissue calcifications, if present, help differentiate scleroderma).
3. *Differential of soft tissue calcification* is very extensive, including dermatomyositis, HPTH, hypoparathyroidism, tumeral calcinosis, metabolic abnormalities involving vitamin D, and HA crystal deposition disease.
K. Suggested survey films: PA and lateral hands.

Polymyositis/Dermatomyositis

Key Concepts

Soft tissue calcifications, subcutaneous or sheetlike in fascial planes; usually no joint abnormalities despite arthralgias.

A. Definition: A disease of unknown etiology that produces *inflammation and muscle degeneration*. In polymyositis the symptoms of proximal muscle weakness and arthralgias predominate; with dermatomyositis, a typical diffuse rash is an additional finding.

B. Epidemiology:
 1. Gender: *Females affected more than males.*
 2. Age: Third through fifth decades; dermatomyositis may also be seen in children, associated with severe systemic symptoms.
C. Clinical signs:
 1. *Muscle weakness,* tenderness, and eventually contracture with atrophy (50%).
 2. *Rash* (50%).
 3. *Raynaud's phenomenon* (33%).
 4. *Arthralgias* (20% to 50%).
D. Laboratory tests: Elevated muscle enzymes during active disease.
E. Extra-articular manifestations:
 1. Pulmonary fibrosis.
 2. Pericarditis.
 3. Abdominal pain, dysphagia.
F. General radiographic description:
 1. *Soft tissue: Muscle edema early, followed by atrophy and calcification.*
 2. Calcification:
  a. *Subcutaneous calcification* is most commonly seen and is nonspecific.
  b. *Sheetlike calcification along fascial or muscle planes* is less common but nearly pathognomonic for the disease; classically, it is seen in the proximal large muscles.
  c. Periarticular calcification may also occur.
 3. Bone density: Transient periarticular osteoporosis occasionally.
 4. Cartilage destruction: Not seen.
 5. Erosive change: If present, generally indicates an overlap syndrome; sporadic reports of erosions in dermatomyositis exist.
 6. Subchondral cysts: None.
 7. Periostitis: None.
 8. Ankylosis: None.
 9. Ligamentous abnormalities: May get flexion deformities.
G. Joints most commonly affected with arthralgias: Hands, wrists, knees; *radiographic abnormalities in joints are rare.*
H. Bilateral symmetry: Common.
 I. Other features: When dermatomyositis develops in older males, it may be associated with malignancy.
J. Differential diagnoses: If calcification is not sheetlike: scleroderma, SLE, overlap syndrome, HPTH.
K. Survey films: Symptomatic sites.

Amyloidosis

Key Concepts

Nodular synovitis that is very bulky. Erosions are better marginated than in RA. Wrist, elbow, shoulder most commonly involved. Chronic hemodialysis is also associated with amyloid deposits, primarily in the hand, wrist, and spine (resulting in the spondyloarthropathy of hemodialysis).

A. Definition: An infiltrative disorder that may be either *primary or secondary* (associated with other disease processes such as multiple myeloma, long-term hemodialysis, rheumatoid arthritis, familial Mediterranean fever, chronic infection, spondyloarthropathy, and connective tissue disorders such as SLE, scleroderma, and dermatomyositis). *Five to 13% of patients with amyloid have bone or joint involvement; this may consist of deposition in bone, synovium, and surrounding soft tissues.*

B. Epidemiology:
   1. Gender: *Males* affected more commonly than females.
   2. Age: Fourth through eighth decade.

C. Clinical signs of the arthropathy: Pain, stiffness, and soft tissue swelling; joint contractures and carpal tunnel syndrome may occur.

D. Laboratory tests: Biopsy often required to confirm the diagnosis.

E. Extra-articular manifestations:
   1. Kidney infiltration: Most common site of involvement; causes the greatest morbidity.
   2. Organomegaly.
   3. Pericardial and myocardial infiltration may lead to cardiac failure.
   4. Pulmonary septal infiltration.
   5. GI tract may be involved from the tongue to anus. Submucosal thickening and decreased peristalsis are observed.

F. Radiographic description of the arthropathy:
   1. *Soft tissue: Bulky nodules,* especially about *wrists, elbows, and shoulders* (*shoulder pad sign:* bulky nodules superimposed on atrophic musculature).
   2. Abnormal calcifications: None.
   3. Bone density: May be diffusely or focally osteoporotic.
   4. Cartilage destruction: *Joint space may actually widen* due to infiltration.
   5. Erosions: *Well-marginated erosions* occur with intra-articular disease.
   6. Subchondral cysts: May occur; appearing as well-defined juxta-articular lytic lesions.
   7. Periostitis or enthesopathy: None.

8. Ankylosis: None.
9. Ligamentous abnormality: *Joint contractures* occur.
10. *MR shows SI intermediate between fibrocartilage and muscle on all sequences,* helping to distinguish amyloid deposits from cellular or water-containing processes such as inflammation, synovitis, or Brown tumors of HPTH.[11]
G. Joints most commonly affected: Wrist, elbows, shoulder; knees and hips less commonly. *In chronic hemodialysis, the spine, wrist, and hands are most commonly affected. The spondyloarthropathy is usually in the cervical spine and appears as disk space narrowing and endplate irregularity.* The obvious differential diagnosis is infection; the absence of a paravertebral soft tissue mass and clinical signs of infection help make the correct diagnosis.[12]
H. Bilateral symmetry: Common.
J. *Differential diagnosis* of the arthropathy: *RA is the prime consideration, but the well-defined erosions, preservation of joint space, and nodular soft tissue may help to differentiate amyloidosis from RA. Remember the association of amyloidosis with multiple myeloma.*

III. RHEUMATIC FEVER

Key Concepts

Nonerosive, but deforming arthropathy (especially at MCP joints) occurs uncommonly.

A. Definition: Rheumatic fever is a syndrome that follows a group A β-hemolytic streptococcal infection (usually of the throat) and produces fever, various systemic symptoms, valvular heart disease, a polyarthritis and, in a few cases, Jaccoud's arthropathy (a deforming nonerosive arthropathy).
B. Epidemiology: Not useful.
C. Clinical signs: The most common *polyarthritis* presents with joint pain, sometimes accompanied by signs of inflammation and swelling. *Large joints* (knee, ankle) are involved most commonly, and the pattern is often *migratory. Radiographs are normal except for occasional nonspecific soft tissue swelling and juxta-articular osteoporosis resulting from the local inflammation.* The arthritis is *self-limited,* disappearing after a few weeks. The much less common *Jaccoud's arthropathy* generally occurs following multiple episodes of polyarthritis and is *clinically asymptomatic.*
D. Laboratory tests: RF is negative.
E. Extra-articular manifestations: Fever; valvular heart disease.

F. *General radiographic description of Jaccoud's arthropathy* (*nonerosive but deforming*):
   1. Soft tissue: Normal.
   2. Abnormal calcifications: None.
   3. Bone density: Usually normal, though juxta-articular osteoporosis may occur.
   4. *Cartilage destruction: Does not occur until very late and then is secondary to mechanical wear due to subluxation.*
   5. *Erosions:* The disease is *nonerosive until very late, when hook erosions on the radial aspect of the metacarpal heads, away from the articular margin, may occur secondary to mechanical pressure.*
   6. Subchondral cysts: Rare.
   7. Periostitis or enthesopathy: None.
   8. Ankylosis: None.
   9. *Deformity: The primary feature of the arthropathy is a reversible deformity* (*ulnar deviation and flexion of the MCPs and fibular deviation and flexion of the MTPs*); occurs secondary to capsular and tendon fibrosis.
G. Joints most commonly affected: By *polyarthritis: knees and ankles;* by *Jaccoud's arthritis: MCPs and MTPs.*
H. Bilateral symmetry: Often occurs, but not prominently.
I. Other features: None.
J. *Differential diagnoses* for Jaccoud's arthropathy:
   1. *SLE:* May be indistinguishable radiographically in the hands or feet.
   2. *RA:* The deformity is identical, but RA rarely causes the deformity without accompanying erosions and cartilage damage. When erosions occur in Jaccoud's they are not the typical marginal erosions seen in RA.
   3. Ehlers-Danlos syndrome: May rarely appear similar.
K. Suggested survey films: PA and ball-catcher (oblique) views of hands: The reversibility will be demonstrated since the hands appear nearly normal on the PA (where they are supported by the cassette) but the deformities are marked on the unsupported oblique views.

IV. OSTEOARTHRITIS (OA)

Key Concepts

Most common locations: DIPs, first CMC, scaphoid-trapezium-trapezoid, lower cervical spine, lumbar facets, hips, knee, first MTP. Normal bone density, focal (weight-bearing) loss of cartilage, sclerosis, osteophyte formation—productive changes are prominent.

A. Definition: Degenerative joint disease stimulated by one or a combination of the following factors (Note: In most cases, osteoarthritis is believed to be secondary, with an underlying cause which usually can be found):

1. Abnormal mechanical forces on the joint (joint deformity, obesity, occupational stresses).
2. Normal forces on abnormal cartilage (due to a pre-existing arthritis such as RA, loose bodies in the joint, osteochondral fracture, or a meniscal abnormality in the knee).
3. Collapse of subchondral bone (due to osteoporosis, avascular necrosis, or hyperparathyroidism).

B. Epidemiology:

1. The most common arthritis.
2. Gender: Males and females are affected equally though the disease often presents earlier in males.
3. Age: Incidence increases with age.

C. Clinical signs:

1. Pain (on bearing weight, relieved with rest).
2. Limited range of motion.
3. Crepitus.
4. Subluxation, most commonly genu varus.
5. Heberden's (DIP) and Bouchard's (PIP) nodes.
6. The radiographic severity of disease does not always correlate strongly with amount of pain.

D. Pertinent laboratory tests: None.

E. Extra-articular manifestations: None.

F. General radiographic description:

1. Soft tissue alterations:
   a. *Heberden's (DIP) and Bouchard (PIP) nodes* are actually the osteophytes formed at these sites.
   b. Effusions occur but are unusual.
2. Abnormal calcifications:
   a. May develop *chondrocalcinosis*.
   b. May develop HA depositions in periarticular sites.
   c. *Loose bodies* may form from synovial metaplasia or fractured osteophytes.
3. *Bone density:* Normal.
4. *Cartilage destruction:* Always present and tends to be focal, predictably in the primary *weight-bearing portion* of the joint.
5. Erosive versus productive bony change: *No erosions.* Three types of *productive change* are commonly seen:

    a. *Osteophytes* may be intra-articular but occur primarily in *non-weight-bearing sites,* due to capsular or ligamentous traction.

    b. *Subchondral sclerosis* due to vascular invasion after abnormal mechanical forces and deposition of new bone in a reparative attempt.

    c. *Cortical buttressing,* another reparative attempt in response to abnormal mechanical forces, is seen primarily in the *medial and lateral aspects of the femoral neck.*

6. *Subchondral cysts:* Common; microfractures in the subchondral bone and synovial fluid pressure probably combine to form cysts, but many do not communicate with the joint. Some ''cysts'' are areas of fibrocartilaginous metaplasia. The cysts tend to occur in *weight-bearing* areas and generally have a *sclerotic margin* (unlike RA erosions). *Eggar's cyst* is found in the weight-bearing portion of the acetabulum and may be the first sign of hip OA.

7. *Enthesopathy is common,* especially on the anterior aspect of the *patella* and the *pelvic and hip apophyses.* It is not distinguishable from that seen in AS and other rheumatoid variants.

8. Ankylosis: Rare in absence of trauma; in erosive OA the DIP joints occasionally may fuse.

9. *Ligamentous abnormality: Commonly seen secondary to the underlying joint OA;* the focal cartilage loss leads to joint deformity, which in turn promotes ligamentous contractions and laxity. These deformities lead to instability, which in turn promotes further arthropathy.

G. Joints most commonly affected:

  1. Hand:

    a. *Multiple IP joints* are often involved with uniform cartilage narrowing, subchondral sclerosis, and osteophyte formation.

    b. Generally, the IP joints are not painful and function is retained.

    c. Occasionally flexion or even radial or ulnar deformity is seen.

    d. Heberden's and Bouchard's nodes represent the underlying osteophytes and not soft tissue swelling.

    e. MCPs are less commonly involved than IPs, and never are involved in the absence of IP joint OA; subchondral cysts may be prominent in MC heads.

    f. Differential diagnosis for IP disease: Rheumatoid variants, such as psoriatic arthritis, that have a combination of erosive and productive changes; erosive OA (see Section I, below).

    g. Differential diagnosis for MCP disease: Pseudogout and hemochromatosis have prominent hooklike osteophytes and cysts, generally seen in the second and third MCPs and often with chondrocalcinosis seen in the triangular fibrocartilage.

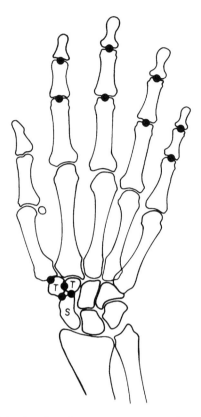

Fig. 2-9 Joints of the hand and wrist most commonly involved with osteoarthritis.

2. Wrist (Fig 2-9):
   a. Typical changes of sclerosis, osteophyte formation, and cartilage loss involve the *first CMC joint,* often with radial subluxation of the thumb.
   b. The second most common site is the *scaphoid-trapezium-trapezoid* complex.
   c. OA at the radial carpal joint is unusual and, if present, is usually related to trauma. Examples include productive change in the adjacent radial styloid after malunion of a scaphoid fracture, or an ulnar plus variant resulting in an ulnar impaction syndrome and subchondral cyst/osteophyte formation on the adjacent lunate.
3. Elbow: Only posttraumatic involvement.

4. Glenohumeral: OA unusual in absence of previous trauma. When present, there are *marginal osteophytes around the glenoid,* as well as *ring osteophytes around the anatomic neck of the humerus,* largest inferiorly. *If there is no history of trauma, pseudogout* should be considered.
   a. A chronic rotator cuff tear (seen as elevation of the humeral head and a sclerotic concave acromion articulating with the humeral head) may lead to OA of the shoulder.
   b. Shoulder impingement syndrome gives a different appearance, with sclerosis of the top of the greater tuberosity and a subacromial spur, seen well with an ''outlet'' view.
5. Acromioclavicular joint: Common; typical changes of OA.
6. SI joint: Subchondral sclerosis and osteophytes are commonly seen in two sites—*anteroinferior to the SI joint and anterosuperior to the synovial portion of the joint* (mid to upper third of SI joint as seen on AP films). Large *osteophytes bridge the joint anteriorly;* this appearance is easily identified as an osteophyte on CT but may be *misinterpreted as focal blastic metastases* on plain film.
   a. *Differential diagnoses:*
      (1) Metastases.
      (2) Ankylosing spondylitis.
      (3) Osteitis condensans ileii (a triangular sclerotic lesion on the iliac side of the inferior SI joint, seen most often in multiparous women).
7. Hip: A common site of OA that is often painful with weight bearing and has a restricted range of motion. Eggar's cyst of the acetabulum and calcar buttressing may be early signs of OA; otherwise expect to see typical signs of focal cartilage narrowing, sclerosis, and osteophyte formation (lateral acetabulum, lateral and especially medial subcapital region). The hip *migrates superiorly in 80%* of patients, usually superolaterally, though sometimes the migration appears to be superomedial due to cartilage narrowing and huge inferomedial osteophytes. *Medial migration with protrusio acetabuli is seen in 20%.*
   a. *Differential diagnoses:*
      (1) If medial migration, look for reasons to differentiate it from RA or the *rheumatoid variants,* which should have combined erosive and productive changes and/or SI joint abnormalities.
      (2) Superior flattening of the femoral head, accentuated by the presence of large inferomedial osteophytes simulates the appearance of *avascular necrosis;* the latter disease process

has normal cartilage width, differentiating it from OA, but if secondary OA occurs, the differentiation is not always possible.

(3) If large cysts are present, *pseudogout or PVNS* should be considered.

(4) An early ring osteophyte in the subcapital position may be difficult to differentiate from an *impacted subcapital fracture.*

(5) An unusual variant of OA in the hip is rapidly destructive hip disease (RDHD). Seen mostly in elderly females, this process results in atrophic destructive changes in the femoral head and acetabulum over a few months. Other joints are less commonly involved. Differential diagnosis includes infection and Charcot joint.[13]

8. Knee: A common site of involvement, with pain on weight bearing; may involve one, two, or all three compartments (medial, lateral, patellofemoral). If single-compartment disease, it is likely to be medial. Specific compartment involvement should be evaluated since unicompartmental OA may be treated with a unicompartmental prosthesis or with a high tibial osteotomy (most commonly a closing wedge tibial metaphyseal osteotomy, which transfers much of the weight bearing to the lateral compartment and may lead to regeneration of fibrocartilage in the medial compartment). With medial compartment predominance, one sees a *typical varus knee deformity and lateral subluxation of the tibia.*

   a. Osteophytes tend to be marginal in all three compartments, as well as on tibial spines.

   b. Enthesopathy of the anterior (nonarticular) surface of the patella at the quadriceps insertion is common and not related to OA.

   c. *Differential diagnoses:*

      (1) If subchondral cysts are especially prominent, consider PVNS or pseudogout.

      (2) If patellofemoral disease is prominent, with little or no medial or lateral compartment disease, consider pseudogout and look for chondrocalcinosis.

9. Ankle: OA rare in the absence of trauma.

10. Foot: Most common in first MTP and first tarsometatarsal (TMT).

11. Spine: Various manifestations are seen that have distinct terminology. These manifestations are often interdependent and therefore coexistent.

   a. *Degenerative disc disease:* Late manifestations are *decreased disc height and disc vacuum sign.* The disc may herniate posteriorly (seen by CT, magnetic resonance imaging (MRI), or myelogram), centrally into an adjacent vertebral body (*Schmorl's nodes*), or anteriorly, resulting in a *limbus vertebra* if it occurs prior to skeletal maturity. (A limbus vertebra results from separation of a ring apophysis from the underlying vertebral body by a herniated disc producing a separate triangular ossicle, usually located at the anterosuperior border of the vertebral body, seen on the lateral film.) Degenerative disc disease often results in reactive sclerosis of the adjacent end-plates termed *discogenic sclerosis* or *idiopathic segmental sclerosis.* Discogenic sclerosis may be difficult to differentiate radiographically from a disc space infection, but the end-plate remains intact in the former process. In addition, the sclerosis of the superior end-plate is distinctive, being triangle-shaped anteriorly. This should also be distinguished from blastic metastatic tumor.

b. *Spondylosis deformans* results from bulging of the anulus fibrosus, stretching of Sharpey's fibers (the attachment of the anulus to the vertebral body), and *traction osteophyte formation* on the anterior and lateral vertebral body, arising several millimeters from the end-plates. These osteophytes may bridge the disc spaces in a bulky fashion, clearly distinct from the thin vertical syndesmophytes of AS. Since spondylosis deformans does not involve a joint, it is not a manifestation of OA but rather a degenerative disease of the spine.

c. *True osteoarthritis* involves the apophyseal joints (facets) and most commonly involves C_{5-7}, L_{4-5}, and S_1 vertebrae. Typical degenerative changes are seen (sclerosis and osteophyte formation) by plain film, but the extent and severity of the resultant stenosis is best judged by CT[14] or MR. The facet OA often results in *spondylolisthesis without spondylolysis* and certainly *contributes to stenosis.*

d. *Uncovertebral* joints (*joints of Luschka*) are found only in the C_{3-7} *bodies,* located posterolaterally. Osteophytes may form and are seen on AP or lateral films, but neuroforaminal encroachment is best evaluated on oblique films.

e. *Spinal stenosis* may be seen on plain film as a decreased interpediculate distance or short AP pedicle length; however, these bony measurements have a very wide range of normal and, so, are useful only infrequently. Furthermore, soft tissue abnormalities often contribute to spinal stenosis (disc bulge, ligamentum flavum hypertrophy). The total picture of congenitally short pedicles modified by soft tissue abnormalities and facet OA is best evaluated by CT or MRI.

H. Bilateral symmetry may be present but is much less common than in RA.

I. Other features:

Erosive (inflammatory) OA: An arthropathy found primarily in *middle-aged women* who experience *distinct inflammatory episodes,* similar to RA, with swollen red joints. ESR and RF are normal. *DIP and PIP* joints are involved, with loss of cartilage, sclerosis, and combined *erosive and productive bony changes.* The erosions on the proximal side of the joint tend to be central and the osteophytes, marginal, giving a distinctive *gull-wing* appearance.[15]

Fusion is seen occasionally.

The *differential diagnosis includes psoriatic arthritis, adult Still's disease, and septic joint (if monarticular). Typical OA of the first CMC joint and STT joints* (usually without erosions) *is often present* and is greatly helpful in arriving at the correct diagnosis.

J. *Differential diagnoses:* Discussed in Section G; varies according to the joint involved; includes RA, AS, psoriatic arthritis, PVNS, and pseudogout.

K. Suggested survey films: PA hands, AP pelvis, AP and lateral knees.

V. NEUROPATHIC (CHARCOT) JOINTS

Key Concepts

Severe destructive arthropathy may be hypertrophic or atrophic. Distribution helps determine etiology: shoulder, syringomyelia; foot (talonavicular or TMT Lisfranc fracture dislocation), diabetes; knee, tabes dorsalis; spine, paraplegia.

A. Definition: A severely destructive arthropathy, usually monostotic, with several etiologies. The *most common etiologies include diabetes, tabes dorsalis, and syringomyelia.* Other etiologies include myelomeningocele or spinal cord injury, multiple sclerosis, Charcot-Marie-Tooth disease, alcoholism, amyloidosis, intra-articular steroids, congenital insensitivity or indifference to pain, and dysautonomia (Riley-Day syndrome). The primary *pathogenesis* is disputed, but most agree that an *initial alteration in sympathetic control of bone blood flow leads to hyperemia and active bone resorption. A neurotraumatic mechanism is usually important secondarily,* with a destructive cycle of (1) blunted pain sensation and proprioception; (2) relaxation of skeletal supporting structures and chronic instability; (3) recurrent injury with normal biomechanical stresses but abnormal joint loading; (4) bony fragmentation and joint disorganization. Progression may be rapid.

B. Epidemiology: Depends on etiology.
C. Clinical signs: Swollen, unstable joint. *The diagnosis may not be clinically obvious since 30% have pain* and the neurologic changes may be difficult to elicit.
D. Laboratory tests: Depends on etiology, VDRL for syphilis, etc.
E. Extra-articular manifestations: Depends on etiology. There may be typical findings of syphilis or diabetes. A syrinx may widen the cervical canal and is best seen on MR. Congenital insensitivity or indifference to pain may be manifest by multiple scars on hands and by intraocular foreign bodies.
F. General radiographic description: The classical description is of *five Ds*—increased *density,* joint distension, bony debris, joint disorganization, and dislocation. This describes the *hypertrophic* variety well, but only 20% of Charcot joints are purely hypertrophic. Forty percent *are primarily atrophic* with such distinctive bone resorption that there often is a sharp transverse cut-off of the bone in the metadiaphysis, with complete resorption of the articular portion, that appears almost surgical. Another 40% are combined hypertrophic and atrophic.[16]
   1. Soft tissue: *Large effusions.*
   2. Abnormal calcifications: Much *bony debris and fragmentation. The effusions may decompress down fascial planes, carrying bony debris far from the joint itself.*
   3. *Bone density: Normal to increased* (except in diabetics).
   4. Cartilage destruction: Prominent early finding.
   5. *Erosive and productive changes coexist;* one or the other may predominate, depending on whether it is an atrophic or hypertrophic form.
   6. Subchondral cysts: May be present.
   7. Periostitis or enthesopathy: Not present.
   8. Ankylosis: Rare; in fact, surgical arthrodesis is difficult.
   9. Ligamentous abnormality: Prominent finding, with *laxity and joint subluxation or dislocation.*
G. Joints most commonly affected: In many cases, the etiology of the neuropathic joint may be suggested by which joint is involved.
   1. *Knee* involvement is usually due to *tabes dorsalis,* which may also involve other joints of the lower extremity or the lumbar spine. Changes are usually hypertrophic.
   2. *Foot* involvement is most commonly due to *diabetic arthropathy,* specifically if the *talonavicular* and TMT joints are involved (the latter often *resembles a Lisfranc fracture dislocation.* Diabetic neuroarthropathy in fact is a more common etiology for Lisfranc fracture dislocation than is trauma). These are often the atrophic or mixed form of Charcot joints. Superimposed infection is a diag-

nostic problem. Alcoholism may rarely result in neuropathic foot joints.[17]

3. *Shoulder* neuroarthropathy is most commonly secondary to *syringomyelia*. It is almost always *atrophic*, with resorption of most or all of the humeral head and neck. This gives the appearance of a clean surgical resection of the humeral head. Watch particularly for subtle collection of debris, superimposed over the axillary or subscapularis bursae or the bicipital tendon groove of the shoulder. The location of these calcifications should allow identification as debris in a joint process, but they are often mistakenly believed to represent tumor matrix and, together with the destruction of the humeral head, chondrosarcoma is (mis)diagnosed.

4. *Spine* neuroarthropathy may be seen in patients with *spinal cord trauma* who have undergone instrumentation and fusion. The *first mobile segment* adjacent to the fusion is most commonly involved.

H. Bilateral symmetry: Rare.

I. Other features: In patients with decreased pain sensation an undetected fracture may occur (probably initiated as a stress fracture). Exuberant periostitis and callus formation may even suggest a bone-forming tumor.

J. Differential diagnoses:
   1. Hypertrophic form: Severe osteoarthritis.
   2. Atrophic form: Joint sepsis.

K. Survey films: Based on clinical suspicion.

VI. BIOCHEMICAL ABNORMALITIES
Gout

Key Concepts

Long interval between onset of clinical disease and radiographic findings: Para-articular erosions with overhanging edges and adjacent tophi with amorphous calcifications are pathognomonic. Bone density is normal, and erosion margins, sclerotic. Hands and feet most commonly are involved.

A. Definition: A *sodium urate* crystal-induced synovial inflammation that may be limited to occasional acute attacks or may be a chronic arthropathy with crystal deposition in capsular and synovial tissues, periarticular soft tissues, articular cartilage, and subchondral bone. This crystal deposition and inflammatory reaction provoke very specific degenerative changes. Disease is (1) idiopathic, (2) secondary to enzyme defects, or (3) secondary to chronic disease processes such as myeloproliferative disorders, renal disease, hyper- or hypoparathyroidism, psoriasis, or diuretic therapy.

B. Epidemiology:
  1. Occurs mostly in *middle-aged or elderly males* (extremely rare in premenopausal women), with fairly strong hereditary factors. May also be relatively frequently seen in young Polynesian males.
  2. Onset at an early age is most often due to renal disease or a myeloproliferative disorder.
  3. Caucasians affected more commonly than blacks.
  4. *Gouty attacks typically occur for several years* (average 12) *before radiographic abnormalities are seen.*

C. Clinical signs: Red, swollen, *extremely painful joints;* usually monarticular or oligoarticular.

D. Pertinent laboratory tests:
  1. Hyperuricemia determination.
  2. *Sodium urate crystals* may be seen in synovial fluid by polarizing microscope.

E. Extra-articular manifestations:
  1. *Tophus in bursa* (olecranon or prepatellar bursa most commonly).
  2. Tophus in the helix of the ear and occasionally other soft tissue sites.

F. General radiographic description:
  1. *Soft tissue* alterations: *Tophi* are eccentric soft tissue nodules adjacent to a joint, often containing amorphous calcification.
  2. Abnormal calcifications: Amorphous calcification within tophi; occasional focal increased density within bone. Chondrocalcinosis may occur but is much less common than in pseudogout.
  3. *Bone density: Normal,* with osteoporosis only in extremely longstanding disease due to disuse.
  4. Cartilage destruction: *Cartilage often remains intact, even late in the disease process and with adjacent erosions.* This may be an important discriminating feature.
  5. Erosive versus productive changes: *Erosions* may be *intra-articular* (*often marginal*) *or para-articular* (often beneath tophi). The para-articular erosions are almost pathognomonic for gout and may show the additional feature of an "overhanging edge," a bony lip, or excrescence extending out toward the tophus, beyond the normal bony margin. Occasionally, with long-standing disease, the erosions may be as mutilating as those of psoriatic arthritis or RA. One helpful feature is that the *erosions usually have a sclerotic margin. Productive changes* are in the form of enlargement of the ends of phalanges and secondary osteoarthritis with osteophyte formation.

6. Subchondral cysts: Not usually present, but the sclerotic marginated erosions give a similar appearance. Occasionally, large subchondral cysts are seen.
7. Enthesopathy: May be present.
8. Ankylosis: Very rare.
9. Ligamentous abnormality: Occasional ligament rupture, but laxity
   is not a common feature.
10. MR appearance: When gout has an atypical clinical and radio-
    graphic presentation, MR may be performed. *With MR, a solitary
    tophus may mimic a bone or soft tissue neoplasm.* A tophus will
    have *low SI on T1 imaging, but variably low to high SI on T2,
    depending on the amount of amorphous calcification present in
    the tophus.* It may be inhomogeneous and appear infiltrative, and
    thus be confusing. *Remember—gout can look like anything, and
    is relatively common, so should always be kept in mind!*

G. Joints most commonly affected: In general, *lower extremity is more
   commonly involved than upper extremity,* and small joints more often
   than large joints.
   1. Foot and ankle: First MTP most common; other MTPs, IPs, mid-
      foot, and hindfoot may also be involved.
   2. Knee: May see marginal erosions or erosions on the articular sur-
      face of the *patella* (which may simulate neoplasm or the normal
      variant dorsal defect of the patella).
   3. *Hand and wrist: DIPs, PIPs, intercarpal* joints are most com-
      monly involved; MCPs less frequently.
   4. Elbow: Extensor surface disease (olecranon).
   5. SI joint involved occasionally.

H. Symmetry: Asymmetric.

I. Other features: *Tophi and erosions are rarely seen until after several
   years of chronic disease.* Remember also that gout is an easy diagnosis
   when it follows all the above rules (pauciarticular, with tophus and
   overhanging edges). However, it may also present as a polyarticular
   disease, without obvious tophi, but with multiple well-marginated erosions. This appearance in an older male patient should always be suspect for gout, but is often misdiagnosed as RA.

J. Differential diagnoses:
   1. Early, nonclassic gout may be mistaken for rheumatoid or psoriatic
      arthritis.
   2. Gout may be confused clinically with pseudogout, but site of in-
      volvement should help differentiate the two.
   3. Xanthomatosis gives soft tissue masses on tendons, sometimes
      with associated bony erosion.

K. Suggested survey films: Feet: AP, lateral; hands: PA.

Calcium Pyrophosphate Dihydrate (CPPD) Crystal Deposition Disease

---

Key Concepts

Intra-articular crystal deposition; pyrophosphate arthropathy often demonstrates chondrocalcinosis and a pattern of degenerative joint disease (DJD) in very specific joints (knee, wrist, second and third MCPs, hip, elbow) as well as in a specific distribution within a joint (e.g., patellofemoral compartment in knee, radiocarpal compartment in wrist). Subchondral cysts are a very prominent feature.

A. Definition:
1. A relatively *common* arthropathy resulting from CPPD crystal deposition (usually intra-articular) with *radiographically distinctive features.*
2. Various terminology relating to this disease is often loosely and incorrectly applied. Resnick suggests the following strict terminology:
   a. *Chondrocalcinosis: Nonspecific cartilage calcification;* the crystals deposited usually are, but may not be, CPPD, and there may or may not be an associated arthropathy.
   b. *CPPD crystal deposition disease:* More specific form of chondrocalcinosis due to CPPD crystal deposition; there may or may not be an associated arthropathy.
   c. *Pyrophosphate arthropathy: Pattern of structural joint damage occurring in CPPD deposition disease that has the appearance of DJD.* However, it occurs in *specific sites that are unusual for DJD but specific for pyrophosphate arthropathy.* Although pyrophosphate arthropathy is associated with CPPD deposition, it *may or may not be manifest as chondrocalcinosis. Pyrophosphate arthropathy may or may not present clinically as pseudogout.*
   d. *Pseudogout:* The *clinical presentation of CPPD deposition disease which resembles gout* (intermittent acute attacks). This is only one of several clinical manifestations of CPPD deposition disease but is often used loosely in lieu of "pyrophosphate arthropathy" in describing the radiographic findings of the latter disease.
B. Epidemiology:
1. *Middle aged or elderly male or female.*
2. May coexist with gout.

C. Clinical signs: Several common patterns.
1. Pseudogout (10% to 20%): Acute self-limited attacks simulating gout or infection.
2. Pseudo-RA (2% to 6%): More continuous acute attacks simulating RA.
3. Pseudo-DJD (35% to 60%): Chronic, progressive arthropathy but with acute exacerbations.
4. Pseudo-DJD without acute exacerbations (10% to 30%).
5. Asymptomatic (10% to 20%).
6. Pseudoneuropathic (rare): Rapidly destructive form.

D. Laboratory tests:
1. Joint aspiration, with calcium pyrophosphate crystals seen in synovial fluid under polarizing microscope.
2. No associated biochemical abnormality.

E. Extra-articular manifestations: None.

F. General radiographic description of pyrophosphate arthropathy:
1. Soft tissue alterations: Local swelling.
2. Abnormal calcifications: Usually intraarticular.
   a. *Chondrocalcinosis is seen in either hyaline or fibrocartilage, most commonly in the knee (menisci)* hyaline cartilage of the knee or carpus, *triangular fibrocartilage complex of the wrist, symphysis pubis, and acetabular labrum.* Other sites include the glenoid labrum, acromioclavicular joint, sternoclavicular joint, and anulus fibrosus.
   b. Crystals may also be deposited in the synovium, capsule, tendons, and ligaments.
3. *Bone density: Normal.*
4. Cartilage destruction: Present.
5. Erosive versus productive bony change: *primarily productive,* with *sclerosis,* osteochondral fragments, and osteophytes (especially notable at MCP heads).
6. *Subchondral cysts:* A distinctive feature, they are *common and tend to be very large, sometimes simulating neoplasm.*
7. Periostitis or enthesopathy: Not present.
8. Ankylosis: Rare.
9. Ligamentous abnormalities: Occasional crystal deposition; instability pattern may be seen in the wrist (see Section G, below).

G. *Joints most commonly affected: The most distinctive feature of pyrophosphate arthropathy—knee, wrist, and second and third MCPs are involved most often.*
1. *Knee: Chondrocalcinosis in menisci as well as hyaline cartilage.* The degenerative features may be seen in all three compartments

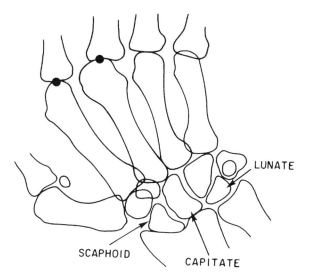

Fig. 2-10   Calcium pyrophosphate arthropathy pattern in the hand: radiocarpal disease, with scapholunate dissociation and SLAC wrist deformity; arthropathy with prominent osteophytes is seen typically at the second and third MCP joints.

but are *often much more prominent in the patellofemoral compartment than the medial or lateral compartment.*

2. *Wrist (Fig 2-10): Chondrocalcinosis in the TFCC and/or intraosseous ligaments and hyaline cartilage (especially in the lunate-triquetral region). Degenerative changes are specifically found in the radiocarpal joint,* often with scapholunate dissociation and scaphoid erosion into the distal radial articular surface. Proximal migration of the capitate between the dissociated scaphoid and lunate may result in a scapholunate advanced collapse (SLAC) wrist pattern. Note however that SLAC wrist deformity may occur in the absence of CPPD and certainly is not pathognomonic for that disease process. This distribution is significantly different from that seen in typical DJD.

3. Hand: *Second and third MCPs* specifically involved; IPs are spared.

4. Hip: If large subchondral cysts are seen with ''DJD,'' consider pyrophosphate arthropathy and look for labral chondrocalcinosis.

5. Shoulder and elbow: A DJD pattern should suggest pyrophosphate arthropathy since DJD is rare in these joints in the absence of trauma. Chondrocalcinosis should be sought.

6. Spine: Uncommon site of CPPD deposition, though perhaps often

overlooked. Reports of CPPD within the ligamentum flavum relate its deposition to enlargement of that structure and subsequent spinal stenosis.[18]

H. Symmetry: Often bilateral but not necessarily symmetric disease.

I. Other features: Several other diseases are seen in association with CPPD crystal deposition: DJD, trauma, gout, HPTH, hemochromatosis, Wilson's disease (documentation questionable), ochronosis.

J. Differential diagnoses:
   1. For chondrocalcinosis:
      a. Other diseases associated with CPPD deposition (see Section I, above).
      b. Scleroderma.
      c. HA crystal deposition.
      d. Periarticular calcification: Renal osteodystrophy, collagen vascular disease, vitamin D metabolic abnormalities.
   2. For the arthropathy:
      a. DJD, but site of involvement differs significantly and reliably.
      b. Others, such as RA or gout, may be suggested clinically but not radiographically since pyrophosphate arthropathy is not an erosive disease.

K. Survey films:
   1. For chondrocalcinosis: AP knees, PA hands and wrists, AP symphysis pubis.
   2. For arthropathy: Add lateral knees to films for chondrocalcinosis, above.

Hemochromatosis Arthropathy

Key Concepts

Nearly identical arthropathy to that of pyrophosphate arthropathy with degenerative-type changes at specific sites: patellofemoral predominance at knee; radiocarpal and second or third MCP joints in hand. Osteoporosis may be present.

A. Definition: An arthropathy that develops in up to *50% of patients who have hemochromatosis,* presumably due to *accumulation of iron and/or CPPD crystals in joints.* Hemochromatosis itself may be either primary (increased GI absorption of iron) or secondary (increased intake of iron by means of blood transfusions, alcoholism, or excess ingestion).

B. Epidemiology:
   1. Age: *Onset in middle age.*
   2. Gender: *Males* affected much more often than females.

C. Clinical signs: Usually mild pain, swelling, and stiffness, but acute attacks may occur.
D. Laboratory tests: Increased serum iron and iron-binding capacity.
E. Extra-articular manifestations: *Clinical triad of bronze skin, cirrhosis, and diabetes.* Heart disease is also seen.
F. General radiographic description of arthropathy: *Nearly identical to pyrophosphate arthropathy.*
   1. Soft tissues: Mild swelling.
   2. Abnormal calcifications: *Chondrocalcinosis* is common but not always associated with joint disease.
   3. Bone density: *Osteoporosis* common.
   4. Cartilage destruction: Present focally.
   5. Erosive versus productive changes: Primarily *productive, with large beaklike osteophytes, noted especially on MCP heads.*
   6. *Subchondral cysts: Prominent,* as in pseudogout arthropathy.
   7. Periostitis or enthesopathy: None.
   8. Ankylosis: None.
   9. Ligamentous abnormality: No deformity.
G. *Joints most commonly affected: Same as pyrophosphate arthropathy.*
   1. *Second and third MCPs.*
   2. *Radiocarpal joint.*
   3. *Knee, especially patellofemoral compartment.*
   4. *Hip.*
   5. *Shoulder.*
H. Symmetry: Usually present.
 I. Other features: None.
 J. Differential diagnosis: Pyrophosphate arthropathy: distinctive features of hemochromatosis include osteoporosis, especially prominent beak-like osteophytes on MCP heads and involvement of more carpal areas.
K. Survey films: PA hands and wrists; AP and lateral knees.

Wilson's Disease

Key Concepts

Osteopenia in young males is suggestive; irregular subchondral bone and fragmentation resembling osteochondritis.

A. Definition: An autosomal-recessive disease associated with abnormal accumulation of *copper.*
B. Epidemiology:
   1. *Males* more often affected than females.

2. Manifest in adolescents and young adults, but arthropathy may develop later.
C. Clinical signs: The articular abnormalities are often asymptomatic. Otherwise, mechanical degenerative symptoms are present.
D. Laboratory tests: Evidence of renal tubular abnormalities.
E. Extra-articular manifestations: Basal ganglia degenerative changes, cirrhosis, Kayser-Fleischer rings in cornea.
F. General radiographic description of the arthropathy:
  1. Soft tissues: Normal.
  2. Abnormal calcification: *Chondrocalcinosis* may be present. There may be an association of Wilson's disease and CPPD crystal deposition disease due to pyrophosphatase inhibition by copper.
  3. Bone density: *Osteopenic*, perhaps due to renal tubular disease.
  4. Cartilage destruction: Present, indicated by decreased width.
  5. Erosive versus productive change: *Indistinct, irregular subchondral bone, with several small fragments or ossicles; this may give the appearance of osteochondritis.* Sclerosis may be present.
  6. Subchondral cysts: Present.
  7. Periostitis or enthesopathy: May be present.
  8. Ankylosis: None.
  9. Ligamentous abnormality: None.
G. Joints most commonly affected: *Wrist and hand (especially MCPs)*, foot, hip, shoulder, elbow, knee.
H. Bilateral symmetry: Often present.
I. Other features: None.
J. Differential diagnoses:
  1. CPPD/hemochromatosis: *The distribution of the arthropathy is the same but the irregularity and fragmentation of the subchondral bone is distinctive.* Chondrocalcinosis may be present in both.
  2. *DJD:* Osteopenia as well as joint distributions make DJD unlikely.
K. Survey films: PA film of hands.

Calcium Hydroxyapatite (HA) Deposition Disease

Key Concepts

Periarticular calcification; shoulder most common site; underlying bone usually normal.

A. Definition: Periarticular calcifications due to HA crystal deposition, generally monarticular, and with an inflammatory reaction but usually without structural joint abnormality. Etiology is unknown, but may relate to repeated minor trauma and deposition in necrotic tissue.

B. Epidemiology: Middle to old age; affects men and women equally.
C. Clinical signs: Generally painful single joint, though may also be poly-articular and/or asymptomatic.
D. Laboratory tests: HA crystals seen by light microscopy with Wright's stain or by electron microscopy, not via polarizing microscope.
E. Extra-articular manifestations: None.
F. General radiographic description:
   1. Soft tissue: May be swollen.
   2. Abnormal calcification: The finding that suggests the diagnosis: The *calcification* is usually *cloudlike and homogeneous,* occurring *periarticularly* (*tendons, ligaments, capsule, bursa*). Occasionally it is intra-articular, producing chondrocalcinosis. The calcification may change over time, enlarging or even disappearing.
   3. Bone density: Normal to partly sclerotic.
   4. Cartilage destruction: Usually none.
   5. Erosive or productive bone changes: None.
   6. Subchondral cysts: Small cysts may be seen.
   7. Periostitis or enthesopathy: None.
   8. Ankylosis: None.
   9. Ligamentous abnormality: Calcification.
G. Joints most commonly affected:
   1. *Shoulder: Calcification located at sites of tendon insertion* (i.e., along the greater tuberosity [supraspinatus, infraspinatus, teres minor], lesser tuberosity [subscapularis], origins of biceps tendons, as well as *subacromial and subdeltoid bursae).* The complex is often called the *Milwaukee shoulder.*
   2. Elbow: Triceps and collateral ligament insertions.
   3. *Wrist:* Any tendon insertion, but especially that of the *flexor carpi ulnaris* adjacent to the pisiform.
   4. *Hand: Periarticular deposits around the MCPs and IPs.*
H. Bilateral symmetry: Not expected.
 I. Other features: None.
J. Differential diagnoses: Other conditions in which HA crystal deposition occurs:
   1. Renal osteodystrophy.
   2. Hypoparathyroidism.
   3. Hypervitaminosis D.
   4. Milk-alkali syndrome.
   5. Collagen vascular disease.
   6. Tumoral calcinosis.
   7. Dystrophic calcification secondary to inflammation or tumor.
   8. Myositis ossificans (progressiva or secondary to trauma).
   9. Parasitic calcification.

10. Enthesopathy.
11. Gouty tophus.
12. CPPD crystal deposition.
K. Survey film: AP film of shoulder and other symptomatic sites.
L. Painful HA deposits may be treated by aspiration under fluoroscopic control or injection of steroids.

Alkaptonuria (Ochronosis)

Key Concepts

Dystrophic dense calcification, most commonly involving the vertebral discs, with degenerative disc signs. Extraspinal manifestations resemble those of DJD.

A. Definition: A hereditary metabolic abnormality due to absence of homogentisic acid oxidase and consequent accumulation of homogentisic acid in various organs, including connective tissues.
B. Epidemiology:
   1. Gender: Affects males and females equally.
   2. Age: Pigmentation occurs in early adulthood and arthropathy, later.
C. Clinical signs: Mild pain and decreased ROM, usually not requiring intervention.
D. Laboratory tests: Urinary homogentisic acid.
E. Extra-articular manifestations: Pigmentation seen in helix of ear.
F. General radiographic description:
   1. Soft tissues: Normal.
   2. Abnormal calcifications: *Dystrophic (HA crystal) calcification most commonly involving the discs, but also cartilage, tendons, and ligaments.*
   3. Bone density: *Osteoporotic.*
   4. Cartilage destruction: Becomes brittle and fragmented.
   5. Erosive versus productive changes: *Sclerosis and small osteophytes.*
   6. Subchondral cysts: Present.
   7. Periostitis and enthesopathy: Not present.
   8. Ankylosis: None.
   9. Ligamentous abnormality: Calcification and rupture.
G. Joints most commonly affected:
   1. *Spine: Osteoporotic with dense disc calcification.*
   2. Extraspinal: *SI joints, symphysis pubis, and large peripheral joints*

may be involved (usually after spine) and show changes of mild DJD.
H. Bilateral symmetry: Often present.
I. Other features: None.
J. *Differential diagnosis:*
 1. *Dystrophic calcification of the nucleus pulposus:* AS or CPPD.
 2. DJD: Osteophytes are not as prominent in ochronosis.
K. Survey films: Lateral spine.

VII. MISCELLANEOUS DISORDERS
Pigmented Villonodular Synovitis (PVNS)

Key Concepts

Monarticular, hemorrhagic effusions, often with erosions, most often occurring in knee or hip.

A. Definition: A proliferative disorder of the synovium with hemosiderin deposition in the synovial tissues; of unknown etiology; it may be extra-articular (giant cell tumor (GCT) of the tendon sheath, seen as soft tissue swelling with or without adjacent bony erosions) or intra-articular, which is described in this section.
B. Epidemiology: Wide range, from adolescent to elderly.
C. Clinical signs: Variably painful effusion.
D. Laboratory tests: None.
E. Extra-articular manifestations: *Giant cell tumor of the tendon sheath is histologically indistinguishable from intra-articular PVNS.*
F. General radiographic description:
 1. Soft tissues: *Hemorrhagic effusion.*
 2. Abnormal calcifications: Very rare calcific metaplasia.
 3. Bone density: Normal to mild osteoporosis.
 4. *Cartilage: Preserved until late in the disease process.*
 5. Erosive versus productive changes: *Erosions on both sides of the joint are common findings.*
 6. Subchondral cysts: May be present, and may be large.
 7. Periostitis or enthesopathy: Absent.
 8. Ankylosis: Absent.
 9. Ligamentous abnormality: Absent.
 10. MR appearance: *MR of PVNS is not specific, but may be extremely useful. Osseous erosions are often more apparent,* especially in the intercondylar notch. *The synovial nodules, with a combination of fibrosis and hemosiderin deposition, usually show low SI on both T1 and T2 sequences.* This classic appearance, however, is

not always present, due to various proportions of lipid, fibrous tissue, hemosiderin, pannus, fluid, cyst formation, and cellular elements. Intravenous gadolinium may more completely define the extent of the lesion.[19] Accurate localization of the entire lesion is important since it will affect choice of therapy: lesions posterior to the cruciate ligament, superior to the femoral condyles, or inferior to the tibial plateau are not accessible to arthroscopic synovectomy and must go to an open procedure. If radiation synovectomy is planned, accurate localization of the abnormality is required as well.

G. *Joints most commonly affected: Knee, hip, elbow* (80% involve the knee).
H. Bilateral symmetry: Usually monarticular.
 I. Other features: Filling defects on arthrography.
J. Differential diagnoses: Infection and other monarticular arthritides; the MR SI may be similar to that seen in synovial chondromatosis, gout, or chronic infection.
K. Survey films: Only as clinically suggested; MR helps direct the diagnosis.

Synovial Chondromatosis

Key Concepts

Synovial metaplasia producing multiple round cartilaginous or osseous intra-articular loose bodies, most often in the knee or hip.

A. Definition: A *synovial metaplasia* of unknown etiology in which *cartilaginous nodules* arise from projections of the synovium. If the pedicle remains intact and a blood supply continues, *osseous bodies* may form. If the bodies become loose, cartilaginous bodies that are nourished by the synovium may continue to grow, whereas osseous bodies may resorb and grow only if they become reattached to the synovium.
B. Epidemiology: Males affected more often than females; third to fifth decades.
C. Clinical signs: Usually pain and limited ROM, though it may be asymptomatic.
D. Laboratory tests: None.
E. Extra-articular manifestations: None.
F. General radiographic description:
  1. Soft tissues: Effusion may be present.
  2. Abnormal *calcifications: Generally, multiple round bodies similar in size and variable in mineralization, sometimes appearing lamel-*

lated and even trabeculated. Note: The bodies may not be mineralized and therefore may be invisible by plain film and seen only on MR. The individual body size may range from 1 mm to 2 cm in different presentations, but are uniform within a single joint.
3. Bone density: Normal.
4. *Cartilage: Normal, though eventually loose bodies may lead to secondary mechanical cartilage destruction.*
5. Erosive versus productive change: Loose bodies may cause mechanical erosions and may also eventually promote DJD with concomitant productive changes.
6. Subchondral cysts: Only with secondary DJD.
7. Periostitis or enthesopathy: None.
8. Ankylosis: None.
9. Ligamentous abnormality: None.
10. MR appearance: Multiple round bodies following the signal of bone on all sequences, surrounded by joint fluid and confined to the expected joint space. May be seen on MR when not apparent on plain film, depending on degree of mineralization.
G. *Joints most commonly affected: Knee, hip, elbow, shoulder.*
H. Bilateral symmetry: *Monarticular.*
I. Other features: Filling defects on arthrography.
J. Differential diagnoses: Loose bodies in DJD.
K. Survey films: As indicated clinically.

Osteochondroses

Key Concepts

Fragmentation of epiphyseal or apophyseal surfaces, which are usually convex; most commonly affects skeletally immature patients. Trauma is the most common etiology. Differential diagnosis usually includes normal variants.

A. Definition: *The osteochondroses represent an inelegant and artificial grouping of disease processes, all once believed to represent necrosis. Only a few are true necroses; most are traumatically induced. Several are normal variants included only because they are "named" disease processes.*
B. Epidemiology:
1. Age: Skeletally immature persons or young adults.
2. Gender: Males more often affected than females (except Freiberg's necrosis, see below).
C. Clinical signs: Pain, decreased ROM.

D. Laboratory tests: None.
E. Extra-articular manifestations: None.
F. *General radiographic description: Increased density, with bony fragmentation in a lucent bed; flattening of a convex surface may occur, though the overlying cartilage is usually intact.* Secondary degenerative change may occur much later.
G. Joints affected:
   1. *Hip: Legg-Calvé-Perthes* disease:
      a. *A true necrosis, seen at ages 4 to 8, when the vascular supply to the femoral head is most at risk.*
      b. *Males* affected more often than females.
      c. *Rare in blacks.*
      d. Asymmetric, *10% bilateral.*
      e. *First radiographic sign* may be *effusion.* Later, *fragmentation and flattening* of the ossification center develop. Metaphyseal irregularity and "cysts" are manifestations of a growth abnormality that results in a short, wide femoral neck.
      f. *Older patients* at time of diagnosis and *females* (skeletally more mature) have a *poorer prognosis.* Gage advocated several "head at risk" signs, but all relate to *lateral extrusion of the femoral head ossification center* (calcification lateral to the acetabular rim), which indicates a lack of coverage of the femoral head and *has a poor prognosis since the head and acetabulum will not be congruent.* Surgical treatment is varied, but the objective is to contain the femoral head within the acetabulum, thus attaining congruity as the hip matures.
      g. MR can be valuable in assessing femoral head coverage in two planes. It is also useful in diagnosing early bone bridging across cartilaginous physeal and metaphyseal abnormalities that are relatively common and may result in growth arrest.
      h. *Differential diagnosis is hypothyroidism* since the "cretinoid hip" gives a similar appearance.
   2. *Lunate malacia: Keinbock's* disease: A true necrosis, believed to be related most often to trauma but commonly also to ulnar minus variant.
   3. *Freiberg's* disease:
      a. A true necrosis, involving the *second and third metatarsal heads* most commonly (fourth and first less commonly).
      b. More common in teenage females; may be related to the trauma of bearing weight in high-heeled shoes.
   4. *Knee: Osteochondritis dissecans affects the lateral portion of the medial femoral condyle* most commonly, but other articular loca-

tions are now recognized, including other sites on the femoral condyles and on the patella.

a. Believed to be related to trauma.

b. Must be differentiated from *spontaneous necrosis*, which affects an *older* patient, has an *acute onset* with *severe pain,* demonstrates *flattening on the weight-bearing (more medial) aspect of the medial femoral condyle,* and may be associated with a medial meniscal tear.

c. *If osteochondritis is symptomatic, it is important to demonstrate whether the "body" is loose (or if the cartilage overlying it is intact). This can be shown on MR if effusion tracks around the body, or by MR arthrography, again looking for tracking of fluid. Alternatively, if there is high SI around the margin of the fragment, this represents granulation tissue around an unstable fragment.*

5. *Tibial apophysis: Osgood-Schlatter's disease:*

a. Several ossification centers may normally be seen in this apophysis, *so soft tissue swelling and pain should be present in addition to bony fragmentation to* suggest this disease process.

b. Thought to be a traumatically induced avulsion; bilateral in 75%.

c. Rare complications include either nonunion of the tibial tubercle or premature closure of the tibial tubercle with secondary genu recurvation.

6. Sinding-Larsen-Johanssen disease: Avulsion and fragmentation of the inferior pole of the patella in this same age group.

7. *Blount's* disease: Osteochondrosis of the *medial aspect of the proximal tibial epiphysis, with resultant genu varus.*

a. *Infantile type is most common,* especially among *blacks.* It *evolves when the normal physiologic bowing of the lower extremity worsens with weight bearing, especially* in early walkers. There is no true necrosis, but the persistent microtrauma of weight bearing and abnormal pressure causes fragmentation of the medial metaphysis, which in turn causes epiphyseal deformity. More than 50% bilaterality.

b. Adolescent type is unilateral and relates to trauma or infection causing bony bridging of the medial growth plate.

8. *Talar dome osteochondritis dissecans:* Develops on medial or lateral convex surfaces of the talus and is probably related to trauma and *ankle laxity.*

9. *Kohler's disease: A dense, fragmented tarsal navicular may be a normal variant* of ossification that is a self-limited process and proceeds to normal ossification; Thus, Kohler's disease should be

suggested only when there is fragmentation of a previously normal tarsal navicular in the presence of pain.

10. *Panner's disease: Capitellum,* most commonly seen in adolescent fast-ball pitchers; self-limited with normal regeneration in most cases; however, hyperemia may lead to acceleration of maturation of the capitellum and radial head; one of the two ''Little League elbows.''

11. *Scheuermann's* disease: Strict definition requires abnormalities in *three contiguous vertebral bodies with at least 5 degrees anterior wedging* in each, resulting in a *dorsal kyphosis.* (Normal kyphosis is 20 to 40 degrees, measured between T_4 and T_{12}). *The end-plates are usually irregular* and often associated with Shmorl's nodes. The etiology is unknown but is not necrosis. Hypotheses include congenital end-plate weakness. *Males and females* are affected equally, especially teenagers; *Lower thoracic spine* is involved in 75%.

12. *Normal variants* that have fragmented ossification centers and *simulate osteochondroses:*
    a. *Femoral condyle* (more posteriorly located than osteochondritis dissecans, seen best on notch view) in skeletally immature persons.
    b. *Calcaneal apophysis* (''Sever's disease'').
    c. *Trochlea.*
    d. *Lateral epicondyle.*
    e. *Anterior tibial apophysis* (Osgood-Schlatter's disease).
    f. Tarsal navicular (Kohler's disease).
    g. Ischiopubic synchondrosis (Van Neck's disease).

H. Bilateral symmetry: Rare.

I. Other features: Arthrography usually demonstrates intact cartilage and, therefore, development of loose bodies is rare.

J. Differential diagnoses:
   1. Normal variants (see above).
   2. Vascular events.
   3. Epiphyseal dysplasias.

Hypertrophic Osteoarthropathy (HOA)

Key Concepts

Presents clinically as arthritis; radiographically has normal joints but thick periosteal reaction; may be primary or secondary.

A. Definition: A disease process of unknown etiology that *presents clinically as arthritis* with painful, swollen joints. Radiographically, the *joints appear nearly normal:* there are only soft tissue swelling and occasional effusions, no erosive or productive changes. The major abnormality is found in the corners of the film—a *symmetric periosteal reaction.* The reaction may show onion skinning, irregularity, or waviness; its *thickness and extent probably depend on the duration of the disease.*

B. HOA may be primary or secondary:

1. Primary HOA (pachydermoperiostitis) is a spectrum of diseases ranging from mere periostitis to the complete process of periostitis, clubbed digits, and thickening of the skin (facial and hands), resulting in pawlike hands. It is often familial and is much more common in males than females. The onset is in adolescence, and there is usually spontaneous arrest of the process in young adulthood.

2. Secondary HOA is periostitis in the extremities noted in patients with a number of disease processes (usually intrathoracic): bronchogenic carcinoma (most common), other malignant, benign, or chronic suppurative diseases of the lung, cyanotic heart disease, liver or biliary cirrhosis, and IBDs. The mechanism of the reaction is entirely unknown. Interestingly, a thoracotomy may lead to clinical remission almost immediately, with slower radiographic resolution.

C. Differential diagnosis of the periostitis:

1. Although it has been observed that primary HOA may have irregular excrescences extending to the epiphyses, it is unlikely that primary and secondary HOA can be differentiated radiographically in the individual case.

2. *Thyroid acropachy:* Generally a feathery, spiculated reaction, predominantly on the hands and feet; clubbing of the digits is often present.

3. *Vascular insufficiency* may also produce symmetric periosteal reaction, usually restricted to the lower limbs.

4. Tuberous sclerosis.

Avascular Necrosis (AVN)

Key Concepts

Early changes of sclerosis, followed by subchondral fracture, bony fragmentation, flattening of weight-bearing surfaces, but cartilage remains intact.

A. Definition: Necrosis of bone, restricted, in this section, to epiphyseal locations. Etiologies are usually related to trauma (vessel interruption), vascular compression, or intraluminal obstruction. The following etiologies are listed in approximate descending order of occurrence:
   1. *Idiopathic.*
   2. *Trauma:* Due to delayed reduction of a hip *dislocation or to subcapital fracture.*
   3. *Steroids:* Exogenous or endogenous (Cushing's disease); thought to be due to an increase in fat cell size and resultant increased pressure.
   4. *Alcoholism:* May be due to fat emboli and increased marrow pressure.
   5. *Sickle cell disease:* Vascular occlusion from sickled cells.
   6. *Gaucher's* disease: Sinusoids are packed with Gaucher's cells.
   7. *Caisson* disease: Nitrogen embolization following rapid decompression, causing an increase in marrow pressure.
   8. *Radiation:* Direct toxic effect on vascular supply to bone.
   9. SLE: The vasculitis may be additive to the steroid therapy in causing AVN. AVN in unusual sites (talus, humerus) should suggest SLE as an etiology.
   10. Pancreatitis: Fat necrosis as well as probable relationship to alcoholism.
B. Epidemiology: Relates to etiology.
C. Clinical signs: Pain with weight bearing, decreased ROM.
D. Laboratory tests: None.
E. Extra-articular manifestations: None.
F. General radiographic description:
   1. *Cartilage is normal* since it is nourished by synovial fluid.
   2. *First radiographic sign is sclerosis,* which is due to different processes at different times. In the hip, this is located centrally in the femoral head. *Initially* it is a *relative sclerosis* (necrotic bone initiates an inflammatory response in the surrounding vascularized bone; the resultant hyperemia causes osteoporosis). Later, a *reactive interface* develops, with bone formation causing increased density.
   3. Later may develop a linear subchondral fracture (*crescent sign*), best seen on a frog-leg film. With further subchondral fragmentation, *flattening and bone deformity* occur. Sclerosis may be increased due to impacted fragments.
   4. Still later, with revascularization, repair and remodeling in the avascular segment occurs; this "*creeping substitution*" also causes sclerosis.
   5. Secondary DJD may occur later.
G. Sites of most common occurrence: *Femoral head, lunate, proximal pole of the scaphoid, and body of the talus* are all at risk for posttrau-

matic AVN. *Humeral head and talar involvement are seen with sickle cell or SLE.* AVN of the spine may be nonspecific, with increased density of the vertebral body and collapse. However, *if air is seen within the vertebral body, this is virtually pathognomonic for AVN.* With MR, this air vacuum shows high SI on T2 imaging since, over the duration of the scan, a transudate crosses into this space.[20] Watch also for the *"H"-shaped vertebra* where the midportion of the superior and inferior end-plates is impacted, *seen in sickle cell and Gaucher's disease.*

H. Bilateral symmetry: With systemic processes, often bilateral but usually not symmetric.

I. Other features:

    1. MRI is the most sensitive imaging tool for detection of AVN[21,22] but is nonspecific. To evaluate early changes of AVN, one must understand the normal *age-related changes seen in marrow. Children normally have fatty marrow only in their epiphyses, but red marrow elsewhere. Adults under age 50 show gradual replacement by fatty marrow in the metaphyses, but hematopoietic marrow predominates. In older adults, fatty marrow predominates.* Patients with *AVN* show *earlier conversion of the metaphyses to fatty marrow.* The *early edema stages of AVN are nonspecific* and diffuse as seen on MR. *After initial edema, the classic appearance may be seen: abnormality in the weight-bearing area with a peripheral low SI rim on both T1 and T2 sequences (sclerosis) and an adjacent inner rim of increased SI on T2 (reactive interface—"double rim" sign).* The central signal within this rim is used to classify AVN: Class A, central signal isointense to fat: Class B, central signal isointense to hemorrhage; Class C, central signal isointense to fluid; Class D, central signal isointense to fibrous tissue or bone. These classes are roughly equivalent to radiographic stages I through IV (I, normal; II, trabecular changes without collapse; III, collapse; IV, DJD).[22] Later, necrosis may present as a diffuse signal abnormality, without the segmental location or double rim sign.

    2. Radionuclide bone scan initially shows a photon deficit, followed by increased activity with revascularization and repair.

J. Differential diagnosis: DJD may simulate advanced AVN of the hip since a large inferomedial osteophyte may make the head appear flattened; intact cartilage should differentiate AVN from DJD until the AVN develops secondary DJD.

K. *Survey films for AVN from systemic causes: AP and frog-leg pelvis films* (the frog-leg view is usually more sensitive). *MR screening includes T1 (or equivalent) coronal and T2 sagittal.* It is not clear whether enhancement gives valuable information about tissue viability.

Remember that MR has 98% specificity in differentiating normal from abnormal, but only 85% specificity in differentiating AVN from non-AVN disease.[23]

L. Treatment of AVN includes osteotomy and realignment of the femoral head to a noncollapsed weight-bearing portion, core decompression either with or without vascularized graft, and prosthesis placement. The treatment decision depends on the portion of head involved with AVN as well as amount and location of collapse. Therefore, a preoperative MR should evaluate both collapse and location of AVN in coronal and sagittal planes, referring to locations with a clock-face description.

M. Clinically occult AVN is interesting. One study of 100 asymptomatic renal transplant patients taking steroids showed 6% to have MR evidence of AVN.[24] In another study, 14% had AVN by MR, but 33% of these resolved over 24 months.[25] The value of screening at-risk asymptomatic patients has not been established since treatment is not clear.

Transient Regional Osteoporosis

Definition: A disorder of unknown etiology that presents clinically as an arthritis and radiographically demonstrates only *osteoporosis involving both sides of a joint. Cartilage remains normal,* and there are neither erosive nor productive changes. *Self-limited disease.* Males affected more commonly than females; usually large joints of lower limbs; *may be migratory.* See also Chapter 4.

MR in transient regional osteoporosis shows SI of diffuse edema. This is not distinguishable from the edema pattern of early AVN, and some have suggested this could be the initial phase of nontraumatic AVN. Since treatment may be different (conservative for transient regional osteoporosis but perhaps core decompression for early AVN), diagnosis is important. With the MR pattern of bone marrow edema in the femoral head, plain films and timing may help make the distinction; with very recent onset, waiting a few weeks and repeating plain films may show the osteoporosis typical of transient osteoporosis.

DISH: Diffuse Idiopathic Skeletal Hyperostosis (Forestier's Disease)

Key Concepts

Severe productive changes of the soft tissues surrounding the vertebral bodies, forming large bulky, flowing osteophytes; predominantly in the thoracic spine, though the entire column may be involved. Clinical signs are mild compared to the radiographic appearance. Strict radiographic criteria should be adhered to in order to avoid an incorrect diagnosis.

A. Definition: *Severe productive bone changes of the spine,* including the *anulus fibrosus, anterior longitudinal ligament,* and even paravertebral connective tissues, of unknown etiology. *Three strict radiographic criteria* must be fulfilled to suggest the diagnosis.[26]
   1. Flowing ossification of the anterolateral aspect *involves at least four contiguous vertebral bodies.* (Note that this rules out spondylosis deformans.)
   2. There is relative *preservation of disc height* over the involved segments, and degenerative disc disease (as manifest by vacuum signs or discogenic sclerosis) is not present.
   3. *Sacroiliitis and facet ankylosis are not present* (eliminating AS from consideration).
B. Epidemiology: *Very common abnormality* in middle-aged and elderly persons; *males* more commonly affected than females.
C. Clinical signs: *Milder than the extent of ossification suggests:* mild back pain, little deformity, and mild decrease in ROM.
   a. With cervical disease, may develop dysphagia.
   b. More peripherally, may have tendinitis.
D. No laboratory abnormality.
E. Extra-articular manifestations: None.
F. General radiographic description:
   1. Soft tissue alterations: Calcification of the anterior longitudinal ligament, paravertebral soft tissue, and occasionally the posterior longitudinal ligament.
   2. Abnormal calcifications: See 1, above.
   3. Bone density: Normal.
   4. Cartilage destruction: None.
   5. No erosive changes: Purely productive; the osteophytes on the spine may be extremely large (up to 2 cm), irregular, and are located at the level of the disc. There may be lucent defects between the vertebral body and the ossifications at the discs, due to disc extrusion.
   6. Subchondral cysts: None.
   7. *Enthesopathy: Common,* especially in the *pelvis, calcaneus* (Achilles and plantar aponeurosis insertions), and anterior surface of the *patella* (quadriceps insertion).
   8. Ankylosis: Rare.
   9. Ligamentous abnormality: *Pelvic ligaments* may become *calcified* as may the anterior and posterior longitudinal ligaments.
G. Most common distribution:
   1. *Thoracic spine: Most commonly* involved; the osteophytes are usually found *anterolaterally, on the right side* (thought to be due to the pulsating aorta on the left).

2. *Cervical spine* is also commonly involved, *usually on the anterior aspect. Ossification of the posterior longitudinal ligament (OPLL) may be seen* and may cause neurologic symptoms. Such posterior ligament ossification may be concurrent with DISH or may be a solitary finding; there is an overlap between the two disease processes. OPLL may have not only the posterior longitudinal ligament ossification, but also bulky anterior osteophyte formation. OPLL predominately involves the cervical spine, while DISH more frequently is thoracic.

3. *Lumbar spine* may also be involved, especially L_{1-3}.

4. Superior (nonarticular portions) SI joints are often bridged by ligamentous calcification, but the lower two thirds of the SI joints are rarely affected.

H. Bilateral symmetry: Often absent in the thoracic spine.

I. Other features: If there are long segments of ankylosis, these may fracture with minor trauma. As with AS, the fracture may be extremely subtle.[27]

J. Differential diagnoses: Abiding by the strict radiographic criteria should eliminate the differentials:

1. Spondylosis deformans.

2. Discogenic sclerosis or degenerative disc disease.

3. Ankylosing spondylitis.

4. Retinoid arthropathy: Patients using retinoic acids for skin disease (chemically similar to vitamin A) often develop skeletal hyperostoses similar to those seen in DISH. The cervical spine is the most common site, but thoracic and lumbar spine involvement is seen as well. Eventually, anterior and posterior longitudinal ligament calcification may be seen. Symptoms are usually mild.

K. Survey films: AP and lateral spine.

Lead Arthropathy

Bullets lodged in bursal and joint spaces can result in lead poisoning due to dissolution of the lead by synovial fluid. With progressive degradation, the fragments are spread throughout the joint, lining the synovium and cartilage. Synovial inflammation and foreign body mechanical damage to cartilage lead to productive change and secondary OA. Clinical lead poisoning requires sufficient breakdown of fragments for a large surface area of lead to be resorbed. Removal of a bullet within a joint may not be necessary if it is not in a position to develop significant mechanical breakdown.[28]

Lyme Arthritis

Radiographic findings are nonspecific, the most common being large knee effusion. Large bands of hypertrophied synovium may be seen within the distended joint. Enthesopathy may be present. Less frequently, erosion or even osteophytes are found; mixed erosive-productive changes may be seen as well. Since these inflammatory changes are nonspecific, typical clinical features are required to suggest the diagnosis (characteristic rash at the site of the tick bite, and a flu-like illness occurring over the summer).[29]

REFERENCES

1. Recht M, Resnick D: MR imaging of articular cartilage: current status and future direction. *AJR* 1994;163:283–290.
2. Schaller J: Spondyloarthritis and other forms of chronic arthritis affecting children. In Jacobs JC, editor: *New Frontiers in Pediatric Rheumatology,* New York, 1986, World Health Communications, Inc.
3. Bywaters E: Still's disease in the adult. *Ann Rheum Dis* 1971;30:121–133.
4. Bjorkgren A, Pathria M, Sartoris D, et al.: Carpal alterations in adult-onset Still's disease, juvenile chronic arthritis, and adult-onset rheumatoid arthritis: comparative study. *Radiology* 1987;165:545–548.
5. Azouz EM, Duffy CM: Juvenile spondylarthropathies: clinical manifestations and medical imaging. *Skeletal Radiology* 1995;24:399–408.
6. Murphey MD, Wetzel CH, Bramble JM, Levine E, Simpson KM, Lindsley HB: Sacroiliitis: MR imaging findings. *Radiology* 1991;180:239–244.
7. Bollow M, Braun J, Hamm B, Eggens U, Schilling A, König H, Wolf K: Early sacroiliitis in patients with spondyloarthropathy. Evaluation with dynamic gadolinium-enhanced MR imaging. *Radiology* 1995;194: 529–536.
8. Bjorkengren A, Resnick D, Sartoris D: Enteropathic arthropathies. *Radiol Clin North Am* 1987;25:189–198.
9. Weissman BW, Rappaport AS, Sosman JL, et al: Radiographic findings in the hands in patients with systemic lupus erythematosus. *Radiology* 1978; 126:313–317.
10. Basset L, Blocka KL, Furst DE, et al: Skeletal findings in progressive systemic sclerosis (scleroderma). *AJR* 1981;136:1121–1126.
11. Cobby M, Adler R, Swartz R, Martel W: Dialysis-related amyloid arthropathy: MR findings in four patients. *AJR* 1991;157:1023–1027.
12. Rafto S, Dalinka M, Scheibler M, Burk D, Kricun M: Spondyloarthropathy of the cervical spine in long-term hemodialysis. *Radiology* 1988;166: 201–204.
13. Bock G, Garcia A, Weisman M, Major P, Lyttle D, Haghigai P, Greenway G, Resnick D: Rapidly destructive hip disease: clinical and imaging abnormalities. *Radiology* 1993;186:461–466.
14. Pathria M, Sartoris D, Resnick D: Osteoarthritis of the facet joints: accuracy of oblique radiographic assessment. *Radiology* 1987;164:227–230.
15. Martel W, Stuck K, Dworin A, Hylland R: Erosive osteoarthritis and psoriatic arthritis: a radiologic comparison in the hand, wrist and foot. *AJR* 1980; 134:125–135.
16. Brower A, Allman R: Pathogenesis of the neurotrophic joint: neurotraumatic vs neurovascular. *Radiology* 1981;139:349–354.

17. Bjorkengren A, Weisman M, Pathria M, Zlatkin M, Pate D, Resnick D: Neuro-arthropathy associated with chronic alcoholism. *AJR* 1988;151:743–745.

18. Brown T, Quinn S, D'Agostino A: Deposition of CPPD crystals in the ligamentum flavum: evaluation with MR imaging and CT. *Radiology* 1991;178: 871–873.

19. Hughes T, Sartoris D, Schweitzer M, Resnick D: Pigmented villonodular synovitis: MRI characteristics. *Skeletal Radiol* 1995;24:7–12.

20. Malghem J, Maldague B, Labaisse M, Dooms G, Duprey T, Devogeloer J, Van de Berg B: Intravertebral vacuum cleft: changes in content after supine positioning. *Radiology* 1993;187:483–487.

21. Mitchell D, Kressel H, Argen P, et al: Avascular necrosis of the femoral head: morphologic assessment by MR imaging, with CT correlation. *Radiology* 1986;161:739–742.

22. Mitchell D, Rao V, Dalinka M, et al: Femoral head avascular necrosis: correlation of MR imaging, radiographic staging, radionuclide imaging and clinical findings. *Radiology* 1987;169:709–715.

23. Glickstein M, Burk D, Schiebler M, Cohen E, Dalinka M, Steinberg M, Kressel H: Avascular necrosis versus other diseases of the hip: sensitivity of MR imaging. *Radiology* 1988;169:213–215.

24. Tervonen O, Mueller D, Matteson E, Velosa J, Ginsburg W, Ehman R: Clinically occult avascular necrosis of the hip: prevalence in an asymptomatic population at risk. *Radiology* 1992;182:845–847.

25. Kopecky K, Braunstein E, Brandt K, Filo R, Leapman S, Capello W, Klatte E: Apparent avascular necrosis of the hip: appearance and spontaneous resolution of MR findings in renal allograft recipients. *Radiology* 1991; 179:523–527.

26. Resnick D, Niwayama G: Radiographic and pathologic features of spinal involvement in diffuse idiopathic skeletal hyperostosis (DISH). *Radiology* 1976;119:559–568.

27. Hendrix R, Melany M, Miller F, Rogers L: Fracture of the spine in patients with ankylosis due to diffuse skeletal hyperostosis: clinical and imaging findings. *AJR* 1994;162:899–904.

28. Peh W, Reimus W: Lead arthropathy: a cause of delayed onset lead poisoning. *Skeletal Radiology* 1995;24:357–360.

29. Lawson J, Rahn D: Lyme disease and radiographic findings in lyme arthritis. *AJR* 1992;158:1065–1069.

3

Trauma

GENERALIZATIONS

The radiologist confronts two dilemmas in the trauma patient. The first is recognition of injury. While this sounds simple, in practice, we quickly learn that it may indeed be quite difficult. It requires a detailed knowledge of gross anatomy and of normal variants that may be mistaken for fractures. The radiologist must become familiar with certain predictable mechanisms that produce certain injuries. The radiologist armed with this information is unlikely to miss evidence of significant trauma.

In each of the subsequent trauma sections, categorized by anatomic site, the reader will find discussions of normal anatomy and of common trauma patterns. Because these are, in general, well-known facts and because this handbook is meant to be pedagogical, these discussions are not referenced exhaustively. If the reader wishes further detail, he is referred to Lee Rogers' excellent text, *Radiology of Skeletal Trauma* for plain film analysis. For magnetic resonance (MR) of sports-related injuries, I recommend Stoller's *Magnetic Resonance Imaging in Orthopedics and Sports Medicine* or Berquist's *MRI of the Musculoskeletal System*. This handbook will demonstrate crucial MR anatomy in the imaging planes of interest by line drawings.

After the trauma is recognized, the radiologist must communicate his findings, using standard technology, which is described below.

I. FRACTURE TERMINOLOGY

A. Definition and biomechanical principles.
   1. A fracture is a complete or incomplete break in the continuity of bone or cartilage.
   2. Bone is anisotropic; it has different mechanical properties when loaded in different directions. Adult cortical bone withstands the greatest stress in compression, less in tension, and the least with shear loading.
   3. When force is applied to bone, contraction of muscles alters the stress distribution and may allow the bone to support higher loads than expected.

4. With greater speed of loading, more energy is stored before failure; with fracture, this energy is dissipated rapidly, resulting in extensive soft tissue damage.

5. Repeated loading reduces the amount of total weight a bone can withstand owing to fatigue of muscles that normally redistribute the stress.

6. A surgical defect (e.g., screw hole or site of bone resection) concentrates stress and decreases bone strength significantly: Such lesions are termed stress raisers.

B. Accurate terminology to be applied in all descriptions.

1. *Open* vs. *closed* fracture.

2. Incomplete vs. complete fractures:

   a. *Incomplete* fractures most often are seen in children. The three major types are *torus* (a buckle of the cortex, a failure on the compressive side); *greenstick* (incomplete fracture on the tension side); and *plastic* (bending without angular deformity and without subsequent remodeling).

   b. *Complete* fractures generally can be described as *transverse, oblique,* or *spiral.*

3. *Comminution:* A fracture that produces more than two fragments. Subsets include *segmental* (two fracture lines isolating a discrete segment) and *butterfly* (a wedge-shaped separate fragment formed at the apex of the force). The latter terms should be used appropriately since they have implications for prognosis as well as treatment (e.g., the blood supply may be disrupted substantially, and a large butterfly fragment may lead to telescoping and instability of the fragments).

4. *Position.*

   a. Description of site, either by anatomic landmarks or by dividing long bones into thirds.

   b. A fracture located near an articular cortex should be designated either as intra- or extra-articular.

5. *Apposition:* Contact of the ends of the fracture fragments.

   a. *Anatomic.*

   b. *Displaced:* Anterior, posterior, lateral, or medial, or a combination of these; the degree of displacement is either measured or expressed as a percentage of cross-sectional diameter.

   c. *Lack of apposition:* Complete loss of contact of the bone ends. If the fragments overlap one another, leaving the shafts but not the ends in contact, it is termed *bayonet* apposition. Complete lack of apposition is termed *distraction* (most commonly due to excessive traction, interposed tissue, or resorption of fragment ends subacutely).

6. *Alignment:* Relationship of the long axes of the fracture fragments. *Angulation* is the loss of alignment; the direction of angulation is best termed fracture *apex* (anterior, posterior, etc.). Alternatively, the direction of angular displacement of the distal fracture fragment may be specified.
   a. *Varus angulation:* The distal part of the distal fragment points toward the body midline (the apex points away).
   b. *Valgus angulation:* The opposite of varus; the apex is directed toward the midline of the body.
7. *Rotation:* Both proximal and distal joints must be included on the same film for proper evaluation. Computed tomography (CT) can be utilized for more precise measurement of both malrotation and limb length discrepancies.
8. Additional definitions:
   a. *Chip fracture:* An isolated bone fragment; this is to be distinguished from an *avulsion,* a fragment that is separated by traction from an attached tendon or ligament.
   b. *Dislocation:* Complete loss of articular contact in a joint; *subluxation* is a partial loss; *diastasis* is separation of a slightly movable joint.
   c. *Stress fracture:* Occurs when *abnormal stress,* often in the form of frequent repetitions of normal stress, *is placed on normal bone.* Stress fractures often occur at predictable sites—this knowledge may make a subtle diagnosis easier. These sites will be mentioned in each anatomic section. *Pathologic fractures* occur when *normal stress is placed on bone that is abnormal* owing to tumor, metabolic bone disease, or other disease. *If pathologic fracture is due to osteopenia, it may be termed insufficiency fracture.* The clinical setting and specific site usually lead to plain film diagnosis of stress/insufficiency fractures. Late plain film findings may be specific as well: linear sclerosis, often perpendicular to major trabecular lines. However, early plain film findings may be subtle (periosteal reaction) or nonexistent since these fractures are usually nondisplaced (initial plain films are read as negative 60%–80% of the time). *The plain film is therefore specific but lacks sensitivity. Bone scans are sensitive but nonspecific* and may often detect stress reaction rather than true stress fracture. In some cases, the pattern of uptake on bone scan secures the diagnosis (i.e., H-shaped sign of sacral insufficiency fractures). A negative bone scan excludes the diagnosis of stress/insufficiency fracture (exception: elderly osteoporotic patients or those using steroids may have a false-negative bone

scan for several days post injury). CT with reconstruction and MR are highly sensitive sources of ancillary imaging. *MR is highly specific if the fracture line itself is shown, but nonspecific if only an edema pattern is seen.* A single T1 or STIR coronal screening exam for subcapital fracture in the elderly patient can be made cost efficient. MR should be avoided in sacral insufficiency fracture work-up; it is often confusing with an edema pattern, while CT directly shows the fracture.

C. Treated fractures: Healing and complications:
1. Same descriptive *terms* are used and healing is evaluated.
2. Healing is affected by many factors: Age of patient, amount of local bone and soft tissue trauma, percentage of bone loss, location of the fracture, degree of immobilization, presence of infection, local malignancy, radiation necrosis, avascular necrosis, intra-articular extension, steroid treatment, and multiple systemic factors. Therefore, *delayed union* is a clinical rather than a radiographic diagnosis.
3. *Nonunion,* on the other hand, is a *radiographic* diagnosis: one sees no bridging bone, and the fracture fragment ends are rounded and sclerotic. Nonunions may be *hypertrophic* or *atrophic.*
4. Fracture complications to watch for:
   a. Avascular necrosis: Especially in subcapital femoral, intra-articular femoral condylar, and waist or proximal pole scaphoid fractures. Watch for increased density as an early sign of avascular necrosis (AVN).
   b. Gas gangrene and osteomyelitis (especially pin tract osteomyelitis, manifested as a dense ring sequestrum).
   c. Hardware failure (described more completely in XIV, below).
   d. Reflex sympathetic dystrophy: Severe regional osteoporosis accompanied by soft tissue trophic changes.
   e. Malunion: Displacement may remodel completely. Limb length discrepancy up to 2 cm can be compensated. Anteroposterior (AP) angulation may be compensated in a hinge joint, but varus or valgus angulation is not compensated and the fracture remodels poorly. Rotational malunion does not remodel at all and is only partially compensated for in a ball-and-socket joint; it is totally uncompensated in a hinge joint.
   f. Remember to simply describe the findings rather than using qualitative terms such as ''good'' or ''acceptable''. Different criteria for ''acceptable'' apply to fractures at different sites depending on functionality.

D. Fractures in childhood are unique in three ways:
1. The bones are more porous, often resulting in incomplete fractures.

2. There is a greater potential for remodeling malaligned fractures depending on:
   a. Number of years of growth left.
   b. Fracture near the growing end of the long bone will remodel better.
   c. Whether the angular deformity is in the plane of movement of the adjacent joint.
3. The epiphyseal plate is the weakest, and one of the most easily fractured, sites in the long bone (15% of pediatric fractures). The *Salter-Harris classification* allows easy radiographic classification, is a reasonable indicator of prognosis, and is a guide to treatment.
   a. Salter 1: Fracture through the plate itself, often unrecognized and having minimal displacement.
   b. Salter 2: Fracture through the plate and extending through the metaphysis. This is the most common of these fractures, and prognosis for healing without deformity is good.
   c. Salter 3: Fracture through the plate and extending through the epiphysis.
   d. Salter 4: Fracture through the epiphysis, crossing the plate, and extending through the metaphysis.
   e. Salter 5: Crush injury to the epiphyseal plate, often unrecognized or misdiagnosed as a Salter 1 injury. Salter 4 and 5 injuries are relatively rare, but have very high complication rates, with partial premature epiphyseal plate closure and resultant deformity.

   Plain film remains the primary means of evaluating epiphyseal injury. However, the injury is often better understood (and may even change Salter-Harris classification) if CT with reconstruction or MR is used. CT or MR are also routinely used to quantify amount and location of bone bridging across an epiphyseal plate prior to corrective surgery.

   Recently, stress injuries of the physis have been described, relating to chronic repetitive stress in a skeletally immature patient. These may be considered a very early Salter 1 injury, and are recognized as widening and irregularity of the growth plate. They are seen in the distal radius and ulna of gymnasts; proximal humerus of baseball pitchers; and distal femur, proximal tibia, and distal fibula of runners. Conservative therapy is recommended.

E. The role of other imaging modalities:
   1. Bone scan can detect occult fractures with nearly 100% sensitivity (exceptions may be the very osteoporotic patient and the patient on chronic steroid therapy). Usually they are used to detect acute

and occult subcapital femoral neck, waist of scaphoid, and various stress fractures.
2. Gallium or leukocyte scans may identify chronic osteomyelitis, which may show little specific change on plain films.
3. Polytomography may detect subtle fractures and is used infrequently. CT may also be useful in the individual case, especially with reconstruction. Remember to firmly tape the imaged structure in place, as motion may obscure nondisplaced fractures.
4. MR is especially sensitive for evaluation of occult fractures (see discussion B, 8c above), if T1 or STIR imaging is used in the appropriate plane.

II. HAND TRAUMA

Key Concepts

Avulsion injuries are easily missed and are functionally important. Watch especially for trauma to the dorsal and ventral aspects of the distal and middle phalanges and to the ulnar aspect of the base of the proximal phalanx of the thumb.

A. Tuft fracture.
B. *Shaft fracture:* Usually *dorsally angulated;* degree is underestimated except on lateral film. Rotational malalignment is an important parameter in functional impairment and is often detected only clinically.
C. Avulsion fracture: Usually dorsal or volar aspect (Fig 3-1).
   1. *Baseball (mallet) finger* (Fig 3-2):
      a. Due to flexion of a forcibly extended finger.
      b. Site of insertion of the common tendon of the extensor mechanism.

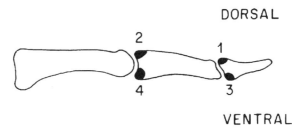

DORSAL

VENTRAL

Fig. 3-1   Usual sites of phalangeal avulsion fractures: *1*, baseball finger; *2*, boutonnière; *3*, flexor digitorum profundus; *4*, volar plate.

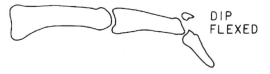

Fig. 3-2   Baseball (mallet) finger: DIP flexion, with or without avulsion of dorsal aspect of the base of the distal phalanx.

    c. Therefore results in either a tendon injury or a dorsal intra-articular avulsion fracture at the base of the distal phalanx.

    d. Clinically, has flexion and volar subluxation of the distal interphalangeal joint (DIP), sometimes with hyperextension of the proximal interphalangeal joint (PIP).

    e. Isolated flexion (the inability to extend the DIP joint while extending the PIP) should raise suspicion of this injury since otherwise this is difficult to do.

  2. Boutonnière (buttonhole) deformity.

    a. Due to PIP flexion with DIP extension and rupture of the middle slip of the extensor mechanism as it passes over the PIP.

    b. The extensor mechanism consists of one middle slip and two lateral slips at the PIP. The middle slip inserts at the base of the middle phalanx, and the two lateral slips join distally to form the common extensor tendon, inserting at the base of the distal phalanx (Fig 3-3).

    c. With rupture of the middle slip, the lateral slips migrate more volarly, forming a buttonhole through which the PIP flexes. The DIP is pulled into hyperextension (Fig 3-4).

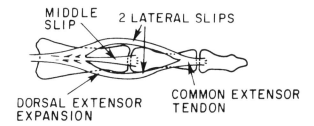

Fig. 3-3   AP view of the extensor mechanism, with the middle slip shown inserting at the base of the middle phalanx and the two lateral slips joining to insert at the base of the distal phalanx.

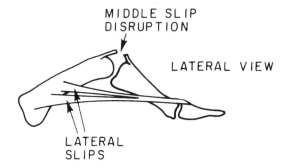

Fig. 3-4 Lateral view of a boutonnière deformity, with PIP flexion and DIP extension, with or without avulsion of the dorsal aspect of the base of the middle phalanx.

    d. Avulsion of the dorsum of the base of the middle phalanx is unusual but may occur.

    e. Boutonnière deformity often occurs some time after the initial injury, as the lateral slips may migrate volarly slowly to form the buttonhole.

    f. It is important to diagnose the injury early on the basis of area of tenderness, soft tissue swelling, and possible avulsion fragment to facilitate early splinting and healing without development of the deformity.

  3. Avulsion of a volar fragment of the proximal base of the distal phalanx (Fig 3-5).

    a. Forced hyperextension of a flexed finger avulses the flexor digitorum profundus from the volar aspect of the distal phalanx.

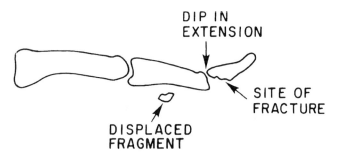

Fig. 3-5 Avulsion of flexor digitorum profundus, with DIP hyperextension, with or without avulsed fragment.

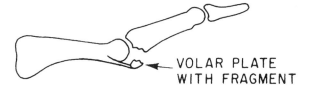

Fig. 3-6   Volar plate fracture with PIP hyperextension.

    b. May be either a pure tendon injury (which requires a stress film for diagnosis) or may produce an intra-articular avulsion fracture.

    c. If a fragment is present, it may be retracted proximally to the volar side of the middle phalanx.

    d. Clinically, the DIP cannot be flexed.

4. Volar plate fracture.

    a. Volar plate: A fibrocartilaginous structure crossing the metacarpophalangeal (MCP) and PIP joints that has a weak proximal attachment but a stronger distal attachment at the base of the middle phalanx volarly.

    b. Hyperextension will avulse this distal attachment, yielding a fragment from the volar side of the base of the middle phalanx (Fig 3-6).

    c. May be seen in conjunction with mallet finger.

5. Collateral (radial and ulnar) ligaments are found at all MCP, PIP, and DIP joints.

    a. May be ruptured or may avulse fragments.

    b. Most common is avulsion of the *ulnar collateral ligament of the MCP of the thumb—"gamekeepers thumb"*—due to a valgus injury (today, commonly due to *ski pole* injury), may give an intra-articular avulsion fragment at the base of the proximal phalanx (ulnar side). If not, stress views are required for diagnosis. After rupture, the edge of the torn ligament (or ligament and avulsion fragment) may be minimally retracted; this may be treated conservatively with casting. Alternatively, the end may become displaced and lock superficial to the adductor aponeurosis (which normally overlies it). This is termed a *Stener lesion,* and usually requires surgical intervention. MR is the most accurate means for evaluating tendon retraction and placement relative to the adductor aponeurosis.[1]

    c. Stress views of the thumb must be truly AP (requiring full pronation of the wrist) and should be compared with the opposite, normal side.

D. Boxer's fracture.
1. Usually neck of fifth metacarpal.
2. Apex dorsal angulation is best appreciated on the lateral view.
3. Volar comminution makes a stable reduction difficult, so watch for reestablishment of the apex dorsal angulation in the follow-up films.
E. Thumb: Note: Standard *hand* films *do not* give true AP and lateral views of the *thumb* and, so, are inadequate for evaluation of thumb trauma. Standard hand films demonstrate the thumb only in varying degrees of obliquity, often giving a false appearance of subluxation at the carpometacarpal (CMC) and MCP joints. Standard thumb views are obtained as follows:
1. AP: Hand fully pronated with the dorsal surface of the thumb held against the film.
2. Lateral: Hand pronated 15 degrees.
F. Fracture of the first MC.
1. It is important to differentiate between intra- and extra-articular fractures, since the former may require open reduction and the latter may be treated closed.
2. One third of first MC fractures are *Bennett* variety—a fracture dislocation with an oblique intra-articular fracture at the base of the MC and dorsal dislocation or subluxation of the MC (the smaller fragment retains its articulation with the trapezium). These are usually treated by open reduction and internal fixation.
3. Far fewer are *Rolando* fractures—comminuted Bennett's fracture with dorsal subluxation and a separate dorsal fragment. These are usually treated closed with casting since pin fixation is not successful in the presence of much comminution.
G. Dislocations.
1. Phalanx: Usually dorsal dislocation, produced by hyperextension.
   a. Volar plate disruption with or without associated volar avulsion.
   b. May be unreducible owing to joint capsule or volar plate interposition. The only radiographic sign of this complication is an interposed sesamoid at the MCP.
2. CMC[2]:
   a. Uncommon site of dislocation.
   b. Fifty percent involve the fifth MC.
   c. Twenty-five percent involve the second MC.
   d. Eighty percent are multiple, usually involving the fifth MC plus another.
   e. Two thirds dislocate dorsally.
   f. The posteroanterior (PA) view is very useful: The palm must

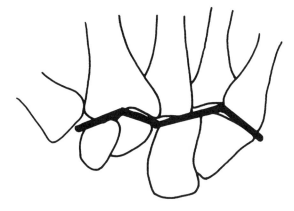

Fig. 3-7   Articulation of the carpometacarpal joints.

be *flat* on the cassette; flexion of the fingers gives a false appearance of overlap at the CMC joints.

g. On the PA view, the CMC joint spaces are of an even width, the opposing carpal and MC joint surfaces are parallel, and there is a zig-zag pattern of articulation (parallel M; Fig 3-7).

h. First MC articulates only with the trapezium.

i. Second MC articulates with the trapezoid. A styloid process is located at the base of the second MC on the ulnar side, which articulates with the trapezoid, capitate, and third MC in a lock-and-key configuration.

j. Third MC articulates with the capitate.

k. Fourth MC articulates with the hamate (radial side).

l. Fifth MC articulates with the hamate (sloping ulnar side).

m. A fracture at the base of an MC or involving the distal carpal row should stimulate a search for an occult dislocation.

III. WRIST TRAUMA

Key Concepts

A fall on an outstretched hand can result in different injuries, depending on age of patient: fracture of both bones of the forearm in a young child; Salter II distal radial fracture in an older child; scaphoid fracture in a teenager or young adult; and Colles' fracture in an older adult. Wrist fractures often are not displaced and therefore, are occult. The PA film must always be examined carefully for continuity of the three arcs. The lateral film is essential for diagnosis of carpal dislocations and instability patterns. The coaxial arrangement of the radius-lunate-capitate must always be demonstrated.

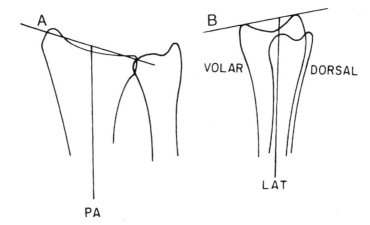

Fig. 3-8 **A,** Normal ulnar tilt of the distal radial articular surface on the PA film. **B,** Normal volar tilt of the distal radial articular surface on the lateral film. Note that the distal ulna is slightly shorter and posteriorly placed with respect to the radial articular surface on a well-positioned lateral film.

A. Distal forearm:
  1. PA film: Normal anatomy.
     a. Distal radial articular surface tilts 17 degrees toward the ulna (Fig 3-8,*A*).
     b. Distal radial epiphyseal line may remain a linear density, with a spurlike projection laterally simulating an avulsion.
     c. Medially, the radius articulates with the head of the ulna at the ulnar notch. The head of the ulna is usually 1 to 2 mm shorter than the radius and either touches or slightly overlaps the radius at the distal radioulnar joint.
  2. Lateral film: Normal anatomy.
     a. Pronator quadratus bulge may be a soft tissue clue to injury.
     b. Distal radial articular surface is angled 10 to 15 degrees volarly (Fig. 3-8,*B*).
     c. On a true lateral film, the dorsal surface of the distal ulna lies 1 to 3 mm posterior to the dorsal surface of the distal radius.
  3. Distal forearm abnormalities:
     a. *Ulnar-plus variant:* An unusually long ulna bears more of the axial load; this is associated with *lunate-triquetral ligament or triangular fibrocartilage complex (TFCC) damage or ulnar impaction syndrome,* with sclerosis and subchondral cyst and eventual osteophyte formation on the ulnar portion of the lunate.

    b. *Ulnar-minus variant:* An unusually short ulna bears less of the axial load; this is associated with lunate osteomalacia (*Keinbock's* disease).

4. *Distal radioulnar dislocation:*
    a. Suggested by an abnormal position of the head of the ulna in the ulnar notch.
    b. Diagnosis is best made by a *CT* axial image through the distal radioulnar notch (both wrists for comparison, *in full supination, neutral, and full pronation*).
    c. May be seen as an isolated injury or may be part of a more complex injury (*Colles'* fracture, *Galleazzi's* fracture-dislocation, or *Essex-Lopresti injury*).

5. Fractures of the distal forearm:
    a. The most common injuries of the skeletal system.
    b. Most result from a fall on the outstretched hand.
    c. Age alone is a very good predictor of the injury:
       (1) 4–10 years: Transverse fracture of the metaphyses of the distal radius and ulna.
       (2) 11–16 years: Salter 2 fracture of the distal radial epiphysis.
       (3) 17–40 years: Fracture of the scaphoid.
       (4) >40 years: Colles' fracture.
    d. Transverse metaphyseal fractures seen in children:
       (1) May be complete or incomplete.
       (2) When incomplete, may be greenstick or torus (buckle).
    e. *Salter fractures of the distal radial epiphysis.*
       (1) *Salter 2* most common.
       (2) Usually displaces dorsally, so often are seen *only on the lateral film.*
       (3) *Gymnasts* may suffer a *repetitive stress injury to the distal radius and ulna,* resulting in epiphyseal plate widening and irregularity; some consider this a type of Salter 1 injury.
    f. Distal radial fractures in the adult:
       (1) Colles' fracture:
          a Most common.
          b The injury is more common in females than in males owing to the higher incidence of senile osteoporosis in women.
          c Associated with fractures of proximal humerus and hip due to falls in osteoporotic patients.
          d Apex volar angulation with dorsal impaction.
          e May or may not have an intra-articular component.

    f May or may not have an associated ulnar styloid fracture.

    g Complications visible on postreduction films:

       i Apex volar angulation and consequent loss of the normal volar tilt of the radial articular surface.

      ii Loss of radial length due to impaction and consequent ulnar plus variant.

    iii Intra-articular diastasis with loss of the normal ulnar tilt of the radial articular surface.

(2) Smith: Reverse Colles', with apex dorsal angulation.

(3) Barton's: Intra-articular fracture of the dorsal lip of the radius; the carpus follows the dorsal fragment. This is an unstable fracture that often requires internal fixation or even placement of an external fixator.

(4) Reverse Barton's: Intra-articular fracture of the volar lip of the radius.

(5) Hutchinson's or chauffeur's: Intra-articular fracture of the radial styloid process. (Do not be fooled by the normal notch at the distal radial epiphysis.)

B. Carpus.

  1. Frequency of carpal injuries.[3]

    a. Forearm injuries are 10 times as frequent as carpal injuries.

    b. Carpal injuries are rare in patients under 12.

    c. Of carpal injuries, 60% to 70% are scaphoid fractures; 10%, dislocations and fracture-dislocations; 10%, dorsal chip fractures (usually triquetrium); and 10%, others.

  2. Normal anatomy of the carpus (PA).

    a. Proximal and distal rows bridged by scaphoid.

    b. Width of intercarpal joints is uniform, about 2 mm.

    c. Three parallel arcs have been described by Gilula[4] to aid in evaluation (Fig. 3-9):

      (1) Along the proximal articular margins of the proximal carpal row.

      (2) Along the distal articular margins of the proximal carpal row.

      (3) Along the proximal articular margins of the distal carpal row.

    d. Fifty percent to 70% of the lunate articulates with the radius.

    e. The lunate is trapezoidal on the PA film. If the shape is triangular, the lunate is rotated abnormally. (This may be seen as an artifact with the hand held in flexion or extension, however.)

    f. The hook of the hamate is normally seen *en face* in the PA

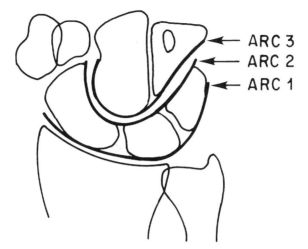

Fig. 3-9   Normal PA carpal view demonstrating particularly the normal shapes of the scaphoid and lunate as well as the three continuous arcs of the proximal and distal carpal rows. Continuity of these arcs assures carpal row integrity.

film overlying the hamate. Its absence indicates fracture, hypoplasia, or an ununited os hamuli proprium.

g. Radial or ulnar deviation can alter the appearance of the PA carpus.
   (1) With radial deviation, only 25% of the lunate articulates with the radius, the scaphoid is foreshortened and distorted. Patients with painful wrists normally hold the hand in radial deviation, so scaphoid fractures may easily be missed!
   (2) With ulnar deviation, 100% of the lunate articulates with the radius and the scaphoid appears elongated.

h. Normal variants of carpus, PA view:
   (1) Multiple accessory ossicles; the most common may be adjacent to the ulnar styloid process and may be indistinguishable from a previous ununited fracture. Others are outlined in Theodore E. Keats' *Atlas of Normal Roentgen Variants That May Simulate Disease.*
   (2) Carpal fusions (most commonly lunate-triquetrum; these may be only partially fused and may simulate fracture).
   (3) Bipartite scaphoid; these may be old nonunions.

3. Normal anatomy of carpus, lateral view (Fig 3-10).
   a. Confusing overlap, but the coaxial relationship between the

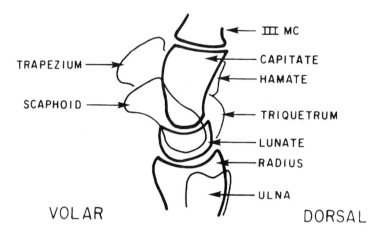

Fig. 3-10   Normal lateral carpal view, in which one must pick out the articulating distal radius, lunate, capitate, and third MC (*bold outline*).

        articular surfaces of the radius, lunate, capitate, and third MC *must* be picked out. An exact linear relationship here is uncommon, but a coaxial relationship is essential.

    b. The scaphoid arches out on the palmar side.

    c. In a true lateral view, the dorsal carpal surface is formed by the triquetrum.

  4. Normal anatomy of the carpus, carpal tunnel view:

    a. The pisiform and hook of the hamate are projected on the ulnar side; the scaphoid and trapezium (with a small hook) are projected on the radial side. Either the lunate or the capitate is seen centrally, depending on how the beam is angled.

    b. The view may be useful to search for calcifications or osteophytes in a patient with carpal tunnel syndrome (CTS). It has been suggested to diagnose *fracture of the hook of hamate,* but since these fractures are usually at the base of the hook and the patients usually cannot hyperextend the hand for the carpal tunnel view, the diagnosis may be difficult in injured patients. A *supinated oblique view,* limited CT, or lateral tomograms seem to be more useful in the diagnosis.

C. Carpal fractures.

  1. *Scaphoid fractures.*

    a. *Seventy percent are at the waist and nondisplaced;* if clinically suspected but not seen, films may be repeated in 7 to 10 days, when sclerosis or resorption about the fracture line may be seen.

b. If it is essential to make the diagnosis acutely, CT with cuts through the long axis of the bone is accurate.

c. The blood supply to the distal pole is separate, so *distal pole fractures heal quickly.*

d. The blood supply to the proximal pole enters at the *waist,* so it may be cut off by a fracture through the waist of the scaphoid. Such fractures are *at risk for delayed union, nonunion, and avascular necrosis of the proximal pole fracture fragment.*

e. A waist of scaphoid fracture may take up to 2 years to unite. It may, in fact, develop radiographic signs of nonunion (rounded, sclerotic fracture fragment edges) yet go on to unite after several months; 90% of scaphoid fractures unite eventually.

f. Scaphoid fractures with delayed union are commonly treated with bone grafting (harvested from the dorsum of the radius) and placement of a *Herbert screw* (two sets of threads at different pitch, designed to compress the two fracture fragments together).

g. When following scaphoid fractures, watch for development of a "dorsal hump" (i.e., apex dorsal angulation at the fracture site). CT is especially useful to evaluate anatomic reduction as well as fracture healing; if the cuts are directed along the long axis of the scaphoid, this is also the direction of the screw and metal artifact will be minimized.

2. Lunate fractures: It is unusual to see an acute fracture, but the lunate is vulnerable to AVN (Keinbock's disease or lunate malacia), so collapse and increased density may be seen. This is felt to be secondary to trauma (though the incident may not be recalled) and has been associated with the ulnar-minus variant. Early AVN may be detected by MR.

3. Triquetrum fractures: Dorsal chip fractures are usually triquetral and are seen only on the lateral film.

4. Capitate fractures: Isolated fracture is rare, but as a part of a complex fracture-dislocation, a transverse fracture of the capitate may be seen; in this case, the proximal fragment frequently rotates 180 degrees.

5. Hamate fractures.

a. Hook of the hamate fracture is best detected on PA films (by its absence) and confirmed by a carpal tunnel view, CT, or supinated oblique view.

b. Proximal pole fractures may be seen as part of a perilunate or lunate fracture-dislocation complex.

D. Carpal dislocations.

1. Most fracture-dislocations of the carpus fall within the vulnerable

zone outlined by Yeager.[5] The inner arc roughly outlines the disrupted ligaments around the lunate, as seen in a pure dislocation, while the outer arc outlines the fractures commonly associated with carpal fracture-dislocation (radial styloid, waist of scaphoid, proximal capitate, base of hamate, lunar surface of triquetrium, and ulnar styloid).

2. With progression from the radial to the ulnar side of the arch, the severity of the injury increases (i.e., a scapholunate dissociation is less severe than a perilunate dislocation, which in turn is less severe than a lunate dislocation).

3. With progression from the radial to ulnar side, the frequency of the injury decreases (i.e., a scapholunate dissociation may be a less severe injury than a perilunate dislocation, but it is also much more common; perilunate dislocations are more common than lunate dislocations).

4. Fracture dislocations are more common than pure dislocation, so look carefully for these fractures.

5. Radiographic analysis: On the PA film, Gilula's first and second arcs are disrupted; on the lateral film, the coaxial radius-lunate-capitate arrangement is disrupted (Fig 3-11,*A*).

6. Perilunate dislocation: The capitate articular surface is dislocated from the lunate (almost invariably dorsally); the lunate maintains its normal articulation with the radius (Fig 3-11,*B*).

7. Midcarpal dislocation: The lunate tilts volarly but is not dislocated from the radius. The capitate is dislocated from the lunate but is not as dorsally placed as in a routine perilunate dislocation. This may be a carpus in transition from a perilunate to a lunate dislocation (Fig 3-11,*C*).

8. Lunate dislocation: The lunate has lost its articulation with both the capitate and radius and is displaced volarly with 90 degrees' rotation. The capitate remains aligned with the radius but sinks proximally (Fig 3-11,*D*).

E. Carpal instabilities.
   1. Ligamentous injury can give instability patterns without frank dislocations.
   2. Radiographic examination.
      a. PA: Look especially for a diastasis at the scapholunate joint (normal scapholunate gap is 2 mm) and lunate tilt.
      b. Lateral: Note the previously discussed coaxial relationships. Also, evaluate the lunate-capitate angle (normally <20 degrees) and the scapholunate angle (normally 30 to 60 degrees; under 30 degrees and over 80 degrees definitely are abnormal; see Fig 3-12,*A*).

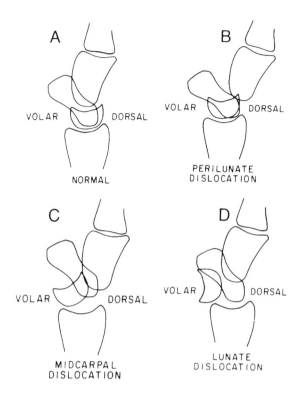

Fig. 3-11   Carpal dislocation patterns as seen on the lateral film. The progression from normal (**A**), to perilunate (loss of articulation of the capitate with the lunate) (**B**), through midcarpal (dislocation of the capitate from the lunate, and subluxation but not dislocation of the lunate from the radius) (**C**), to lunate (**D**) (dislocation of the capitate from the lunate and of the lunate from the radius) demonstrates increasing severity of injury as well as the possible sequence of injury patterns in a single person. A patient who presents initially with a perilunate dislocation may go on to a midcarpal dislocation, and convert to a lunate dislocation if there is sufficient ligamentous disruption.

3. Fluoroscopy: Occasionally wrist instability patterns are transient and can be seen only under fluoroscopy. This is especially true in patients who have midcarpal pain, normal plain films, and audible clicks.
4. Standard fluoroscopy (with videotaping) includes:
    a. PA: Radial to ulnar deviation with fist clenching.
    b. Lateral: Dorsiflexion and palmar flexion.
    c. AP: Fist clenching.
    d. Anything else to elicit and define a click.

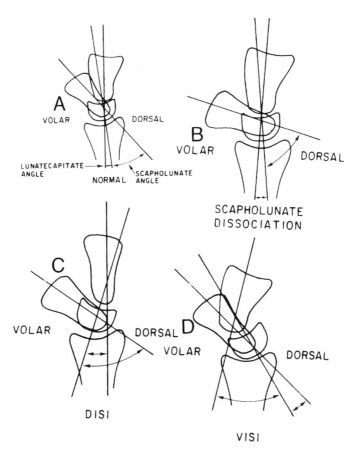

Fig. 3-12   Carpal instability patterns. **A,** Normal, with lunate–capitate angle less than 20 degrees and scapholunate angle of 30 to 60 degrees. **B,** Scapholunate dissociation with rotary subluxation of the scaphoid (normal lunate–capitate angle, abnormally large scapholunate angle). **C,** Dorsiflexion carpal instability pattern, with increased lunate–capitate angle, increased scapholunate angle, and dorsiflexion of the lunate. **D,** Volar flexion carpal instability, with increased lunate–capitate angle, often decreased scapholunate angle, and volar flexion of the lunate.

5. Scapholunate dissociation may be accentuated by AP filming with a clenched hand and radial or ulnar deviation, which drives the capitate proximally between the scaphoid and lunate, widening that gap.
6. Capitate-lunate instability may be seen best when pressure is applied to the scaphoid tuberosity and longitudinal traction is maintained while the hand is flexed (both PA and lateral projections).

7. Triquetrum-hamate instability: During radial-to-ulnar deviation, the proximal carpal row snaps from palmar flexion to dorsiflexion once ulnar deviation is obtained.

8. Scapholunate dissociation. Gap at scapholunate joint is greater than 2 mm. (First clenching may help, see discussion above.) Patient may or may not have scaphoid rotation, manifested on PA film by scaphoid foreshortening and ''ring'' sign and on lateral by increase in scapholunate angle without abnormal lunate flexion (Fig 3-12,*B*).

9. Dorsiflexion carpal instability (also termed dorsal intercalated segment instability—DISI; Fig 3-12,*C*).

   a. Increased dorsiflexion of lunate, with consequent increase in lunate-capitate angle on lateral.

   b. Palmar flexion of scaphoid, with consequent increase in scapholunate angle on lateral.

   c. May or may not have scapholunate dissociation.

10. Volar flexion carpal instability (also termed volar intercalated segment instability—VISI; Fig 3-12,*D*).

    a. Volar flexion of lunate and dorsiflexion of capitate, giving a zig-zag deformity and abnormal lunate-capitate angle on lateral.

    b. Often, but not invariably, there is a decrease in scapholunate angle.

    c. Rare instability pattern compared to DISI if secondary to trauma, but relatively common if secondary to ligamentous instability in rheumatoid arthritis (RA).

11. Ulnar translocation: Entire carpus translocates ulnarly from the radial styloid process, usually secondary to an inflammatory process such as RA.

12. Dorsal carpal subluxation: Dorsal subluxation relative to the distal radius, often secondary to a residual fracture deformity such as Colles' fracture with apex volar angulation.

F. Wrist arthrograms.

1. Always examine with fluoroscopy first to look for instability.

2. Objective is usually to rule out disrupted TFCC or interosseous ligaments by watching the flow of contrast from one compartment to another (Fig 3-13).

3. Radiocarpal injection: Dorsal approach, wrist held in slight flexion, needle angulated proximally to avoid the lip of the radius; 25-gauge, 1 1/2-inch needle placed between the scaphoid and radius (and specifically *not* at the scapholunate junction). 2 to 4 milliliters of contrast (60% in 10:1 mixture with epinephrine,

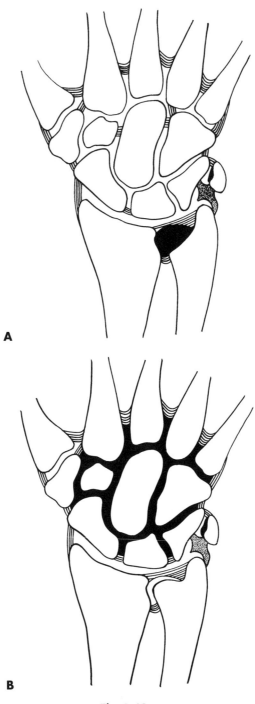

A

B

Fig. 3-13

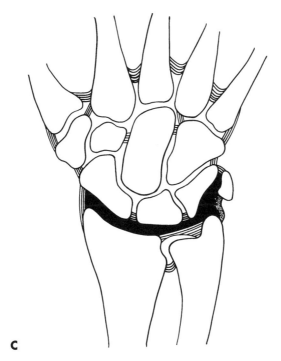

C

Fig. 3-13 *(continued) Compartments of the wrist.* **A,** Distal radioulnar joint, sparated from the radiocarpal joint by the intact TFCC, which stretches between the radius and ulnar styloid. **B,** Midcarpal joint: a large joint, extending between the base of metacarpals 2 to 4, not extending into the first CMC joint, and depending on intact scapholunate and lunate triquetral ligaments as well as radial and ulnar capsules for its integrity. **C,** Radiocarpal joint, located between the other two joint spaces. (Reprinted with permission from the ACR Skeletal Learning File, BJ Manaster, ed., 1993, case #332.)

 1:1000) injected using digital subtraction technique. Follow this with PA, lateral, and oblique films as well as a postexercise series.[6]

4. Contrast normally is retained in the radiocarpal compartment. Communication between the triquetrum and pisiform is a normal variant. The expected distribution of contrast with various injections is demonstrated in Fig 3-13.

5. Contrast entering the distal radioulnar joint indicates TFCC disruption.

6. Contrast entering the midcarpal joint indicates disruption of one of the following interosseous ligaments: scapholunate, lunate-triquetral, triquetral-hamate, scaphotrapezium. Identification of the

exact site of disruption is important if surgery is contemplated; this can usually be accomplished by a frame-by-frame analysis of the digital portion of the study but often is missed otherwise. Scapholunate and lunate triquetral perforations are most common. Capsular disruption may also be demonstrated.

7. Degeneration of these ligaments and the TFCC may occur normally in the older age group. It is also a common finding in patients with erosive arthropathies.

8. If the radiocarpal injection is normal, a distal radioulnar joint injection should be performed as well as a midcarpal injection (at the scaphoid-capitate joint), in order to avoid missing a ball-valve type of ligamentous perforation.

9. Interpreting the clinical significance of wrist abnormalities seen by arthrography is difficult. Studies show that ulnar-side pain correlates with ulnar-side abnormalities much more strongly than does radial-side pain with radial-side abnormalities. Bilateral wrist arthrography studies suggest that bilaterally symmetric and often asymptomatic arthrographic abnormalities occur frequently. This suggests that simply demonstrating ligamentous perforations may not be an adequate screening tool.[7,8] However, there is also great controversy regarding the efficacy of all treatment methodologies for chronic wrist pain, which are unproven in the sense of outcome analysis.

G. MR of the wrist: MR can range from being absolutely useless to being invaluable for chronic wrist pain evaluation. It is not a good survey tool, since specific studies are tailored to demonstrate specific anatomy or disease processes. On the other hand, if MR is tailored to answer a specific question, it can demonstrate anatomy and pathology beautifully.[9] In general, a small field of view and coil system is required. Sequences and planes are adjusted, depending on the tissues and sites to be studied.

1. Ligamentous abnormalities: It remains controversial whether MR or arthrography (or the more expensive MR arthrography) is superior for evaluating the TFCC and intrinsic ligaments of the wrist. Variable MR morphology and signal intensity (both within the ligament and at the insertional site) have been demonstrated making the risk for false positive significant.[10,11] Accuracy claims range from 50% to 95%. The study is extremely technique-sensitive, and requires a reader with extensive experience. Accuracy in diagnosing TFCC tears hovers around 90%, but again is dependent on the reader being fully versed in the variability of the TFCC morphology and signal.[12]

The question may become moot with the increased popularity

of arthroscopy, but if excellent "true-negative" rates are established, the exam may remain clinically efficacious. The external ligaments of the wrist have been demonstrated by MR, but clinical application and accuracy have not yet been established.

2. Tendons: Since they are low signal on all sequences, pathology such as rupture, dislocation, inflammation, and degeneration can be demonstrated if proper attention is paid to imaging technique. De Quervain's disease (fibrosis of the extensor pollicis longus and abductor pollicis brevis tendons) can be shown. The most common tendon subluxation involves the extensor carpi ulnaris being displaced from its groove on the dorsal surface of the ulna, returning to position with a painful snap through a pronation-supination motion.

3. Carpal tunnel syndrome (CTS): This is usually a clinical diagnosis that can be supported by nerve conduction tests. MR can be helpful in atypical presentation. MR is performed in the axial plane. The osseous canal containing the flexor tendons and median nerve (the latter a higher SI than the tendons), contained by the flexor retinaculum, is well seen (Fig 3-14). Median nerve size, shape, and signal are evaluated at the level of the distal radius, pisiform, and hook of hamate. Retinacular bowing is evaluated, as well as

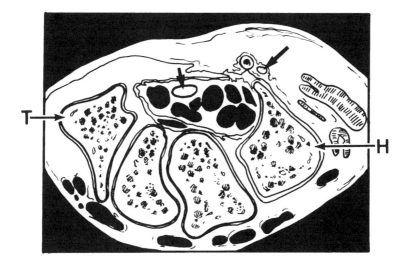

Fig. 3-14 Carpal tunnel, at level of the hook of hamate, note the low signal flexor tendons, the intermediate signal median nerve surrounded by fat (*short arrow*), the flexor retinaculum, and the ulnar nerve (*long arrow*) and vessels outside the flexor retinaculum. H, hamate; T, trapezium.

the presence of osseous fracture or mass lesion contributing to a restricted carpal tunnel. At the level of the distal radioulnar joint, the median nerve is round and has moderate SI. The nerve is slightly flattened within the carpal tunnel normally, with maintenance of the same SI.[13] With CTS there is swelling of the median nerve at the level of the pisiform, flattening at the level of the hamate, palmar bowing of the flexor retinaculum, and increased SI of the median nerve on T2 weighted images.[14] Quantitative measurements are available.[13,14]

4. Osseous abnormalities: Avascular necrosis, occult fractures, and bone bruises are well demonstrated by MR.
5. Miscellaneous masses and nonspecific carpal cysts are well seen.

IV. ELBOW TRAUMA

Key Concepts

For elbow trauma, must evaluate: fat pads (provide a hint that an occult fracture is likely to be present); ossification centers, especially medial epicondyle (knowing the epiphyseal maturation sequence is useful, especially to avoid missing a medial epicondylar avulsion); anterior humeral line (diagnoses occult supracondylar fracture); radiocapitellar line (diagnoses occult radial head dislocation): if there is a dislocation, look for fracture.

A. Normal anatomy.
   1. AP film:
      a. Radius articulates with capitellum.
      b. Ulna articulates with trochlea.
      c. Normal carrying angle 165 degrees (on AP, apex valgus; functionally, this displaces the hand away from the thigh).
      d. Bowman's angle describes the normal cubitus valgus in a child and is used to evaluate for abnormal valgus or varus in the presence of a supracondylar fracture. The angle is formed by a line bisecting the humeral shaft and a second line along the metaphysis of the medial epicondyle. This angle decreases with varus angulation. The abnormal and normal elbows are compared; 5 degrees is considered a significant difference in angulation (Fig. 3-15).
   2. Lateral film:
      a. The condyles of the humerus are normally anteriorly placed with respect to the humeral shaft, described by the *anterior humeral* line: on a true lateral film, a line drawn along the humeral cortex intersects the capitellum in its *middle third* (Fig. 3-16).

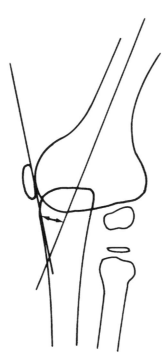

Fig. 3-15   Bowman's angle, decreased in cubitus varus resulting from malignment of a supracondylar fracture.

      b. Radiocapitellar line: With the elbow in *any* position, a line bisecting the proximal radial shaft intersects the capitellum. If it does not, there is a radial head dislocation (Fig. 3-17).

      c. Fat pads: Seen on lateral film, flexed 90 degrees, the anterior fat pad is normally seen in the coronoid fossa as a straight (not convex) lucency. In the absence of effusion, the posterior fat pad is not seen; with an effusion, the posterior fat pad is a convex lucency in the olecranon fossa of the humerus. With a small effusion, an abnormal (convex) anterior fat pad may be seen without a posterior fat pad. In the presence of trauma and abnormal fat pads, a fracture is extremely likely in adults, less likely in children. Multiple views may be necessary to demonstrate subtle nondisplaced fractures.

B. Normal variants.

    1. There is a normal chevron appearance of the trabeculae seen in the lateral humerus in the supracondylar region.

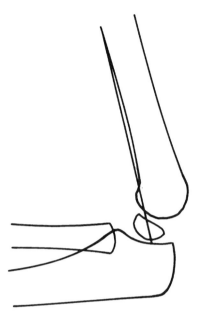

Fig. 3-16 Anterior humeral lines on a true lateral film must intersect the middle third of the capitellum. In a supracondylar fracture, the anterior humeral line usually intersects the anterior third of the capitellum (or none) since the distal fragment is displaced or angulated posteriorly. An abnormal anterior humeral line and abnormal fat pad may be the only clues to a supercondylar fracture since the fracture line itself often is occult.

    2. When the radial tuberosity is seen *en face,* it may present as a well-circumscribed lucency, possibly simulating neoplasm.
    3. Supratrochlear ossicle: A normal variant found in the trochlear fossa, to be distinguished from a chip fracture.
    4. Supracondylar process: A hooklike process arising from the anterior humeral cortex in the supracondylar region that may occasionally fracture and cause a median nerve injury. As an aside, the supracondylar process is almost invariably present in avian species!
C. Epiphyseal maturation sequence. Ossification occurs by:
    1. Capitellum: 1 year.
    2. Radial head: 3 to 6 years.
    3. Medial epicondyle: 5 to 7 years; last to fuse.
    4. Trochlea: 9 to 10 years; ossifies in multiple centers, so may appear fragmented.

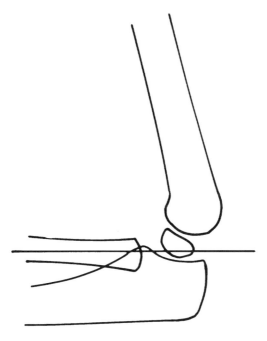

Fig. 3-17 Radiocapitellar line: A line bisecting the proximal shaft of the radius must intersect the capitellum in *any* position of the elbow; an abnormal radiocapitellar line is the best indicator of subtle radial head dislocation.

5. Olecranon: 8 to 10 years; two separate centers of ossification appear markedly separated from the metaphysis.
6. Lateral epicondyle: 9 to 13 years; sliver shape initially, located very lateral to the metaphysis, so may mimic an avulsion.
7. The timing is not as important as the sequences. The crucial part of the sequence can be remembered by the mnemonic ''CRIT'': ''C'' for capitellum, ''R'' for radial head, ''I'' for internal (medial) epicondyle, ''T'' for trochlea. Specifically, note that the trochlea never ossifies before the medial epicondyle. Since the flexor muscles of the forearm arise from the medial epicondyle, with avulsion, the medial epicondyle ossification center is pulled inferiorly and may become trapped in the joint. In a patient who is too young to have an ossified trochlea, this avulsed fragment may be mistaken for the trochlea; thus, the diagnosis is easily missed. Note: The presence of a ''trochlea'' in the absence of a medial epicondylar ossification center is diagnostic of an avulsed and trapped medial epicondyle. This avulsion of the medial epicondyle

is one of the two types of *"Little League elbow"* occurring in curve ball pitchers.

D. *Elbow fracture in children.*[15]

    1. *Supracondylar fractures, 60%:* Almost always have *posterior displacement of the condyles and an abnormal anterior humeral line.* (See discussion above.) The reason for the posterior displacement of the distal fracture fragment is that the injury is usually a result of a FOOSH (fall on outstretched hand). Usually ages 3 to 9.

        a. May be occult except for abnormal fat pads and the anterior humeral line extending abnormally through the anterior portion of the capitellum.

        b. May result in abnormal cubitus varus or valgus; Bowman's angle and the opposite elbow are useful for the evaluation. (See discussion above.)

    2. *Lateral condylar, 15%.*

        a. Usually *Salter 4,* involving the capitellum. (Fig. 3-18).

        b. The extensor muscle mass attaches to the metaphyseal fragment and displaces it distally and posteriorly. Internal fixation is required.

    3. *Medial epicondyle avulsion, 10%: May be trapped in the joint; often unrecognized,* resulting in severe late disability. (See discussion of epiphyseal maturation sequence, C, above.)

    4. Jerked elbow (*nursemaid elbow*): Preschooler who refuses to move his/her elbow from a flexed, pronated position; mechanism is traction, trapping the annular ligament/capsule; plain films are normal or rarely show effusion; reduction by supination (often occurs while filming).

    5. Positive fat pad in elbow of child but no visible fracture: unlike adults, the child often does not have an occult fracture.

E. *Elbow fractures in adults.*

    1. *Radial head* fractures.

        a. *Half of all adult elbow fractures.*

        b. Most common cause of positive fat pad signs in adults.

        c. *Half are undisplaced,* so several views may be required.

        d. *Essex-Lopresti fracture:* A severely comminuted radial head fracture associated with subluxation of the distal radioulnar joint.

    2. *Olecranon fracture: If distal to the triceps insertion, the fracture is widely displaced due to retraction by the triceps.* Strong internal fixation required. The mechanism is a sudden strong contraction of the triceps.

    3. Transcondylar fracture: Generally in older patients with osteoporosis.

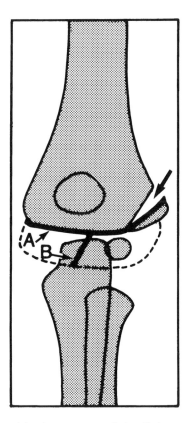

Fig. 3-18 Lateral condylar fractures in a skeletally immature patient. Note that, in this age group, often the capitellum is the only ossified epiphyseal center (dotted lines outline the non-ossified portion of the distal humeral epipysis). In a case like this, the only plain film finding is the metaphyseal fracture (*arrow*). Theoretically, this should continue as either a Salter 2 or 4 injury (*lines A* or *B,* respectively). Statistically, this fracture is almost invariably a Salter 4 (*line B*).

4. Intracondylar T or Y: Most distal humeral fractures in adults are this type or a more comminuted variant. The vertical component is usually at the trochlear ridge. Check for diastasis of the condyles at this site, interrupting the articular surface. These fractures require internal fixation, usually with a transcondylar screw and medial and lateral reconstruction plates. One usually sees an olecranon screw and wiring as well; this is fixation for the olecranon osteotomy required for the posterior surgical approach usually used in these cases.

F. *Dislocated elbow.*
   1. *Eighty percent to 90% are posterolateral, involving both the radius and ulna.*
   2. Often have associated coronoid process or radial head fractures, which may become trapped in the joint.
   3. An isolated dislocated radial head is rare in adults. An ulnar fracture (Monteggia's) must be excluded.
   4. Myositis ossificans is a relatively frequent complication, associated most often with fracture-dislocations. It is usually located in the antecubital fossa, ventrally, in the brachialis muscle. There is an increased incidence of myositis with delay in treatment.
   5. Congenital elbow dislocation: There is associated radial head overgrowth and an abnormally shaped radial head articular surface, so it is easily differentiated from traumatic dislocation.
   6. Separation of the distal humerus in children initially may look like a dislocation. The radial head, however, maintains its normal relationship with the capitellum, and the capitellum is no longer aligned with the humerus. The fragment tends to be displaced medially rather than posterolaterally (as in most dislocations of the elbow).

G. *Forearm fractures.*
   1. Almost invariably include *both bones,* or at least one bone and a dislocation at either the elbow or wrist. The exception to this rule is the *"nightstick"* fracture, a fracture of the ulnar shaft resulting from a direct blow (presumably while the arm is protecting the head).
   2. If there is an isolated radial fracture or mid to distal ulnar fracture, the associated dislocation may be subtle and must be sought out. Three named forearm fracture-dislocations include:
     a. *Monteggia: Ulnar shaft fracture with radial head dislocation.* Use the radiocapitellar line to evaluate for the dislocation.
     b. *Galleazi: Radial shaft fracture with distal radioulnar joint (DRUJ) dislocation or instability.* DRUJ instability is difficult to diagnose, and may require CT with axial cuts through both wrists in supination, neutral, and pronation.
     c. *Essex-Lopresti: Comminuted radial head fracture with distal radioulnar joint dislocation or instability.* This is an easily missed association, since most radial head fractures are isolated processes. However, recognize also that most radial head fractures are not highly comminuted. If significant comminution occurs, there is enough force present to extend down the forearm, disrupting the interosseous membrane, and extend through the soft tissues supporting the distal radioulnar joint. This is a highly unstable situation, but a subtle diagnosis. The

DRUJ may need CT diagnosis (see b above, in Galleazi's discussion). The importance of this diagnosis cannot be overly stressed, since the treatment of comminuted radial head fractures is often simple resection. In an Essex-Lopresti injury, the unstable radial shaft will then migrate proximally. This, in turn, causes a relative ulnar-plus variant. If the etiology of this ulnar-plus is not recognized, it may be treated with ulnar shortening. This, in turn, brings the resected radius in contact with the capitellum—you can see the vicious cycle developing, as the forearm gets shorter!

3. Treatment of both bone fractures in children usually is casting, as they heal and remodel well. Adults usually have both bones plated. Evaluation for malrotation can be difficult since true supinated AP films are rarely obtained. Use this rule of thumb: the radius is not malrotated if the radial tuberosity is on the opposite side of the shaft from the radial styloid process. The ulna is not malrotated if the coronoid process is on the opposite side of the shaft from the ulnar styloid process.

H. Soft tissue injuries and MR of the elbow. MR can be extremely useful in evaluating the following injuries, including overuse syndromes. Remember that small field of view, adequate coils, and thoughtful choice of plane, positioning, and sequence will maximize the value of the exam.[16,17]

1. *Osteochondritis dissecans:* The most common site in the elbow is the capitellum, and injury may range from a chondral defect, through AVN (Panner's disease), and if untreated, eventually progresses to osteoarthritis and intra-articular loose bodies. The injury results from repetitive trauma involving lateral compression from valgus stresses (throwing, racquet sports, gymnastics). *Two normal variants* which may simulate chondral defects must be recognized:

    a. *Pseudodefect of the capitellum* located posterolaterally at the junction of the capitellum and nonarticular portion of the posterolateral distal humerus (Fig 3-19).

    b. A small *groove in the olecranon,* opposite the trochlea, where the coronoid process joins the ulna. Both of these normal variants are seen on sagittal images (Fig 3-19).

2. *Lateral epicondylitis:* Commonly known as ''*tennis elbow*'' but also seen in golfers, carpenters, and other professions or sports requiring repetitive motions of the forearm. MR may show thickening of the common extensor tendon at its lateral epicondylar origin, or high SI. (Before making a diagnosis based on these findings, be certain the patient has not had an injection at this site for at least a month, as this can give the same appearance.) Less

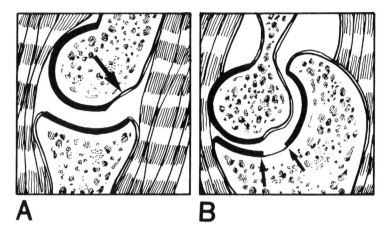

A   **B**

Fig. 3-19   Normal variants on sagittal MR imaging of the elbow. **A,** Pseudo defect of the capitellum, due to the normal junction of the smooth capitellum and the rough nonarticular surface of the lateral epicondyle, frequently seen as a notch like defect (*arrow*). **B,** Normal groove (*arrows*) in the articular surface of the olecranon where the coronoid process joins the olecranon, appears as a defect. Neither of these should be mistaken for an osteochondral defect.

frequently, dystrophic calcification may form at the site. Osseous change is rare.

3. *Medial epicondylitis:* Seen in an older age group, with repeated stress of the forearm flexors. Thickening and edema at the flexor tendon origin are sought in the adult. In professional pitchers and tennis players, large hypertrophic traction spurs may develop opposite the medial epicondyle on the medial aspect of the coronoid tubercle. In children, subtle bone marrow edema and widening or irregularity of the medial epicondylar apophyseal line corresponds to early avulsion of the medial epicondyle[16] (Little League elbow).

4. *Ulnar collateral ligament tear:* The ulnar collateral ligament and joint capsule are the primary elbow stabilizers, and are injured with repetitive flexion and valgus stress (throwing). Of the ulnar collateral ligament complex, it is the cordlike anterior bundle that is best seen on MR (Fig 3-20), and also the most important functionally. The posterior (oblique) bundle and transverse ligaments are generally not seen. Intrasubstance sprain is seen as thickening or increased SI (but question the patient regarding recent injections). Complete disruption is shown as ligament discontinuity.

5. *Radial collateral ligament tear:* This structure extends from the lateral epicondyle to the annular ligament and is much less commonly ruptured. It is part of the lateral complex which includes the supina-

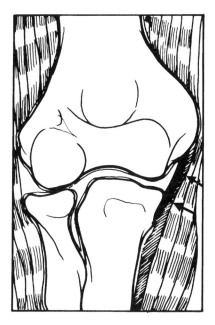

Fig. 3-20   Normal coronal MR appearance of the ulnar collateral ligament (*arrows*). Immediately adjacent to the ligament is the forearm flexor group of muscles, originating from the medial epicondyle.

tor muscle, common extensor tendon, and the lateral ulnar collateral ligament (extending from the lateral epicondyle posteriorly to the lateral side of the ulna, giving posterolateral stability).

6. Median nerve/pronator tunnel syndrome: Rare nerve entrapment due to compression from the pronator teres. Watch for edematous or inflammatory changes.

7. *Cubital tunnel syndrome:* The *ulnar nerve* lies in the cubital tunnel posterior to the medial epicondyle (Fig 3-21). Repetitive valgus stress may cause inflammation. The nerve can sublux in flexion. Neuropathy may be caused by nearby fracture, inflammation and fibrosis of adjacent tissue, thickened retinaculum, or accessory anconeus muscle. More distally, traction osteophytes from the medial side of the corocoid process may compress the ulnar nerve (seen on coronal section or plain film). The ulnar nerve is normally seen surrounded by fat, with SI isointense to muscle; inflammation is seen as thickening and areas of high SI.

8. *Distal biceps tendon rupture:* This is a *rare* injury, representing only 3% of biceps tendon injuries and usually in older males. The rupture occurs at the *level of the radial tuberosity;* the mechanism

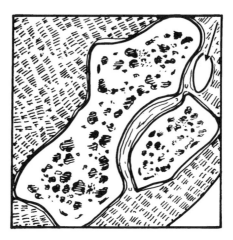

Fig. 3-21 Axial MR appearance of the normal locations of the ulnar nerve (*arrow*) posterior to the medial epicondyle.

is excessive force in extension on a flexed supinated forearm.[18] Clinically, the retracted muscle can often be felt as a lump. The biceps tendon is best seen on axial views, located anterior (volar) to the brachialis tendon (Fig 3-22). Findings of an empty tendon sheath filled with fluid, tendon retraction, and a poorly defined mass obscuring the normal distal portion of the tendon suggest complete rupture. Chronic partial biceps ruptures may be particularly difficult, as they present with an antecubital soft tissue mass, cortical irregularity at the radial tuberosity, and occasional prominent osseous reaction. Misdiagnosis of neoplasm is possible.

9. Triceps tendon tears are extremely uncommon. With enough force, the outer tendinous insertion on the olecranon may be partially torn, but the deeper muscular attachment remains intact. The olecranon itself fails, with transverse fracture, rather than complete triceps rupture.

V. SHOULDER TRAUMA

Key Concepts

Axillary lateral view is essential in evaluating shoulder trauma and may be obtained using only minimal abduction in an injured shoulder. Anterior dislocation of humeral head is much more common, but posterior dislocation is more often missed. The unstable glenohumeral (GH) joint has many soft tissue abnormalities to check for, beyond the rotator cuff tear (RTC) and Hill-Sachs lesion.

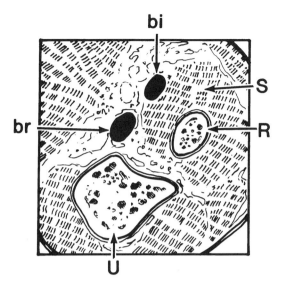

bi

br

S

R

U

Fig. 3-22   Axial view immediately distal to the elbow, demonstrating the expected location of the biceps tendon (*bi*) and brachialis tendon (*br*). R, radial head; U, ulna; S, supinator. Axial views are required for evaluation of distal biceps processes, although sagittal may demonstrate a complete rupture with retraction.

A. *Sternoclavicular (SC) joint.*
1. Fifty percent of the clavicular articular surface extends above the manubrium, so the normal articulation has an unusual (though bilaterally symmetric) appearance.
2. A *"bump"* noted clinically at the SC joint most likely represents a *dislocation or infection (especially in intravenous [IV] drug abusers or elderly patients)*.
3. Either entity is best diagnosed by a *limited CT scan* tailored to the area. This allows definition of both soft tissue and bone detail as well as evaluation of alignment. Only two or three axial cuts are usually required, which certainly is cost effective compared to polytomography.
4. If plain films are requested, an AP with 40 degrees cephalic angulation is likely to be the most useful.
5. The *medial clavicular epiphysis ossifies late* (18–20 years of age) and fuses late (about 25 years of age). As this is the age range in which *most SC dislocations* are seen, it is felt that many of them *are actually Salter 1 or 2 fractures.* Watch for that small ossification center remaining with the manubrium on the CT cuts.

6. Dislocation may be anterior or posterior (the clavicle tends to move slightly superiorly in either case).
7. Anterior is more common than posterior.
8. A posterior dislocation has the potential to compress the great vessels or trachea. Surgical reduction may be required, so accurate diagnosis is mandatory. If evaluation of the great vessels is required, MR may be preferable to CT. It should be noted that the surgical complication rate in this injury is also high.

B. Clavicle.
   1. Rhomboid fossa: Concave and irregular fossa located at the medial clavicle inferiorly; site of attachment of costoclavicular ligaments; may be asymmetric and may appear quite destructive.
   2. Fractures.
      a. Eighty percent involve the middle third. Callus formation may be exuberant.
      b. Fifteen percent involve the distal third. In these cases, the integrity of the coracoclavicular (CC) ligament must be evaluated, just as in an acromioclavicular (AC) separation.
   3. Distal clavicular resorption: Differential diagnosis:
      a. RA.
      b. Hyperparathyroidism (HPTH).
      c. Infection.
      d. Traumatic osteolysis: Fairly massive osteolysis following major or minor repetitive trauma which stabilizes by approximately 18 months and progresses to a reparative phase; associated with weight lifting.

C. AC joints.
   1. Evaluation requires single film demonstrating both AC joints, filmed with and without weights suspended from wrists (not grasped by hands) for stress.
   2. AC separation may involve the AC joint itself (and a tear of the AC ligament) as well as the CC ligaments (conoid and trapezoid).
      a. Type I: Sprain, with intact ligaments and normal radiograph.
      b. Type II: AC ligament disruption with widening of the AC joint; CC ligaments may be stretched slightly but are intact.
      c. *Type III: Both AC and CC ligaments are disrupted,* allowing widening of the AC joint and droop of the scapula (''elevation'' of the clavicle relative to the acromion and coracoid processes).
      d. *Type IV: Posterior dislocation of clavicle* relative to acromion; usually seen only on axillary lateral film since often no AC widening is seen on the AP film, even though both the AC and CC ligaments are disrupted.

3. The width of the AC joint is normally 3 to 5 mm but may occasionally be as wide as 8 mm. The normal difference between sides should be less than 2 to 3 mm.
4. The width of the CC ligament is 11 to 13 mm. The difference between the left and right side should be less than 5 mm.
5. Rule of thumb: These numbers may be difficult to remember, but they translate roughly to a 50% side-to-side difference in width of either the AC or CC being significant.
6. The coracoid apophysis may be avulsed as part of the type III separation.

D. Scapula.
1. Fractures are uncommon and usually are not displaced significantly because of extensive muscular coverage. When evaluating scapular fractures, the most important feature is whether they become intra-articular, extending into the glenoid. These may require surgical reduction.
2. Ossification centers not to be mistaken for fracture: Coracoid, acromion (with occasional os acromiale), glenoid rim, and longer apophyses along the vertebral border and inferior angle.
3. Os acromiale: A normal variant due to persistent lack of fusion of the acromial ossification center. Although it is considered a normal variant, it has been associated with shoulder impingement syndrome, so should be considered worthy of comment in a dictated report.
4. Another normal variant in the scapula is a ''hole'' in the body. Holes develop in thin bone which have large muscles with opposing pulls on either side of the bone. The scapula is a classic example, with the infraspinatus on its dorsal side and subscapularis on the ventral side. Not surprisingly, scapular holes are much more common in species which primarily use their arms for locomotion (the brachiators, including orangutans).

E. Shoulder joint anatomy (Fig. 3-23).
1. Glenoid is shallow, deepened somewhat by the cartilaginous labrum, and maintained primarily by muscular forces and the glenohumeral ligaments (GHL).
2. Glenoid is directed anteriorly, so AP film shows overlap of humeral head and glenoid. A 45-degree posterior oblique film shows the joint in tangent.
3. In external rotation, the greater tuberosity is seen laterally and the lesser tuberosity is superimposed over the humeral head.
4. In internal rotation the head appears more rounded, the lesser tuberosity is superimposed over the humeral head.
5. The axillary lateral is the only true lateral view of the shoulder

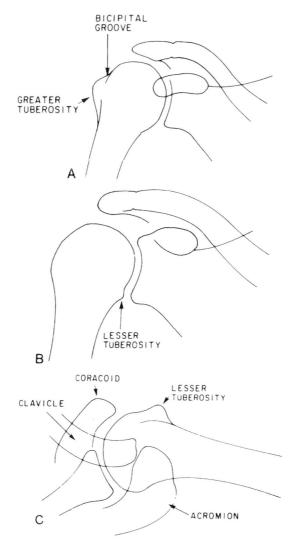

Fig. 3-23   Normal shoulder. **A,** External rotation. **B,** Internal rotation. **C,** Axillary lateral.

joint. The coracoid is seen to be anterior and the acromion, posterior. If properly positioned, the AC joint is centered over the humeral head.

6. The "arch" view can be useful when evaluating for impingement, since it shows the arch of the acromion and coracoid overlying

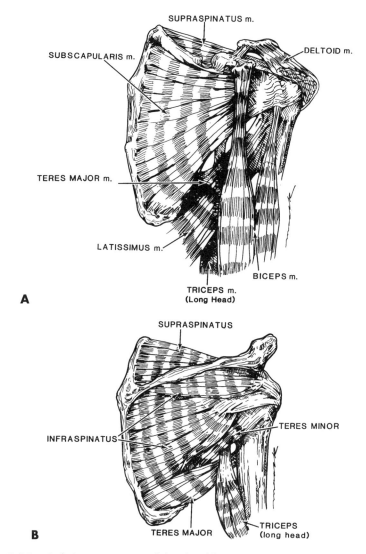

SUPRASPINATUS m.

SUBSCAPULARIS m.

DELTOID m.

TERES MAJOR m.

LATISSIMUS m.

BICEPS m.

TRICEPS m.
(Long Head)

A

SUPRASPINATUS

INFRASPINATUS

TERES MINOR

TERES MAJOR

TRICEPS
(long head)

B

Fig. 3-24   Soft tissue anatomy of the shoulder. **A,** Anterior. **B,** Posterior.

the humeral head. Watch for a downward sloping or "hooked" acromion, as well as subacromial spurs on either this or the AP films.

7. Soft tissue anatomy of the shoulder.
   a. Muscles (Fig 3-24):
      (1) *Supraspinatus:* Originates in supraspinatus fossa of the

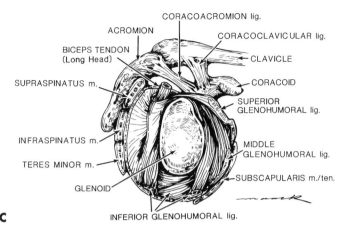

Fig. 3-24 *(continued)* **C,** Sagittal views at the glenoid fossa.

dorsal scapula and extends superiorly over the humeral head to insert on the superior facet of the greater tuberosity, acting as an external rotator of the humeral head and elevator of the arm.

(2) *Infraspinatus:* Originates in the infraspinatus fossa of the dorsal scapula and extends superiorly and posteriorly over the humeral head to insert on the middle facet of the greater tuberosity, acting as an external rotator of the humeral head.

(3) *Teres minor:* Originates at the lateral border of the scapula and extends posterior to the humeral head to insert on the lower facet of the greater tuberosity, acting as an external rotator of the humeral head.

(4) *Subscapularis:* Originates from the subscapularis fossa of the ventral side of the scapula and extends anteriorly to the humeral head to insert on the lesser tuberosity of the humerus; a few superficial fibers continue across the bicipital groove to attach to the greater tuberosity. The subscapularis is the only structure to insert on the lesser tuberosity, and acts to internally rotate the humeral head.

These four muscles (supraspinatus, infraspinatus, teres minor, subscapularis) together form the rotator cuff; the rotator cuff separates the (GH) joint from the subacromial and subdeltoid bursae. The deltoid is superficial to the rotator cuff muscles. It arises from three broad sites (scapular spine, acromion, and clavicle), caps the shoulder, and inserts over the lengthy distance of the deltoid tuberosity.

(5) *Biceps:* Two-heads—the short originates at the coracoid process and the long from the superior glenoid. This long head of the biceps is initially associated with the capsule, labrum, and superior GHLs and is at risk at its origin for trauma-related injury (see Section I and J, SLAP lesions). The biceps tendon then passes between the supraspinatus and subscapularis tendons of the rotator cuff (the biceps interval), and is intra-articular for a short distance, before entering the bicipital groove. This groove lies between the greater and lesser tuberosities; the bicipital tendon is held in the groove by the coracohumeral ligament as well as fibers of the supraspinatus and subscapularis tendons crossing the groove. Since a part of the biceps tendon is intra-articular, it is subject to articular disease processes.

b. *Capsule:* The capsular mechanism of the shoulder is complex and often difficult to image. It *consists of the glenoid labrum, the GHLs, the fibrous capsule itself, and the synovial recesses.* The capsule is divided into anterior and posterior components by the origin of the long head of biceps at the superior glenoid and the long head of triceps at the inferior glenoid. The posterior capsule is not complicated, simply inserting along and blending into the posterior labrum. *The anterior capsule is made more complex by the three GHLs.* These are thick fibrous bands formed within the capsule that are *important stabilizing structures* of the joint and are best seen in a joint that is distended by fluid or air.[19] The superior glenohumeral ligament (SGHL) is best seen in axial images at the level of the coracoid and near the origin of the long head of the biceps (Fig 3-25). The SGHL arises along with the long head of biceps from the superior glenoid, but the SGHL extends anteriorly from the glenoid, forming a ''Y'' with the biceps tendon and then blending into the anterior capsule before inserting on the humerus near the lesser tuberosity. The SGHL is rarely injured. The middle glenohumeral ligament (MGHL) is highly variable in size and may even be absent. It originates adjacent to the anterior glenoid or along the scapular neck, extends at a 45-degree angle to the glenoid, and merges with the capsule lining the subscapularis muscle. The inferior glenohumeral ligament (IGHL) is the largest and structurally most important of the GHLs. It originates from the inferior glenoid labrum near the

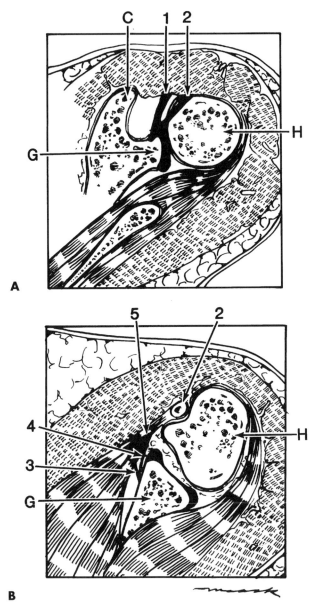

Fig. 3-25 Axial images of a distended GH joint, showing the GHLs. **A,** Superior, at the level of the coracoid. **B,** More inferior, at the level where the glenoid labrum is well seen.

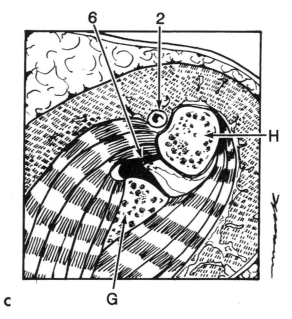

Fig. 3-25   *(continued)* **C,** Most inferior, at the inferior aspect of the glenoid. H, humeral head; C, coracoid; G, glenoid; *1,* SGHL; *2,* long head biceps; *3,* anterior capsule; *4,* MGHL; *5,* subscapularis tendon; *6,* IGHL.

origins of the long head of the triceps and fans out, reinforcing the anteroinferior capsule below the subscapularis muscle.

Three types of capsular insertions at the glenoid have been described. Type I inserts on or near the labrum, type II more medially, and type III even more medially on the scapular neck. A type III insertion is believed by some to be related to instability (either predisposing to or resulting from it); others have not demonstrated such an association.[20]

c. Labrum: The glenoid labrum is a fold of the capsule that is composed of fibrocartilage and dense fibrous tissue. While it serves to deepen the glenoid cavity, this mechanical function may be less important than its function as an attachment site for the GHLs. *Integrity of the labrum itself is difficult to confidently diagnose because of its variability in morphology and appearance.*[21] Anteriorly, the labrum tends to be triangular while posteriorly it is rounded in shape. The shape and size, however, varies with internal and external rotation of the shoulder. Furthermore, the superior glenoid labrum may have various normal clefts and foramina. The articular surface of the labrum is loosely adherent to the articular cartilage of the glenoid, allowing fluid to track between the two, simulating a tear. Furthermore, intralabral signal intensity may be altered due to a number of abnormalities unrelated to a tear and is not useful alone in evaluating this structure.[22] Two normal variants of the anterosuperior labrum are described. The sublabral foramen represents a segment of the anterior superior labrum that is not attached to the underlying glenoid margin. The other variant, termed the Buford complex, is seen as an absent anterosuperior portion of the labrum but thick cord-like MGHL. Both variants are difficult to identify or differentiate from labral tears; normal adjacent superior and anteroinferior labral segments may help suggest the variant rather than a tear of the labrum.

F. Shoulder dislocations and instability.
   1. Common site of dislocation due to the shallowness of the articulation.
   2. *Anterior dislocations (95%)*:
      a. Humeral head moves anteriorly and medially.
      b. The posterolateral portion of the humeral head impacts on the anteroinferior portion of the glenoid.
      c. This wedge-shaped impaction, called a *Hill-Sachs defect,* is best seen on an AP film with internal rotation. The defect may be difficult to see on an axillary lateral film and may be missed entirely on an external rotation film. It is easily seen on MR at the posterolateral aspect of the humeral head on an axial view at about the level of the coracoid. More distal to this, the posterolateral aspect of the humeral head normally flattens as it begins to form the neck of the humerus; this region should not be mistaken for a Hill-Sachs lesion.
      d. The corresponding chip fracture of the anteroinferior rim of the glenoid is called the Bankart lesion. It may be seen on either the AP or axillary views, but often not both. If only the fibrous labrum is involved, it is best detected by double-contrast arthrography with CT or by MR.
      e. The Hill-Sachs or Bankart lesion may be seen either acutely (30% to 40%) or after recurrent dislocation. It does not so much indicate a recurrent dislocation, as a potentially unstable shoulder.
      f. Osseous lesions of course are not the only contributors to shoulder instability. *Patients with clinical signs of shoulder*

instability should be evaluated with cross-sectional imaging (MR, MR arthrography, or CT arthrography), specifically looking for the integrity of the glenohumeral ligaments, joint capsule, subscapularis tendon, bicipital tendon dislocation, glenohumeral subluxation, as well as labral tears and Hill-Sachs/Bankart osseous lesions. These findings may be subtle and easily overlooked. "Redundancy" of the subscapularis bursa and subluxation of the glenohumeral joint are good hints to look more closely for labral, capsular, and GHL injuries. The subscapularis may be torn, atrophied, or even hypertrophied in chronic instability. Remember that a labral tear may manifest as a tear itself, altered morphology of the labrum, a flap, or as imbibation of contrast in a frayed labral structure. Glenoid labral cysts have been associated with labral tears and GH instability.[23] Inferior labral-ligamentous abnormalities seen on MR arthrography are strongly predictive of anterior shoulder instability.[20]

    g. Incidence of dislocation recurrence is inversely related to the patient's age at the time of initial dislocation.

    h. The position of the shoulder at the time of injury determines which of the stabilizers is likely to be injured. Ninety-degree abduction with external rotation stresses the IGHL; 45-degree abduction stresses the subscapularis and MGHL/IGHL. Dislocation in 0-degree abduction or adduction injures the SGHL, coracohumeral ligament, and superior labral attachments.

    i. Surgery for recurrent anterior glenohumeral joint dislocation:

       (1) Bankart: Staple capsulorraphy (staple or sutures secure the capsule and labrum to the glenoid).

       (2) Bristow: Moving the tip of the coracoid to the anterior glenoid, secured with screw.

       (3) Du Toit: Arthroscopic capsular stapling.

       (4) Magnusen-Stack: Subscapularis tendon shortening/transfer.

       (5) Putti-Platt: Subscapularis shortening.

3. *Posterior dislocation (2% to 4%)*:

    a. *Usually secondary to shock therapy or seizures.*

    b. Directly posterior, without superior or inferior change in alignment.

    c. *Fifty percent are not recognized initially* for two reasons: The subtle signs are missed on the AP film, and axillary lateral films are not obtained. The abnormality is very obvious on axillary lateral film, so these should be obtained routinely.

    d. *The humeral head is usually locked in internal rotation. This* is the most reliable sign in the absence of an axillary lateral view.

    e. *Trough sign:* A vertical density parallel to the articular surface corresponding to a ''reverse Hill-Sachs'' impaction on the anteromedial portion of the humeral head. A ''reverse Bankart'' chip fracture of the posterior glenoid may be seen as well.

    f. Rim sign: The humeral head often appears to be slightly displaced laterally, giving a ''widened'' joint space. This appearance is highly dependent on positioning of the film and is less reliable than the others.

  4. Inferior dislocation (luxatio erecta): A rare dislocation in which the articular surface is dislocated entirely inferior to the glenoid with fixed abduction of the shaft.

G. Rotator cuff tear (RCT).

  1. Rotator cuff consists of the supraspinatus, infraspinatus, teres minor muscles (inserting on the greater tuberosity, external rotators), as well as the subscapularis muscle (inserting on the lesser tuberosity, internal rotator).

  2. The supraspinatus and infraspinatus muscles and tendons primarily occupy the space between the humeral head and acromion process (anteriorly and posteriorly, respectively). *It is the supraspinatus tendon that is most commonly torn, near its insertion site on the greater trochanter.*

  3. Rotator cuff tears may be acute or chronic, the latter being common in patients with RA or impingement. Other causes include aging, high levels of overhead shoulder activity, trauma, and GH instability.

  4. *Secondary signs of a chronic tear:*

    a. *Elevation of the humerus* with a decrease in the acromiohumeral distance due to attenuation and retraction of the supraspinatus and infraspinatus muscles.

    b. Inferior surface of the acromion becomes convex and sclerotic owing to the mechanical apposition of the humeral head.

    c. In RA, the complication of medial impaction of the surgical neck of the humerus on the inferior glenoid may occur. This leads to a mechanical erosion and an occasional fracture of the surgical neck.

  5. Diagnosis is made by arthrography or MR. Arthrography is minimally invasive, requires about 15 minutes of physician time, and is highly accurate and cost-efficient if the clinician only wishes to know about the presence or absence of a complete RCT. With arthrography, the needle is placed in the GH joint and contrast normally enters the axillary and subscapularis bursae. *In the pres-*

ence of a tear, contrast enters the subacromial bursa, which com-municates with the subdeltoid bursa. Diagnosis may also be made either by ultrasound or MR.

6. *MR of the rotator cuff.* Sensitivity increases with use of T2-weighted fat saturated images.[24] *The most easily missed tears are of the supraspinatus at its anterior-most insertion on the greater tuberosity.* To find these, make sure to evaluate the more anterior coronal oblique MR cuts, as far anteriorly as the bicipital tendon (Fig 3-26). The presence of *high signal intensity within the tendon on short-TE images (proton density) is sensitive for rotator cuff disease, but not specific. It may be caused by tendon degeneration, the magic angle effect, or normal fat between muscle bundles.*[21,25] *A RCT is more specifically diagnosed with increased signal intensity on T2-weighted images.* The size and location of the tear, the integrity of the remaining tendon tissue, and the degree of muscle atrophy are valuable parameters in surgical planning and should be included in the report. Rarely, an RCT will not show increased T2 signal, presumably due to obliteration of the defect by scar tissue. Positioning the arm in full abduction, external rotation may increase sensitivity for partial tears on the undersurface of the infraspinatus.[26] MR arthrography may further increase sensitivity, both for RCT and other abnormalities relating to instability (inject 0.1 ml gadolinium dilated in 20 ml sterile saline for a total of 15 cc in shoulder).

H. *Shoulder impingement syndrome.*

1. *Impingement of the greater tuberosity and soft tissues on the cora-coacromial ligamentous and osseous arch, generally during abduction of the arm. This requires clinical diagnosis.*

2. May be reproduced under fluoroscopy with abduction, external rotation, or elevation of the humerus, eliciting a sharp pain.

3. Seen in young patients as well as older patients.

4. Presentation similar to that of a RCT.

5. May progress to tendinitis or RCT.

6. The variant os acromiale (unfused acromial ossification center) has been associated with impingement syndrome. Additionally, *anatomic variations in the acromion can lead to inflammation of the subacromial-subdeltoid bursa and to tendon degeneration and tear.* Three types of acromion process have been described, based on the morphology of the undersurface: Type I is flat, type II is gently curved, and type III is hooked anteriorly. The *hooked acromion,* an acromion with an *inferior spur,* or an acromion that *slopes downward* either laterally (seen on coronal views) or anteriorly (seen on sagittal views) may result in impingement syndrome.

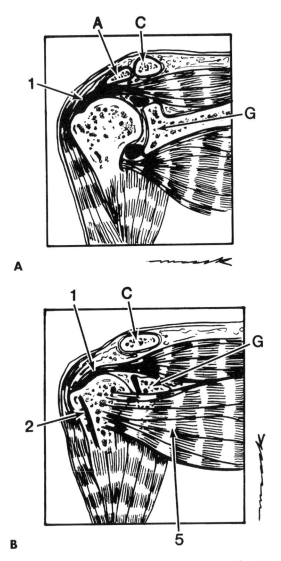

Fig. 3-26 Coronal oblique images of the supraspinatus tendon in its mid-portion (**A**) and anterior-most insertion (**B**). Confirmation of the integrity of the rotator cuff can be sought with the lateral oblique sagittal images, where the cuff forms a low signal "horseshoe" (**C**).

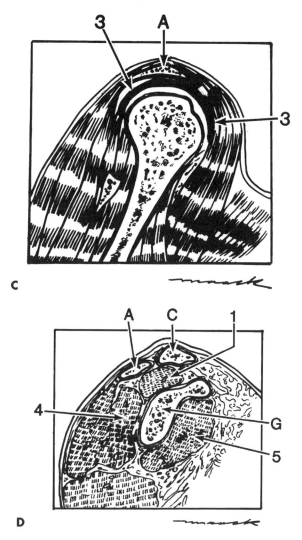

Fig. 3-26   *(continued)* More medially on the sagittal images, one sees the Y portion of the scapula and the muscle bellies of the rotator cuff (**D**). G, glenoid; A, acromion; C, clavicle; *1,* supraspinatus tendon; *2,* long head biceps; *3,* rotator cuff "horseshoe;" *4,* infraspinatus; *5,* subscapularis.

A cautionary note however: apparent acromial shape is sensitive to minor changes in radiographic technique and MR section viewed, and even then shows considerable interobserver variability.[27,28] Actual measurement of an acromial angle on the arch view (intersection of lines drawn along the inferior cortex of the anterior and posterior portions of the acromion) is more reliable in identifying patients with primary impingement (more than 27 degrees correlates with impingement).[29] Acromioclavicular joint osteoarthritis may also impinge on the supraspinatus tendon. Finally, hypertrophy of the supraspinatus muscle itself, seen in a very muscular individual, may cause impingement even with normal osseous anatomy.

7. Surgical procedures for impingement include acromionectomy, horizontal acromioplasty, and sectioning of various soft tissue constraints.

8. Another type of impingement, posterosuperior glenoid impingement, is described as a cause of posterior shoulder pain in throwing athletes. Bone marrow edema and subchondral cyst formation are common MR findings, located deep to the infraspinatus tendon insertion. Infraspinatus tears and fraying are occasionally found, along with supraspinatus tears. MR arthrography with the shoulder imaged with the arm in abduction and external rotation may show subtle infraspinatus flaps or imbibation of contrast.[30]

I. *Biceps tendon pathology.*

1. Long head has a complex course, arising at the superior glenoid labrum (where it is intimately associated with the SGHL), then passing intra-articularly to the bicipital groove; it is retained in the groove by supraspinatus and subscapularis fibers, as well as the coracohumeral ligament.

2. *At its origin on the labrum, the biceps tendon may be avulsed or torn as part of a SLAP lesion* (see Section J).

3. In its *intra-articular portion,* the biceps tendon is *subject to articular processes,* including inflammation, degeneration, and impingement (especially if there is a rotator cuff tear, allowing elevation of the humeral head and impingement against the coracoacromial arch). This may result in biceps tendon hypertrophy, flattening, or rupture.

4. The bicipital tendon sheath may be distended with fluid (underlying tendon may or may not be normal): *Tenosynovitis.*

5. *Bicipital tendon rupture* is uncommon in the absence of rotator cuff disease; with rupture, there is *retraction* of the tendon through the bicipital groove, resulting in an "empty" groove on axial images and a clinically obvious muscular bulge; if the tendon

reattaches and fibroses in the groove, the diagnosis may be clinically occult and difficult by MR.[31]

6. *Bicipital tendon dislocation:* The bicipital tendon acts as one of the anterior shoulder stabilizers; *a dislocated tendon should alert one to other signs of anterior instability.* Conversely, if overlying stabilizers (especially the coracohumeral ligament) are disrupted, the tendon may dislocated. *Most dislocations are extra-articular,* with the tendon subluxing superficially to the subscapularis tendon. *If the subscapularis tendon is torn, the long head of the biceps will slip medially, deep to the subscapularis tendon and remain in an intra-articular position, immediately anterior to the glenoid labrum* (Fig 3-27). In either case, the bicipital groove is empty. The subscapularis may be completely ruptured, or may appear partially intact, held in place by superficial fibers attaching across the groove to the greater tuberosity.

J. *SLAP* lesion: *Injury to the superior glenoid labrum, biceps tendon, or labral-biceps complex, most commonly from a fall or throwing action.* Pain and instability may result. Four types are arthroscopically described.[32] Type I shows fraying of the glenoid labrum and intact biceps (11%); type II shows stripping of the superior labrum and biceps of the bony glenoid (41%); type III shows a bucket-handle tear of the labrum, with intact biceps anchor (33%); type IV shows a bucket-handle tear of the labrum, with the tear extending into the biceps tendon. MR is helpful, but diagnosis can be difficult, with normal variants of the superior labrum simulating labral injury, and the four types of SLAP lesions difficult to differentiate.

K. Compressive and entrapment neuropathies.

1. *Suprascapular nerve entrapment*[33]: The suprascapular nerve arises from the brachial plexus, passes through the scapular notch, enters the supraspinous fossa, and branches into the supraspinatus and infraspinatus nerves (the latter enters the infraspinatus fossa). Scapular fractures or mass lesions (usually ganglion cysts or cysts associated with labral tears) may compress the nerves at the various locations. Depending on the site of entrapment, weakness and atrophy of the supraspinatus and/or infraspinatus muscles is seen.

2. *Quadrilateral space syndrome*[34]: Axillary nerve compression in the space formed by the long head of the triceps medially, the teres minor superiorly, the teres major inferiorly, and the humerus laterally. Compression of the axillary nerve may result from fracture, mass lesions, or extreme abduction of the arm. Atrophy of the deltoid and teres minor may result.

L. *Proximal humerus fractures.*

1. Relatively common, especially in osteoporotic bones.

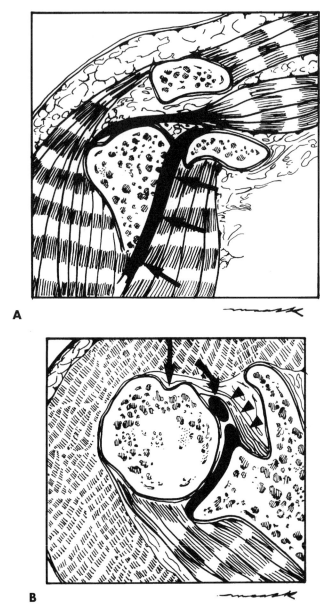

Fig. 3-27 Intra-articular biceps tendon dislocation. **A,** Far anterior oblique coronal, showing the origin of the long head biceps at the superior glenoid, and the medial displacement of the tendon (*arrows*). **B,** Axial image at the level of midglenoid, showing at the labrum, the medially displaced tendon (*curved arrow*), the empty bicipital groove (*straight arrow*), and subscapularis tendon (*arrowheads*), which appears intact through residual attachment of a few fibers crossing the groove to the greater tuberosity.

2. *Neer's four-segment classification* helps assess prognosis and guide treatment:
   a. Four segments are involved: Humeral head, humeral shaft, greater tuberosity, lesser tuberosity.
   b. When any of the segments is displaced more than 1 cm or angulated more than 45 degrees, it is considered significantly displaced.
   c. If one segment is displaced, it is termed a two-part fracture; a three-part fracture has two displaced segments, etc.
   d. If none of the fragments is significantly displaced or angulated, it is termed a nondisplaced fracture, no matter how comminuted it is.
   e. Eighty percent of proximal humeral fractures are nondisplaced. Fragments are held together by joint capsule, periosteum, and rotator cuff muscles.
   f. An axillary lateral film *must* be obtained since the apex anterior angulation is relatively common and is not evaluated by the other views.
3. *Pseudosubluxation of the shoulder* following such a fracture is temporary and is due to hemarthrosis and/or *atony* of the deltoid and rotator cuff muscles.
4. Skeletally immature baseball pitchers may develop repetitive stress-related injury to the proximal humeral physis, seen as a widening and irregularity of the epiphyseal plate; unilateral.
M. Humeral shaft.
   1. Deltoid tuberosity is a normal lateral cortical thickening extending approximately halfway down the shaft.
   2. Shaft fractures generally heal easily and rarely require internal fixation.
   3. Malunion is usually not significant since the shoulder is a ball-and-socket joint, which tolerates some degree of angular, as well as rotational, malalignment.

VI. PELVIC TRAUMA

Key Concepts

In pelvic trauma, all parameters outlined herein must be evaluated since pelvic fractures and dislocations may be extremely subtle. Judet views are very useful, and, for unstable injuries, CT is invaluable. Sacral fractures and/or sacroiliac (SI) joint dislocations are particularly hard to see. Single breaks in the pelvic ring or transverse process fracture at L_5 should alert one to the possibility of a sacral fracture or dislocation.

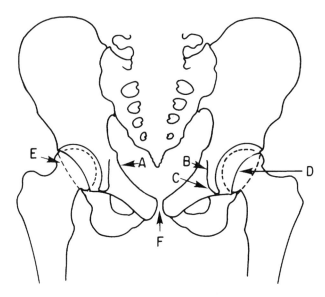

Fig. 3-28   AP pelvis. **A,** Iliopubic line. **B,** Ilioischial line. **C,** Teardrop. **D,** Anterior acetabular rim. **E,** Posterior acetabular rim. **F,** Symphysis pubis.

A. Anatomy: The pelvis is a ringlike structure formed by two arches.
   1. Major arch is posterior and superior, formed by the iliac wings and sacrum, joined at the SI joints.
   2. Smaller arch is anterior and inferior, formed by the pubic and ischial bones, joined at the pubic symphysis.
   3. Three centers of ossification join at the triradiate or Y cartilage of the acetabulum; they may be mistaken for fractures in skeletally immature patients.
   4. *AP:* In a trauma patient it must be demonstrated that the following structures are intact (Fig 3-28):
       a. Iliopubic line.
       b. Ilioischial line.
       c. Teardrop.
       d. Anterior acetabular rim.
       e. Posterior acetabular rim.
       f. Symphysis pubis.
       g. The sacrum, often obscured by bowel gas, must be observed carefully. The sacral foraminal lines should be checked for distortion, interruption, and asymmetry. A fractured L_5 transverse process particularly suggests an occult sacral fracture. The SI joints are normally wide in adolescents but should be only 2 to 4 mm wide in adults. An increase suggests disruption.

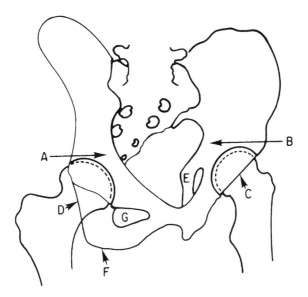

Figure 3-29   Judet (oblique) view of the pelvis. Note that the anterior oblique (*right side*) shows the anterior column and posterior acetabular rim best, while the posterior oblique (*left side*) shows the posterior column and anterior acetabular rim best. **A,** Anterior column and iliopubic line. **B,** Posterior column and ilioschial line. **C,** Anterior acetabular rim. **D,** Posterior acetabular rim. **E,** Ischial spine. **F,** Ischial tuberosity. **G,** Obturator foramen.

    h. The symphysis pubis width may be up to 10 mm in adolescents but is no more than 5 mm in adults. Increased width indicates disruption, as does superior displacement. (Superior displacement of up to 2 mm is normal if the inferior pubic rami remain symmetrically placed.)

5. Judet: The lateral pelvis is divided into anterior and posterior columns. These columns are not easily differentiated on the AP film but are important to distinguish for reasons of treatment and prognosis. Lateral films are impractical because of overlap of structures; 45-degree oblique, or Judet, views are substituted (Fig 3-29), which show the critical anatomy exceptionally well. Note that the posterior (or external) oblique shows the *posterior* column and *anterior* acetabular rim, while the anterior (or internal) oblique shows the *anterior* column and the *posterior* acetabular rim. The SI joints and iliac wings may also be seen to better advantage. Also check the following:

    a. Femoral head subluxation or dislocation (usually posteriorly).

      b. Disruption in dome (superior, weight-bearing portion) of acetabulum.

      c. Medial migration of femoral head (indicating a medial wall acetabular fracture).

   6. CT:

      a. Should not be used routinely in stable pelvic fractures because of cost and radiation concerns but is particularly useful in evaluation for sacral, SI joint fracture-dislocations.

      b. It is also useful in a search for intra-articular loose bodies after acetabular fracture or hip dislocation.

      c. CT has been shown to upgrade the designation of trauma severity in 30% of unstable pelvic fractures[35] over AP film findings. This usually involves demonstration of severe comminution or displacement at the SI joint, demonstration of occult SI joint or sacral injuries, or demonstration of extension of a fracture into the acetabulum. However, even though "severity" of fractures may be upgraded by CT, good plain films, especially in conjunction with Judet or inlet/outlet views, result in only rare misdiagnoses of pelvic fractures. The addition of CT only rarely alters patient management.[36]

B. Sacral fractures.

   1. Isolated traumatic sacral fractures usually are transverse and result from a direct blow.

   2. When they are a part of complex pelvic trauma, sacral fractures are usually vertical, interrupting the sacral foramina and neural arches.

   3. Sacral stress or insufficiency fractures due to osteoporosis are vertical and seen as a dense line, generally extending parallel to the SI joint. They are extremely difficult to see, and a large percentage are missed. They are picked up more frequently by bone scan or CT.

C. Pubic fractures.

   1. Ischiopubic synchondrosis: Usually fuse by 12 to 13 years; bulbous, irregular, and asymmetric so may be confused with neoplasm or healing fracture.

   2. Insufficiency fractures of the superior and inferior pubic rami are common in osteopenic patients. In the presence of osteoporosis, the pubic fractures may become expanded and appear aggressive or neoplastic. In osteomalacia, the pubic rami often develop wide, lucent Looser's zones.

   3. Stress fracture: Occurs at the junction of the pubis and ischium, often during a marathon run. Females more likely to be affected than males.

D. Apophyseal avulsion injuries.

   1. Four apophyses: Appear by puberty, fuse by age 25.

a. Crest of ilium, ending in anterior superior iliac spine (origin of sartorius muscle).

b. Anterior inferior iliac spine (origin of rectus femoris muscle).

c. Ischial tuberosity (origin of hamstring muscle).

d. Inferior pubic ramus (at symphysis, origin of adductor muscle).

2. Generally, avulsion results in amorphous bone formation between the pelvis and avulsed fragment, which gradually matures. In the early stages, this ossification may give the appearance of an osteosarcoma.

3. Adductor avulsion injuries of the pubis generally cause sclerosis and widening of one side of the symphysis but can also be seen bilaterally. This may simulate neoplasm or infection.

E. Stable pelvic fractures.

1. Two thirds of pelvic fractures.

2. Single breaks or breaks along the peripheral margins (i.e., avulsion, iliac wing fracture, sacral fracture, or ischiopubic rami).

F. Unstable pelvic fracture-dislocation.

1. One third of pelvic trauma.

2. Involves pelvic disruption in two places or more (double vertical fracture-dislocation).

a. Most common is vertical shear or Malgaigne; this usually consists of a sacral fracture plus ipsilateral superior and inferior pubic rami fractures. Variants include iliac wing fracture, SI joint disruption, and symphysis pubis disruption.

b. Another form, the straddle fracture, involves both superior and inferior pubic rami on both sides.

3. These unstable fractures are associated with a significant risk of visceral injury and hemorrhage, and often require internal fixation.

4. With unstable pelvic fracture-dislocation, it is common to get an ''open-book'' disruption of the posterior ring (i.e., loss of the normal angulation of the sacrum with the iliac wings and resultant anterior ring diastasis).

5. On the AP view, the iliac wings may appear asymmetric, one being broader and flatter than the other. The true extent of the ''open-book'' disruption is best seen by CT (Fig 3-30). The degree of this open-book displacement, as well as the amount of cephalocaudad displacement, are indicators of stability and prognosis. If these fractures are not reconstructed internally, change in these parameters must be sought in follow-up films.

6. Pelvic fractures may also be classified according to mechanism and direction of injury, a concept that is useful in management

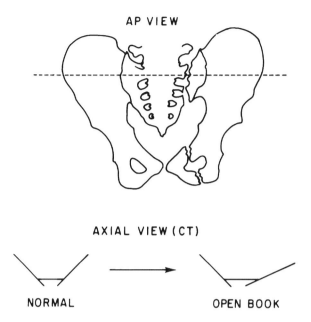

Fig. 3-30   "Open-book" disruption in a vertical shear fracture. The degree of angular asymmetry of the iliac wings may be difficult to assess on AP film (*top*). The difference between the axial view on normal CT (*left*) and CT with fracture and "open-book" displacement (*right*) is much more obvious.

of life-threatening hemorrhage that may be associated with the injury.[37]

a. Lateral compression: The essential elements include horizontal fractures through the pubic rami and crush or buckle fracture of the acetabulum, involving at least the medial wall (type 1); a type 2 variant is described where the lateral compressive force is located more anteriorly, which causes the ipsilateral iliac wing to rotate internally, either disrupting the posterior SI ligaments or extending a fracture through the posterior iliac wing:

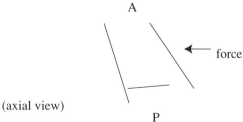

With greater force, a type 3 lateral compression pattern develops, in which there is internal rotation on the side ipsilateral to the force and disruption of the SI joints with external rotation on the contralateral side:

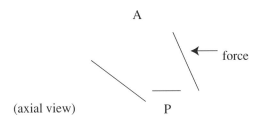

(axial view)

There is a relatively low incidence of significant arterial hemorrhage in lateral compression injury, with the exception of type 3.

b. Anterior-Posterior (A-P) compression: The essential elements include vertical pubic ramus fractures at its simplest (type 1), but with greater force may show symphysis pubis diastasis and disruption of the anterior sacroiliac ligaments (type 2, the classic "open-book" injury); greater A-P force causes complete disruption of both the anterior and posterior pelvis (type 3), with wide diastasis of the symphysis pubis and both anterior and posterior SI ligament disruptions, as well as sacrospinous and sacrotuberous ligament disruption, resulting in not only external rotation but also upward rotation of the hemipelvis; posterior column acetabular fractures are common in type 3 injuries; likelihood of arterial hemorrhage is high in either type 2 or 3.

c. Vertical shear: Due to superior-inferior forces, resulting in vertical fractures of the pubic rami and posterior wing (iliac wing or SI joint/sacrum). The injury may be significantly unstable, with separation and superior migration of the lateral hemipelvic fragment. There is a high incidence of pelvic bleeding.

d. Combined mechanical injury: No single dominant vector.

7. Assessment must therefore include direction of instability (superior-inferior, A-P, external or internal rotation, diastasis), assessment of both anterior and posterior SI ligament disruption, and evaluation for acetabular injury or hip dislocation. Type 3 lateral compression, types 2 and 3 A-P compression, and vertical shear injuries may result in life-threatening pelvic bleeding. Hemodynamically unstable patients often require immediate arterio-

grams and embolization (even prior to CT), so plain film indicators of unstable pelvic fractures should be sought in these patients. Patients who are not hemodynamically unstable can often be treated with external fixation; this stabilization may reduce bleeding and eliminate the need for arteriograms.

G. Acetabular fractures: The most commonly used classification system is Letournet-Judet. This classification system is based on understanding the anterior and posterior columns of the acetabulum. Ten fracture patterns are described in the classification system, but five of them comprise 90% of the fractures seen. These five include posterior rim fractures (17%), transverse acetabular fractures (10%), both anterior and posterior column fractures (29%), transverse-posterior wall fractures (19%), and transverse T-shaped fractures (13%). A reasonable approach is to differentiate between column fractures (which usually end up being both columns), wall fractures, and transverse fractures (which will be one of the three types: transverse, transverse T, and transverse posterior wall). One must carefully evaluate the obturator ring, the posterior rim, the iliac wing, and both the iliopectineal and ilioischial lines. Fracture orientation and comminution, of course, should be evaluated. The following hints may be useful:

1. If the obturator ring is broken, it is either a T or a column fracture.
2. With an oblique fracture of the iliac wing, there is always an anterior column fracture, but often a both-column fracture.
3. The ''spur'' sign, seen on the obturator oblique view as a spur of bone located just superior to the acetabulum at its posterior aspect, indicates a posterior column fracture. This may be very subtle.
4. On axial CT, if the main fracture plane is sagittal, then the fracture is transverse. If the main fracture plain is coronal, then you have a column (usually both-column) fracture. An oblique fracture usually indicates an acetabular rim fracture.

VII. HIP TRAUMA

Key Concepts

Subcapital fractures in the elderly may be extremely subtle but are common and must be suspected. Hip dislocations in the presence of other trauma are easily overlooked and, if unreduced for 24 hours, are complicated by AVN. Hip pain in an adolescent should prompt a search for the subtle changes of slipped capital femoral epiphysis.

A. Anatomy.
   1. AP film must show the hip in slight internal rotation. This allows

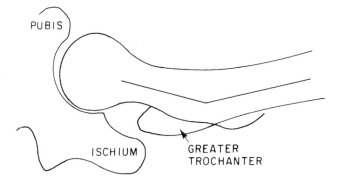

PUBIS

ISCHIUM

GREATER
TROCHANTER

Fig. 3-31   Groin lateral view of the hip, demonstrating the normal anatomy and the normal neck-shaft anteversion.

the neck of the femur to be elongated, the greater trochanter to be seen in profile, and the lesser trochanter (a posteromedial structure) to be less prominent. The normal femoral neck-shaft angle is 115 to 140 degrees.

2. Frog-leg lateral film superimposes the superior border of the greater trochanter over the femoral neck, simulating an impacted fracture line. It is, however, a useful view to confirm a subcapital fracture, AVN, or slipped capital femoral epiphysis.

3. Groin lateral is true lateral (Fig 3-31). The normal neck-shaft anteversion angle is 125 to 130 degrees.

4. Oblique view of the pelvis (Judet) is useful to evaluate acetabular fracture or a dislocated hip. The internal oblique shows the posterior acetabular rim, and the external oblique shows the anterior acetabular rim (see Fig 3-29).

5. Soft tissues: Bulging fat planes may represent a hip effusion, but they are not always present or symmetric. They also require a prefectly positioned patient (external rotation or flexion of a hip causes a false-positive bulging of the fat planes). The three fat planes are iliopsoas, gluteal, and obturator internus. More reliable indicators of effusion may be an increased distance from the teardrop medially, or from the superior acetabulum; in the absence of trauma, a symptomatic hip with evidence of effusion must be emergently aspirated to rule out infection.

6. Normal variant: Herniation pit. This is an ovoid well-marginated defect in the superolateral quadrant of the femoral neck, located anteriorly. Its appearance and typical location should differentiate it from pathological processes.

B. Epidemiology.
   1. Hip fractures are rare in young and middle-aged patients but extremely common in the elderly owing to senile osteoporosis[38]: By age 80, 10% of Caucasian females and 5% of Caucasian males fracture a hip; by age 90, 20% of Caucasian females and 10% of Caucasian males fracture a hip.
   2. Subcapital fractures are twice as common as intertrochanteric fractures.
   3. Femoral neck fractures resulting from falls are highly associated with distal radius and proximal humeral fractures in the elderly.
C. Femoral neck fractures.
   1. Basicervical: Rare; nonunion is a relatively common complication.
   2. Transcervical: Rare.
   3. Subcapital:
      a. Common.
      b. May be impacted or displaced, complete or incomplete.
      c. May be as obvious as a change in angulation or disrupted or angulated trabeculae, or as subtle as a line of increased density (impaction) or an irregularity confined to the lateral cortex at the junction of the head and neck.
      d. Ring osteophytes seen on the AP film or the superior border of the greater trochantar seen on a frog-leg film may be mistaken for a sclerotic impaction fracture line.
      e. If the plain film is not diagnostic for a suspected subcapital fracture, a single coronal T1-weighted or STIR MR sequence may be a cost-effective diagnostic tool. Accuracy is extremely high, and the MR sensitivity is not affected by patient age or osteoporosis, as a bone scan might be.
      f. Garden classification system.
         (1) Stage I—incomplete fracture of the lateral trabeculae.
         (2) Stage II—complete nondisplaced fracture.
         (3) Stage III—complete fracture with partial displacement (mild varus, distal fragment externally rotated); trabeculae of fragments are not aligned.
         (4) Stage IV—complete displacement, with distal fragment externally rotated and proximally displaced with apex varus angulation.
      g. Twenty-five percent to 30% of Garden stage III or IV subcapital fractures have appearance of a lytic lesion at the superolateral portion of the neck due to the rotation and angulation of the fracture; these should not be misinterpreted as pathologic.[39]
      h. If incomplete or impacted in a reliable patient, a subcapital fracture may be treated conservatively with bed rest. Other-

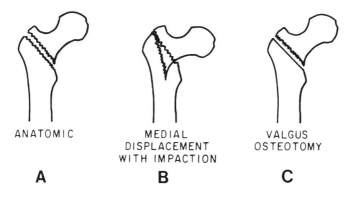

ANATOMIC   MEDIAL   VALGUS
                DISPLACEMENT   OSTEOTOMY
                WITH IMPACTION

A   **B**   **C**

Fig. 3-32 Positions accepted for reduction of an intertrochanteric fracture: **A,** Anatomic. **B,** Medial displacement (of the shaft) with impaction (of the medial spike on the proximal fragment). **C,** Valgus osteotomy.

wise, Knowles pinning is the most common procedure. Depending on the patient's condition and the appearance of the fracture, primary endoprosthesis placement may be elected.

 i. AVN is a complication in 8% to 30% of subcapital fractures.[40]

D. Intertrochanteric fractures.

 1. Common fracture, generally in older age group than subcapital fractures.

 2. Two-, three-, or four-part, depending on involvement of greater and lesser trochanters.

  a. The area of greatest comminution is posteriomedial, in the regions of the calcar and lesser trochanter. The large defect in this region is seen best on a groin lateral film.

  b. The oblique fracture usually angles from the greater trochanter superiorly to the lesser trochanter inferiorly. The reverse diagonal is rare but more unstable.

 3. Fixation.

  a. Usually internally fixed with a sliding or dynamic screw. This allows settling with impaction up to a point. If settling continues before the fracture heals, the screw head cuts out of the osteoporotic femoral head and neck.

  b. The optimal placement of the head of the screw is slightly posterior and inferior in the femoral head, with the tip approximately 6 mm from the articular surface. The screw head specifically should *not* be anterior or superior.

  c. Three common positions are accepted for reduction (Fig 3-32).

(1) Anatomic: If the posteromedial comminution is not severe.

(2) Medial impaction: The shaft is medially displaced and impacted on the spike of the proximal fragment; this gives stability at the expense of a minor loss of length.

(3) Valgus: Osteotomy to reduce shear and thereby stabilize the fracture.

4. AVN is rare in intertrochanteric fractures. The major complications are instability and cutting out of the hardware as the pattern of fixation collapses into a varus configuration in the osteoporotic patient.

E. Avulsion fracture of the lesser trochanter.

1. Not uncommon in children or adolescents, as avulsion of the apophysis by the iliopsoas.

2. If it is found as an isolated fracture in adults, it is usually due to underlying bone pathology (metastatic disease).

F. Femoral shaft fracture.

1. May be fixed internally by compression plate, with or without cerclage wire if highly comminuted.

2. Intramedullary (IM) rod may be used if the fracture is not highly comminuted and does not have a large butterfly fragment. Successful use of an IM rod depends on its filling the width of the medullary canal to stabilize a fracture. If the fracture is at the proximal or distal third (where the canal flares), rotational stability may be lost unless the rod is fixed with an interlocking screw.

3. In evaluating an IM rod, check for distraction of the major fracture fragments, progressive shortening with migration of the rod, and rotation of the fragments.

G. Stress fracture of the femur.

1. In the proximal or midshaft, it usually involves the medial cortex.

2. In the distal third of the shaft, it usually involves the posterior cortex.

3. Stress fractures also occur in the medial femoral neck, just proximal to the lesser trochanter. These present as vague hip or groin pain. If suspected but equivocal on x-ray, MR should be used for confirmation. Continued athletic activity can result in fracture propagation requiring internal fixation.

4. Vertical stress fractures of the femur have been described. These can be quite subtle on plain film and show a confusing marrow edema pattern on MR, but are straightforward on CT with reconstruction.

H. Hip dislocation.

1. A rare result of severe trauma.

2. Often associated with femoral shaft fracture. The dislocation may

be overlooked clinically because of the discomfort of the obvious shaft fracture. It may be overlooked radiographically as well unless a pelvic film is obtained.

3. Posterior dislocation is most common (approximately 90%). The head is usually located superiorly and is held in internal rotation. There is usually an associated posterior acetabular rim fracture. If the dislocation is directly posterior, it may be more difficult to recognize on the AP film: a lack of congruence of the head with the acetabulum may aid in determining diagnosis. Alternatively, the femoral heads may appear to be different sizes: the smaller one is less magnified, closer to the film, and therefore, posterior.

4. In the rare anterior hip dislocation, the head is usually found overlying the obturator foramen.

5. Early diagnosis is imperative since a delay in reduction sharply increases the probability of AVN (approaching 50% if unreduced for 24 hours).

6. After reduction, the hip joint should be studied closely for an increase in teardrop width. Such an increase may indicate the presence of retained fracture fragments, which is easily confirmed with CT. Additionally, impaction fractures may be seen on the femoral head (analogous to the Hill-Sachs lesion in the humeral head after shoulder dislocation). Avulsion fractures of the ligamentum teres may be seen intra-articularly. Posterior acetabular rim fractures are relatively common.

I. Slipped capital femoral epiphysis (SCFE).

1. Epidemiology:

a. Usually 10 to 16 years old. Rarely, it may be seen in younger children in the presence of infection, severe trauma, congenital hip dislocation, or rickets.

b. Males are more often affected than females.

c. Blacks are more often affected than Caucasians.

d. Obese persons are more often affected than nonobese persons.

e. Bilateral (20%) but rarely symmetric.

2. SCFE occurs during the years of rapid growth, which is also the stage at which the femoral neck configuration changes from valgus to varus. This introduces the factor of shear stress in a growth plate weakened by rapid growth; minor trauma may therefore precipitate SCFE.

3. Radiographic appearance on AP film (Fig 3-33) (SCFE is almost always posteromedial):

a. The epiphyseal plate appears wider, with less distinct margins.

b. The epiphysis itself appears shorter.

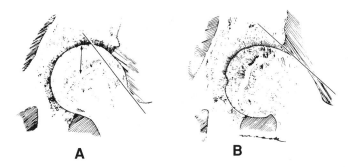

Fig. 3-33 AP of a normal hip (**A**) and slipped capital femoral epiphysis (**B**) showing the medial displacement and "shortening" of the epiphysis, and "widening" of the epiphyseal plate. A line drawn along the lateral aspect of the femoral neck usually intersects a portion of femoral head (**A**) but often does not intersect the femoral head in a slipped capital femoral epiphysis (**B**).

      c. A line drawn along the lateral femoral neck may intersect a smaller portion (or none) of the femoral head.

      d. A frog-leg lateral or groin lateral confirms the findings.

    4. Treated by pinning in situ; this yields a varus deformity with a short, broad femoral head.

    5. Complications.

      a. DJD: Surprisingly, a late occurrence, often 30 years later.

      b. AVN: In about 10%; the probability is greater with open reduction, acute severe slips, and attempted repositioning.

      c. Chondrolysis: Acute disappearance of cartilage in SCFE, chondrolysis has been associated with pin penetration through the articular cortex. In one study, chondrolysis was seen more often in black girls with SCFE; chondrolysis is also seen idiopathically. The differential diagnosis is infection.

J. MR considerations at the hip.

    1. AVN (see full discussion in Chapter 2, AVN).

    2. Cancellous bone of the femur and hip contains marrow; MR signal characteristics depend on the predominant marrow type, which, in turn, depends on patient age:

      a. Birth—red marrow throughout femur except the nonossified epiphysis.

      b. Child—fatty marrow forms within the epiphyses, and, with age, begins to replace the red marrow of the diaphysis; metaphyses retain red marrow.

      c. Adolescence through adulthood—fatty marrow in diaphysis and epiphysis; first replaces red marrow in the distal metaphysis and gradually replaces red marrow in the proximal femoral metaphysis; generally, red marrow predominates in the proximal metaphysis under age 50, and fatty marrow over age 50; it may present as an inhomogeneous pattern in the proximal femoral metaphysis, which should not be mistaken for tumor.

   3. MR arthrography of the hip: Abnormalities of the labrum may be detected, which may be helpful in patients with chronic hip pain of undetermined etiology; osteochondral defects may be seen as well; beware of the large variability in the appearance of a normal labrum.[41]

K. "Snapping hip"[42,43]: Coxa Saltans, external type, is due to a thickened, iliotibial band or the anterior edge of the gluteus maximus snapping over the greater trochanter; intra-articular type may be diagnosed by MR arthrography (see Section J-3); internal type is due to the iliopsoas snapping over the femoral head and capsule as the hip moves from flexion to extension; internal and external types are usually diagnosed clinically, but, occasionally, iliopsoas bursography is used to evaluate the internal type; the needle is placed as for hip arthrography (superomedial part of femoral neck), then retracted 5 to 10 mm and contrast is injected into the iliopsoas bursa.

VIII. KNEE TRAUMA

Key Concepts

Most knee injuries involve soft tissues and show only effusion on plain film. A fat-blood level in suprapatellar pouch demands a careful search for intracapsular fracture. Meniscal anatomy is somewhat complex; this must be borne in mind when interpreting knee arthrograms or MR studies. Knee dislocations have commonly associated arterial injury.

A. Soft tissues in knee trauma.
   1. On lateral film, the fat pad posterior to the quadriceps tendon is divided into anterior and posterior compartments by a soft tissue density, the suprapatellar bursa.
      a. In the absence of effusion, the suprapatellar bursa is less than 5 mm wide.
      b. Suprapatellar lipohemarthrosis indicates an intracapsular fracture, which may be occult.
B. Femoral condyle.
   1. If intra-articular femoral condylar fracture is present, patient is at risk for AVN.
   2. Osteochondritis dissecans.

  a. Etiology uncertain but possibly due to repeated minor trauma.

  b. Most often involves lateral portion of medial femoral condyle but other sites are seen as well.

  c. Most common in adolescents and young adults.

  d. Arthrography demonstrates whether the overlying cartilage is intact; MR may assess this as well (see Chapter 2, Osteochondritis dissecans).

  e. Normal variants in children: In 3- to 6-year-olds, the femoral epiphysis is normally irregular, especially medially. In 10- to 13-year-olds, a femoral condylar irregularity is found on both condyles posteriorly (seen best on a notch view); it is bilateral, asymptomatic, and resolves with maturity. Neither of these entities should be mistaken for osteochondritis dissecans or an erosive arthropathy.

 3. Spontaneous osteonecrosis: An entity distinct from osteochondritis dissecans; affects an older adult age group. Pain is a much more striking feature; found on the medial femoral condyle, but more medial and superior than osteochondritis dissecans; subchondral lucency with subsequent flattening; 75% have associated torn medial meniscus.

C. Tibial fracture.

 1. Tibial plateau fracture:

  a. Often seen in auto-pedestrian accidents since the plateau is at the height of fenders and bumpers.

  b. Eighty percent are limited to the lateral plateau since most result from a valgus stress.

  c. The tibial plateaus are sloped posteriorly 10 to 20 degrees. The AP knee film therefore is not tangential to the tibial joint surface.

  d. Anterior depressed fragments may be overlooked since the anterior margin is projected superior to the posterior margin. Similarly, the extent of posterior depressed fragments may be exaggerated.

  e. Oblique films may be necessary for the initial diagnosis. MR or CT with reconstruction may be required to establish the extent of tibial plateau depression.

  f. In general, depression greater than 1 cm or widely separated (5 mm) vertical split fractures require internal fixation.

 2. Anterior tibial tubercle apophysis: May have multiple ossification centers and appear fragmented. The osteonecrosis Osgood-Schlatters disease should be suggested only in the presence of fragmentation, soft tissue swelling, and pain.

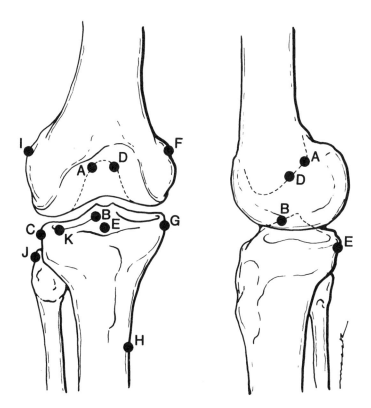

Fig. 3-34 Avulsion sites around the knee: (**A**) ACL origin. (**B**) ACL insertion. (**C**) Lateral capsular attachment. (**D**) PCL origin. (**E**) PCL insertion. (**F**) MCL origin. (**G**) MCL insertion of deep fibers. (**H**) MCC insertion of superficial fibers. (**I**) LCL origin. (**J**) LCL insertion. (**K**) Gerdy's tubercle, insertion of iliotibial band. (Reprinted with permission from Manaster BJ, Andrews CL. *Fractures and dislocations of the knee and proximal tibia and fibula.* Sem Roent. 1994·:113–133.)

3. Anterior tibial spine fracture (see Fig 3-34 for osseous avulsion sites around the knee).
   a. Adjacent to the site of origin of anterior cruciate ligament (ACL) so may be avulsed.
   b. More common in children and adolescents than adults.
   c. May appear hinged, completely detached, or inverted.
4. Avulsion of the posterior cruciate ligament (PCL) may result in avulsion of a sliver of bone from the posterior tibia near the plateau.
5. Lateral capsular sign: Avulsed sliver of bone from the lateral proximal tibia, at site of capsular insertion. Sign associated with ACL

tear. Also termed Segond fracture. Another avulsion fracture may be found more anteriorly at the lateral tibial joint line. Gerdy's tubercle may be avulsed here by the attached iliotibial band. Differentiation between this and the Segond fracture should be made.

6. Proximal fibular fracture or dislocation.
    a. Dislocation is rare.
    b. Normally, the fibular head is located posterolateral to the tibia, so there is slight overlap of the two on both AP and lateral films.
    c. Injury may involve peroneal nerve.
    d. Site of insertion of the lateral collateral ligament, so may be avulsed.

7. Stress fracture.
    a. Common in the proximal tibial shaft.
        (1) Early, may see faint transverse or oblique lucency within the posterior cortex of the proximal tibial shaft.
        (2) Later, may see transverse band of density and callus formation along the posterior (not anterior) cortex.
        (3) Radiographic lag of 2 to 6 weeks.
    b. Ballet dancers and basketball players develop stress fractures in the anterior cortex of the midshaft of the tibia; multiple, partial stress fractures at various stages of healing may be seen.

8. Trampoline fracture: Pediatric fracture, incomplete, due to impaction; located at the proximal tibial metaphysis, anteriorly.

9. Toddler's fracture: Tibial diaphyseal spiral fracture, usually without a specific history of injury, and often difficult to identify on plain film.

10. Stress-related epiphyseal plate injury: Seen in skeletally immature joggers, where repeated stress causes widening and irregularity of the epiphyseal plate. Locations include distal femur, proximal tibia, and distal fibula/tibia.

D. Epiphyseal injury.
    1. Occurrence is relatively rare about the knee, but complications are frequent.
    2. Salter 2: 70%.
    3. Salter 3: 15%: These usually involve the medial condyle and are due to valgus stress. They are undisplaced and often occult. Oblique or valgus stress films are helpful.
    4. The knee is the most common site of Salter 5 fractures: They usually are seen in the proximal tibia, associated with tibial shaft fractures.
    5. A disproportionately large number of significant growth disturbances stem from epiphyseal injuries about the knee, despite the

rarity of epiphyseal injury. Therefore, the prognosis should be guarded, and early diagnosis of bony bridging across the epiphysis should be actively sought. If not obvious by plain films, these bony bars may be diagnosed and even mapped for resection by MR or CT with reconstruction.

E. Patellar trauma.

  1. Patellar fracture:

    a. Sixty percent are transverse, through the midportion. These are due to an indirect force (violent pull of the quadriceps tendon). The transverse fractures may or may not be distracted, depending on whether the medial and lateral retinacula are intact.

    b. Twenty-five percent are stellate, due to direct trauma.

    c. Vertical much less common.

    d. Bipartite or multipartite patella: The fragments are found on the superolateral border and have well-corticated margins. They are frequently, but not invariably, bilateral. The margins of the bipartite patella often appear unmatched at the articular surface.

    e. Dorsal defect of the patella: A rounded lucency on the articular (dorsal) side of the patella is a normal variant, not to be confused with osteochondritis dissecans, and is difficult to differentiate from an erosion.

    f. Osteochondral (flake) fracture: Usually from the medial facet, associated with lateral patellar dislocation and seen on the sunrise view.

  2. Patellar dislocation: Usually lateral; tendency for patellar tracking abnormalities is defined by patellar tilt, lateral patellar displacement (Fig 3-35), and patella alta.

    a. Study of choice is the *sunrise* view: Obtained with the knees flexed 20 degrees. (With more flexion, the patella becomes engaged in the patellofemoral groove, and subtle abnormalities in alignment are not detected.)

    b. In most cases, the lateral facet is slightly longer than the medial facet.

    c. Patella alta: Elongation of the infrapatellar tendon associated with recurrent subluxation. On the lateral flexed (20 to 30 degrees) view of the knee, the ratio of the infrapatellar tendon length (from the inferior pole of the patella to the anterior tibial tubercle) to the length of the patella is 1.0 ± 0.2. If this ratio is greater than 1.2 patella alta exists.

F. Knee dislocation.

  1. Anterior dislocation is more common than posterior or mediolateral.

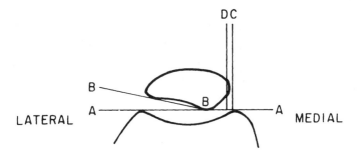

Fig. 3-35 Sunrise view, obtained to evaluate patellar tilt or displacement. *A-A* and *B-B* form an angle that normally is open laterally. If the angle is open medially, this constitutes patellar tilt. *Line C* is perpendicular to *A-A* at the tip of the medial femoral condyle. *Line D* is 1 mm lateral to *line C* (*line D* normally intersects the medial patella). If the patella is lateral to *line D,* it is laterally displaced and subject to subluxation; this position occurs in 30% of patients with condromalacia patellae.

2. Thirty percent have an associated arterial injury (since the popliteal artery is fixed both proximal and distal to the knee joint), so arteriography is mandatory.
3. Cruciate ligaments, collateral ligaments, and the peroneal nerve are often injured as well.
G. Soft tissue injury to the knee: Menisci:
   1. Function to increase the tibiofemoral contact area (properly distributing tibiofibular load), providing shock absorption across the knee, lubrication, and passive stabilization.
   2. Meniscus is at risk for degenerative tear due to its structure, with a middle perforating bundle of horizontal fibers splitting the superior and inferior portions of the meniscus and located in the plane of shear stress; horizontal degenerative tears result.
   3. Menisci are attached to the joint capsule and are mobile, but differentially; with knee motion, the excursion of the posterior horns is not as great as that of the anterior horns, and the excursion of the posterior horn of the medial meniscus is less than that of the lateral meniscus posterior horn; it should not be surprising that the less mobile posterior horns are at greater risk for tear, and the medial meniscus more frequently than the lateral.
   4. MR criteria for meniscal tears: Direct-abnormal signal:
      a. Grade 1: Globular increased signal intensity in the central portion of the meniscus—no clinical significance.
      b. Grade 2: Linear increased signal intensity in the central portion

of the meniscus, not reaching the articular surface—no clinical significance.

c. Grade 3: Increased signal intensity within the meniscus that comes into contact with an articular surface—this is the only direct MR evidence of meniscal tear.

5. MR evidence for meniscal tear: Indirect—abnormal meniscal morphology (size, shape, or capsular attachments); to be aware of abnormal morphology of a meniscus, one must understand the normal variations in shape of different parts of the menisci.

   a. Normal menisci are semicircular in shape, attached around the periphery of the tibial plateau articular surface; the medial meniscus is slightly more C-shaped, while the lateral is more O-shaped (see top line drawing, Fig 3-36).

   b. The menisci taper from a height of 3 to 5 mm at the periphery to a sharp, thin central edge; therefore, they appear triangular in all radial and coronal MR sections and nearly all sagittal sections.

   c. The triangular lateral meniscus does not vary in size or shape in its anterior horns, body, or posterior horn.

   d. The medial meniscus has a predictable variability in its morphology: the body is the smallest portion, shaped as an equilateral triangle (Fig 3-36, A), the posterior horn is a much more elongated triangle (the largest of the sections of either meniscus, Fig 3-36, B), and the anterior horn is sized between these two.

   e. Menisci that do not correspond to these size criteria, or which have frayed or blunted edges, may be considered torn, but the positive predictive value for size and shape criteria alone is less than that of signal criteria alone; therefore, morphologic criteria are important but should be interpreted more cautiously than signal criteria.

   f. Sagittal MR sections may either show the separate anterior and posterior horns (Fig 3-36,E) or the "bowtie" configuration at the far peripheral portion of the meniscus (Fig 3-36,D), which includes part of the body as well as the anterior and posterior horns.

   g. The MR appearance of the lateral meniscus from the body around to the posterior horn is more complicated (Fig 3-36,C); the popliteal hiatus partially interrupts the meniscal attachment to the capsule; the popliteal tendon (arising on the lateral femoral condyle and coursing downward obliquely and medially to the tibia) traverses the popliteal hiatus, with discontinuous superior and inferior struts (fascicles) maintaining a meniscal

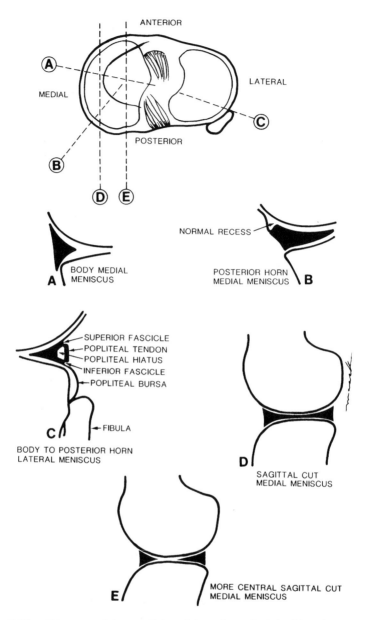

Fig. 3-36 Diagram of the medial and lateral menisci (looking down on the lateral tibial plateau). The labeled lines represent the various planes in which MR sequences are commonly taken. **A** and **B** represent radial planes through the body and posterior horn, respectively, of the medial meniscus. **C** represents a radial cut through the body or posterior horn of the lateral meniscus. **D** and **E** are sagittal cuts through the medial meniscus at different distances from the periphery. (Reprinted with permission from Manaster BJ. *Magnetic resonance imaging of the knee.* Seminars in US, CT and MR. 1990;307–326.)

attachment to the capsule; a torn strut with displaced meniscus should be sought in this region.

   h. Normal variant: Transverse ligament; this structure connects the anterior horns of the medial and lateral menisci and is seen far anteriorly on coronal images (Fig 3-37); it appears in cross-section immediately anterior to the anterior horn; at its confluence with the anterior horn of the lateral meniscus, it may be mistaken for a meniscal tear (Fig 3-37,*B*); follow the structure on adjacent cuts to the intercondylar notch to convince yourself that it is not an anterior horn tear.

   i. Normal variant: Superior recess of the posterior horn, medial meniscus; this smooth vertical recess is normally located only at the site (Fig 3-36,*B*) and should not be mistaken for a partial peripheral meniscal tear.

   j. Normal variant: The normal meniscocapsular junction has fibro-fatty tissue and a moderately high signal that should not be mistaken for a peripheral tear.

6. Discoid meniscus: A variant where the meniscus is abnormally large, approaching a circular shape:

   a. More common in the lateral meniscus.

   b. The body of the meniscus is larger and more elongated than usual.

   c. Easily seen on coronal or radial images; on the sagittal series, one will note the "bowtie" appearance over more than the usual 2 to 3 cuts.

   d. Discoid menisci develop tears easily; an adolescent with signs of knee locking should be evaluated carefully for a discoid meniscus and tear.

   e. If the discoid is partial, diagnosis is more difficult.

7. "Air" arthrogram may occur during MR; the air causes a signal void which "blooms" on gradient echo imaging and may simulate a meniscal tear or a loose body.

8. Types of meniscal tears:

   a. Horizontal cleavage: Degenerative, most common in the general population; oriented parallel to the tibial plateau.

   b. Vertical-radial tear: Perpendicular to the tibial plateau, extending in a radial direction from the central edge towards the meniscosynovial junction.

   c. Vertical-longitudinal tears: Perpendicular to the tibial plateau, propagating circumferentially along the AP extent of the meniscus (bucket handle and flap or parrot beak tears are subsets of this variety; a bucket handle tear has such a long cleavage that the central mobile fragment can sublux into the intercon-

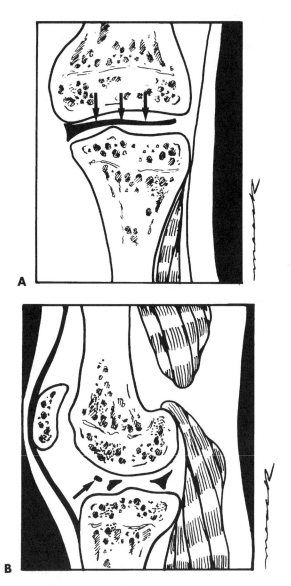

Fig. 3-37 Diagram of the transverse ligament. The structure connects the anterior horns of the medial and lateral mensisci, so is seen far anteriorly on the coronal view (**A,** *arrows*). The ligament is seen in cross-section in and near the intercondylar notch (**B,** *arrow*) and assumes a lentiform shape as it approaches the anterior horn of the lateral meniscus, sometimes simulating a tear (**C,** *arrow*).

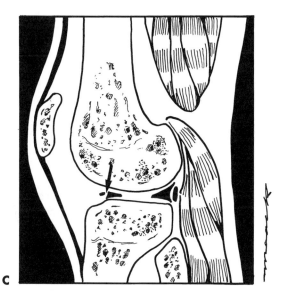

Fig. 3-37 *(continued)*

dylar notch, often interposed between the PCL and the tibial eminence, giving the appearance of a second PCL).

 d. Peripheral tear: Near the meniscocapsular junction.

 e. Complex tears: Different characteristics in different sites.

9. Accuracy: Some highly experienced readers show remarkably high accuracy rates, but more general experience is suggested by a large study including several different radiologists at different MR centers; average diagnostic accuracy in this study was about 90% for meniscal tears.[44] Many believe that the very high true negative rate of MR makes the exam cost-effective in eliminating unnecessary arthroscopy.

10. The equivocal meniscal tear—what to do?

 a. Require seeing the abnormality on more than one image.

 b. Require that the abnormal meniscal signal unequivocally extend to the free meniscal edge, rather than just approaching it.

 c. Do not overcall the various "dots, fissures, and clefts" encountered in both anterior and posterior horns close to the intercondylar notch.

11. Associated findings and statistics may help your accuracy with equivocal meniscal tears:

    a. Posterior horn more frequently injured than body, body is more frequently torn than anterior horn.

    b. Isolated anterior horn tears are rare, though more common in the lateral than the medial meniscus, especially in serious athletes.

    c. Isolated meniscal tears occur 3 to 4 times more frequently in the medial meniscus.

    d. Frequency of lateral meniscus injury increases in the presence of ligament injuries.

    e. Bone bruises often have ipsilateral meniscal injury.

    f. In the presence of ACL and MCL injuries, tears of the medial or lateral meniscus is common; the combination of ACL, MCL, and medial meniscus has been termed O'Donoghue's Terrible Triad; lateral meniscal injuries are actually more common than medial with this ligamentous combination due to the valgus force with external tibial rotation required.

12. Meniscal cysts: Synovial fluid collections that develop secondary to meniscal tears:

    a. Most cysts are parameniscal; true intrameniscal cysts are rare.

    b. Usually anterolateral, along the joint line, related to tears in the anterior horn lateral meniscus.

    c. The less common medial meniscal cyst may dissect into soft tissues distant from the meniscus, making diagnosis difficult.

13. MR evaluation of the postoperative meniscus:

    a. MR fairly unreliable.[45,46]

    b. Following primary repairs, $\frac{2}{3}$ of healed menisci show persistent high signal that reaches the free edge.

    c. Following partial meniscectomy, accuracy of MR varies with the extent of surgery: Menisci with less than 25% resection can be accurately evaluated for re-tear, but accuracy of MR is poor following a larger partial meniscal resection since high signal extending to the free edge remains.

    d. Accuracy postop improves if an effusion is present, tracking into a meniscal tear; in the absence of fluid, MR arthrography will greatly improve accuracy in diagnosing a re-tear.[47]

H. Soft tissue injury to the knee: Hyaline cartilage.

1. Hyaline cartilage is the least well-visualized structure in the knee by MR.

2. The presence of fluid in the joint, or MR arthrography significantly increases the likelihood of diagnosing small cartilaginous defects.

3. With special sequences and high resolution, the mutilaminar appearance of cartilage can be observed.

4. Chondromalacia patellae is best seen on axial views as focal signal intensity changes or surface irregularity or actual defects.

I. Soft tissue injury to the knee: Anterior cruciate ligament.

1. Primary stabilizer of the knee against anterior subluxation of the tibia relative to the femur; collateral ligaments and other soft tissues are the secondary stabilizers.

2. The ACL originates from the noncartilaginous portion of the anterior aspect of the intercondylar eminence of the tibia and courses posteriorly and proximally to insert on the inner face of the lateral femoral condyle (Fig 3-38).

3. Osseous abnormalities associated with ACL injury (see Fig 3-34):

   a. Medial tibial spine: Since it lies adjacent to the site of origin of the ACL, it may be avulsed with ACL injury. However, not all fractures of the tibial spine are related to ACL injury. In children, the ACL is usually stronger than its osseous attachments, and ACL injury involves avulsion and displacement of the tibial spine more frequently than in adults.

   b. Lateral capsular sign (Segond fracture): oval-shaped fragment found adjacent to the lateral tibial plateau; must be differentiated by donor site from an avulsion of the adjacent fibular styloid (by LCL) and from an avulsion of Gerdy's tubercle (iliotibial band); the Segond fracture itself is not of great functional significance, but the mechanism commonly results in an ACL injury as well.

   c. Avulsion of the ACL insertion on the lateral condyle at the intercondylar notch: Very rare.

   d. Posterolateral tibial rim fracture: Rarely detected on plain film, but MR often shows bone bruises in this region, resulting from impaction on the femoral condyle more anteriorly; these two sites impact in the combined valgus and anterolateral rotatory subluxation of the knee that is frequently associated with ACL injury; the anterolateral femoral condyle may show either bone bruise or impaction of the lateral femoral sulcus (deeper than 1.5 mm).

   e. Radiographic anterior drawer sign: Anterior displacement of the tibia relative to the femur; implies not only ACL disruption but also injury to the secondary restraints (collateral ligaments, capsule, menisci).

4. ACL rupture (intrasubstance):

   a. Degree of pain and disability is variable.

   b. Hemorrhagic effusions common (75% of acute hemarthroses are associated with ACL rupture, even in the absence of demonstrable laxity).

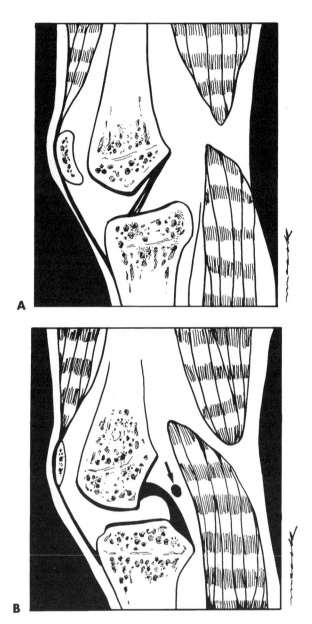

Fig. 3-38 Diagram of oblique sagittal views through the intercondylar notch, at the lateral aspect (**A**) showing the ACL and the medial aspect (**B**) showing the PCL. The *arrow* shows the ligament of Wrisberg, one of the meniscofemoral ligaments, in cross-section. This meniscofemoral ligament is seen in its entirety on a posterior coronal view (**C**) where the ligament (*arrowheads*) parallels the PCL (*arrow*).

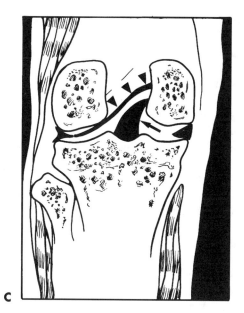

Fig. 3-38 *(continued)*

c. Rupture is far more common than avulsion; rupture most often is near the femoral condylar insertion.

d. ACL is normally a thin but solid dark band on MR, appearing taut and paralleling the dark intercondylar line. The fibers are arranged in a spiral configuration, and several distinct bundles of fibers may be seen at the origin near the tibial intercondylar eminence (Fig 3-38); these may be separated by fibro-fatty tissues, which may be seen as high signal on T2 images (therefore, high signal in this region is not a reliable indicator of a tear).

e. Acutely, an ACL rupture may have high signal intensity, but this rapidly dissipates. Small foci of high signal intensity should be ignored if the fibers appear intact.

f. Reasonable criteria for intrasubstance ACL rupture: Discontinuity of fibers, concavity at the anterior margin of the ACL, a ''mass'' consisting of hematoma and torn fibers near the femoral attachment (but do not be fooled by the partial volume effect of the femoral condyle near the edge of the notch!).

g. Secondary criteria: Failure to locate an ACL within two cuts lateral to the PCL; excessively ''bowed'' PCL in the absence of other signs of PCL injury.

    h. If the diagnosis of ACL rupture is equivocal on sagittal images, check the coronal section (Fig 3-39); a discordant appearance usually indicates an intact ligament at arthroscopy.[48]

    i. Partial ACL tears are not reliably differentiated from complete tears on MR.

    j. Chronic ACL rupture may be difficult to diagnose since the fibers may attach and fibrose to the PCL, appearing intact.

  5. ACL repair/reconstruction:

    a. Arthroscopic repair may be made via suture or staples.

    b. Tendon reconstructions are seen with tunnels and various fixation devices.

    c. Bone-patellar tendon-bone composite reconstructions (either autograft or cadaver): The tendon is placed along the course of the ACL, and secured by placing the bone wedges in osseous tunnels in the lateral femoral condyle and mid tibial plateau; plain film evaluation includes site of the osseous tunnel (opening should be the origin/insertion of the ACL) (Fig 3-40), hardware failure, graft fracture or migration, patellar fracture at the site of graft harvest, and eventual graft rejection[49]; if necessary, MR may be used to evaluate location and integrity of the graft.

J. Soft tissue injury to the knee: Posterior cruciate ligament.

  1. Primary restraint against posterior tibial translation; most common mechanism of isolated PCL injury is blunt trauma to the anterior proximal tibia ("dashboard injury").

  2. The major portion of the tibial attachment of the PCL lies posteriorly behind the joint surface, in a depression behind the intercondylar region of the tibia; the thick ligament courses proximally and anteriorly to insert on the most distal and anterior aspect of the inner force of the medial femoral condyle (Fig 3-38).

→

Fig. 3-39. Diagram of oblique coronal views, far posterior (**A**), showing the biceps femoris (*curved arrow*) and popliteus muscle (*arrow*); posterior (**B**) showing the PCL (*long arrow*) and the biceps tendon insertion (*short arrow*) at the femoral head. The next cut anteriorly (**C**) (though still quite posterior in section) shows the LCL (*arrowheads*) originating at the lateral femoral condyle and inserting along with the biceps femoris on the fibular head. A mid-coronal cut (**D**) shows the thin ACL spiraling to the tibia (*arrow*) and the MCL with its deep fibers inserting near the tibial plateau and superficial fibers inserting several centimeters more distally (*arrowheads*). A more anterior cut (**E**) shows the insertion of the iliotibial band on Gerdy's tubercle (*arrow*). An even more anterior cut in the same series is seen in Fig 3-37,*A*, showing the transverse ligament.

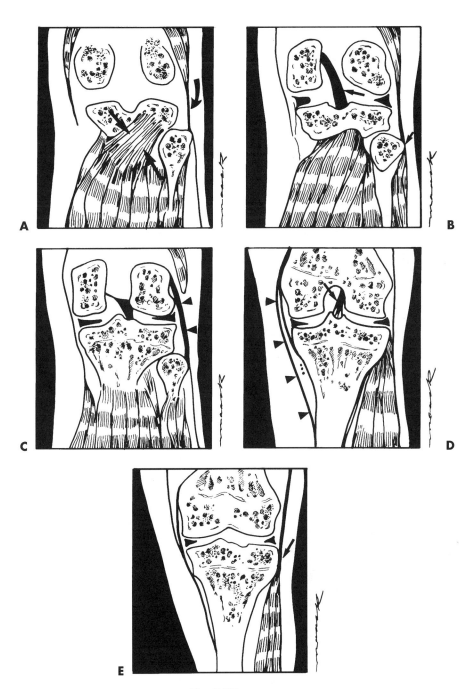

Fig. 3-39

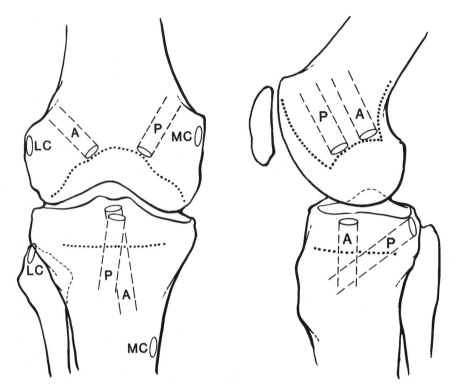

Fig. 3-40 Diagrams showing anatomic sites for the tunnels for ACL and PCL reconstructions (*A* and *P*, respectively), as well as isometric points for attachments of the LCL and MCL. Tunnel positioning or ligament attachment should roughly parallel the sites shown on these diagrams. (Reprinted with permission from Manaster BJ, *Imaging knee ligament reconstructions.* RSNA Categorical Course in Musculoskeletal Radiology 1993;211–218.)

 3. Osseous abnormalities associated with PCL injury (see Fig 3-34):
    a. Avulsion at the medial femoral condyle, midaspect of the inter-condylar notch: Rare.
    b. Avulsion of the posterior tibial insertion, with the fragment usually retracted slightly proximally above the line of the tibial plateau.
    c. Posterior displacement of the tibia relative to the femur ("sag") suggests not only PCL, but also disruption of secondary stabilizing soft tissue structures of the knee.
 4. PCL rupture (intrasubstance):
    a. Uncommon due to its size and strength.

      b. Hemorrhagic effusion less constant or tense compared with ACL.

      c. In the extended knee (position for MR), PCL is slightly convex posteriorly, and located one or two sagittal cuts medial to the ACL; expect to see it in its entirety on two contiguous cuts.

      d. Criteria for rupture: Lack of continuity, increased signal intensity (valid with PCL, but often not with ACL), or irregularity of contours.

      e. A sharply bowed PCL indicates laxity, either from PCL rupture/avulsion, or as a secondary sign of an ACL tear.

  5. PCL reconstruction: As with ACL, may be soft tissue or bone-patellar tendon-bone composite; in the latter case, tunnel positions are as indicated in Fig. 3-40 and complications are as outlined in the ACL section (I, 5.)

K. Soft tissue injury to the knee: Medial collateral ligament.

  1. MCL is the primary restraint to valgus laxity; mechanism of injury is a valgus force, with or without a rotational element.

  2. MCL is a long structure, located external to the capsule (Fig 3-39). The femoral attachment is just distal to the adductor tubercle. The superficial portion courses distally and slightly anteriorly to insert on the anteromedial face of the tibia, distal to the level of the tibial tubercle about 5 cm below the joint line. The deep portion arises with the superficial portion, is contiguous with the joint capsule and the medial meniscus, and inserts on the tibial condyle just distal to the plateau. There is a variable amount of fat between the superficial and deep fibers; they may or may not appear as separate structures.

  3. Osseous abnormalities associated with MCL injury: Pelligrini-Steada (calcification in and around the MCL due to previous trauma) is common, but true avulsions are rare; the most common plain film sign of MCL injury is joint line gapping; lateral bone bruise or plateau fracture should raise suspicion for MCL injury.

  4. MCL rupture (intrasubstance): Two distinct types of injury:

      a. Edema and hemorrhage in adjacent soft tissues, indicating a sprain.

      b. Ligamentous thickening, discontinuity, or alteration in signal intensity, indicating a rupture.

  5. Frequently associated injuries: ACL rupture, meniscal tears, contralateral bone bruise.

  6. MCL repair is usually either not performed or is primary and not seen radiographically; if rupture is near the ligament origin or insertion, staple placement is evaluated (Fig 3-40).

L. Soft tissue injury to the knee: Lateral collateral ligament.
  1. The biceps femoris and LCL both contribute to lateral joint stability, and join together at their insertion on the fibular head (Fig 3-39).
  2. Osseous abnormalities associated with LCL injury: Avulsion at the lateral condylar origin is rare. Either the biceps femoris or LCL may fail by avulsing the fibular styloid. The third lateral structure, the iliotibial band, may avulse this insertion on Gerdy's tubercle (Fig 3-34). LCL disruption may be indicated by lateral joint line gapping. Medial bone bruising may suggest LCL injury.
  3. LCL rupture (intrasubstance):
    a. LCL is an uncommon injury, usually seen in combination with other injuries of the knee, including biceps femoris and popliteal injuries.
    b. Peroneal nerve injury may be suggestive.
    c. Intrasubstance tears seen as discontinuity, increased signal, and fiber retraction.
  4. Repairs are primary if the tear is intrasubstance; fibular styloid process fractures may be stabilized with a screw.
M. Soft tissue injury to the knee: Patellar tendon.
  1. Injuries include complete interruption or avulsion, diffuse interstitial tear with multiple foci; focal increased signal without discontinuity (partial tear or degeneration), and bursitis.
  2. Most common site of inferior patellar tendon rupture is the junction of the tendon with the lower pole of the patella; plain film findings are patella alta, retraction of the quadriceps tendon, or a small avulsion. Tibial tubercle disruptions have an extremely low incidence.
  3. Jumper's knee: Patellar tendinitis or partial patellar tendon tears; usually proximal patellar tendon, but, occasionally, the distal quadriceps tendon is involved; seen on MR as focal thickening with increased signal.
N. Soft tissue injury to the knee: Cysts.
  1. Popliteal cysts most commonly found in the semimembranosus-gastrocnemius bursa, but can dissect into other planes.
  2. Meniscal cysts: Uncommon, communicate with meniscal tears; usually lateral and adjacent to the joint line; if medial they may be forced posteriorly to mimic a popliteal cyst.
  3. Ganglion cysts may be difficult to distinguish as such.
  4. Pes anserine bursitis: Fluid beneath the tendons of the pes anserinis (conjoined tendons of the sartorius, semitendinosus, and gracilis at the anteromedial tibia near the joint line).

IX. ANKLE TRAUMA

Key Concepts

Occasionally lateral malleolar fractures are seen only on the lateral film. Impaction at the corners of the plafond is an easily missed injury. Anatomic reduction (including normal length of fibula) is crucial for an acceptable result. With an isolated medial injury and widened mortise, proximal fibular fracture should be sought. Two special cases are found in the maturing skeleton—juvenile Tillaux and triplane fractures.

A. Anatomy.
1. The medial malleolus has two colliculi. The anterior one is longer than the posterior one, giving it a double density on an AP film.
2. The lateral margin of the tibia has the fibular notch. The fibula normally fits the notch snugly. If, after a fracture, the fibula is shortened, the more bulbous distal fibula does not articulate properly in the fibular notch. This leads to lateral shift of the talus, decreased surface contact between the tibia and talus, and early DJD (see Fig 3-41); therefore, only 2 to 3 mm of fibular shortening is acceptable.
3. The lateral malleolus is located 1 cm distal and 1 cm posterior to the position of the medial malleolus.
4. The tibial joint surface is termed the plafond (ceiling).
5. A 15- to 20-degree internal oblique film brings the malleoli parallel to the horizontal plane for evaluation of the ankle mortise. Joint space should be an even 3 to 4 mm over the entire talar surface. Two millimeters' widening of the mortise is abnormal.
6. The articular surface of the talus narrows posteriorly. This prevents

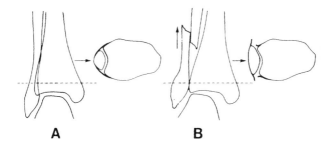

A   **B**

Fig. 3-41 AP view of the normal ankle (**A**) with axial cut through the fibular notch. After fracture and fibular shortening, the larger distal fibula does not articulate as well with the fibular notch and ankle mortise widening occurs (**B**).

posterior dislocation, which requires disruption of the ankle mortise.

7. The base of the fifth metatarsal is included on the lateral ankle film since it is a common site of a fracture that may be mistaken clinically for ankle trauma.

8. For stress films, varus and valgus stress is applied to the calcaneus. An anterior drawer stress may also be performed. There is a wide range of normal ankle laxity (normal talar tilt with stress is 10 to 12 degrees but may increase to 20 degrees in lax ankles), so comparison ankle stress films are recommended.

9. Normal variants include the os trigonum posterior to the talus (fused or unfused) and irregular and multiple accessory ossicles at both medial and lateral malleoli.

10. Ankle effusion is seen on lateral film as an anterior convex soft tissue density at the tibiotalar joint. The pre-Achilles fat triangle lies between the Achilles tendon and the deep muscles of the leg and is sharply defined in the absence of effusion or inflammation. The fat density extends 2 mm distal to the posterior tubercle of the calcaneus.

B. Trauma:

1. Structures to be examined:

   a. Soft tissues, for swelling or effusion; soft tissue swelling distal to the malleoli suggests ligamentous injury.

   b. Malleoli and posterior tibia, for fractures.

   c. Mortise, for disruption.

2. In general, oblique or spiral fractures of the malleoli are due to impacting (pushing) forces, while transverse fractures are due to avulsing (pulling) forces. However, rotational forces are usually a complicating factor to simple inversion or eversion injuries.

3. Lauge-Hansen classification is based on the mechanism of occurrence and may be useful to focus the search for less obvious injuries. It is not useful for treatment or prognosis.

4. Weber (AO) classification is the one most used by surgeons since it correlates well with both treatment and prognosis. It uses the level of the fibular fracture to deduce the injury to the tibiofibular ligaments.

   a. Weber A: Transverse avulsion fracture of the lateral malleolus at or distal to the tibiofibular joint. This injury spares the tibiofibular ligament complex. It may be associated with an oblique fracture of the medial malleolus.

   b. Weber B: Spiral fracture of the lateral malleolus beginning at the level of the ankle joint. This leads to a partial disruption of the tibiofibular ligament, and diastasis of the ankle mortise depends on the extent of injury. It may be associated with a transverse or slightly oblique avulsion fracture of the medial malleolus below the ankle joint or with a deltoid ligament rupture.

    c. Weber C: Fibular fracture proximal to the ankle joint. This invariably tears the tibiofibular ligament complex and leads to lateral talar instability. It may be either a pure ligamentous tear or an avulsion of the anterior (Tillaux-Chaput) or posterior (Volkmann) tubercles of the distal tibia or, more rarely, a flake from their fibular attachment. The medial malleolus is avulsed just below the level of the ankle joint, or the deltoid ligament may be torn.

  5. *Pylon (pilon) fracture*[50]: Results from *axial compression,* with or without rotation; results in severe distal tibia comminution (intra-articular) along the plafond; the malleoli, whether or not fractured, maintain their relationship to the talus; talar fractures may be present as well; classification of pylon fractures includes type 1 (non-displaced), type 2 (moderate displacement), and type 3 (severe displacement and impaction of fragments).

C. Postoperative evaluation: Exact anatomic and stable reconstruction of the ankle mortise is necessary to prevent traumatic arthritis:

  1. Correct length of fibula and its exact position in the fibular notch of the tibia.

  2. Restoration of the ankle mortise.

  3. Less than 1- to 2-mm displacement of either a posterior malleolar fragment or posterior displacement of the distal fibular fragment. When present, these are signs of persistent subluxation of the ankle joint.

D. Other fractures of ankle:

  1. Watch for *impaction of the plafond* at its junction with the medial malleolus in an inversion injury. This may indicate a severe injury and may be quite occult, as may be osteochondral fractures of either the medial or lateral dome of the talus.

  2. With an eversion injury and isolated transverse medial malleolar fracture or isolated widening of the ankle mortise there may be a tibiofibular ligament tear and fracture of the proximal third of the fibula (*Maisonneuve* fracture). The entire fibula should be examined radiographically in such a circumstance since the pain of the proximal fibular fracture may be masked by the pain of the ankle injury.

  3. *Insufficiency* fractures may be seen simultaneously in the distal tibia and fibula, usually within 3 to 4 cm of the plafond.

  4. *Stress* fractures are seen in the fibulas of runners 3 to 7 cm from the

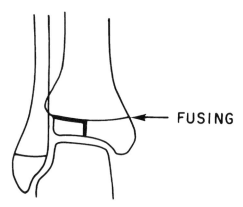

Fig. 3-42 Juvenile Tillaux fracture: Salter 3 injury occurring at the last portion of the epiphysis to fuse.

tip of the lateral malleolus. Stress injuries in skeletally immature runners are seen as widening and irregularity of the distal fibular growth plate.

5. Fusion of the distal tibial epiphysis starts at 12 to 13 years of age. It begins centrally and proceeds medially and finally laterally. This pattern may be confused on radiographs with a fracture. The *juvenile Tillaux* fracture is seen secondary to this fusion pattern; it is a Salter 3 fracture of the lateral portion of the distal tibial epiphysis that occurs after fusion of the medial portion of the epiphysis (Fig 3-42).

6. The *triplane* fracture is another juvenile pattern of ankle fracture. It involves the lateral half of the distal tibial epiphysis and a posterior triangular metaphyseal fragment. "Triplane" indicates the three planes of the fracture: vertical through the epiphysis, horizontal through the epiphyseal plate, and oblique through the metaphysis (extending from anterior and inferior at the epiphyseal plate, posteriorly and superiorly; Fig 3-43). There are two types. If a triplane fracture occurs after the medial portion of the epiphysis has fused, the medial malleolus remains intact and it is a two-fragment triplane fracture. If the triplane fracture occurs before the epiphysis starts to fuse, a three-fragment fracture occurs; it gives the appearance of a Salter 2 involving the posterior metaphysis and a Salter 3 involving the medial epiphysis. With reconstruction, CT is very useful in completely delineating the extent of fractures and displacement.

E. Soft tissue injuries of the ankle and foot: Tendons. Excellent overall reviews of this topic are found in References 51 and 52.

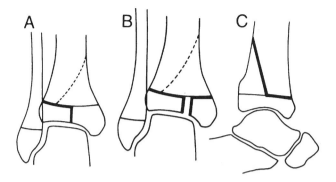

Fig. 3-43 Triplane fractures. **A,** Two-part triplane, with fusion of the medial portion of the epiphysis. **B,** Three-part triplane occurring prior to fusion of the medial portion of the epiphysis. **C,** Lateral appearance of either variety of triplane fracture, which in this view looks like a Salter 2.

1. *Flexor tendons:* In order of position from anteromedial to postero-lateral on the ankle, *posterior tibial, flexor digitorum longus, flexor hallucis longus (known popularly by the mnemonic "Tom, Dick, and Harry")* (Fig 3-44).

   a. *Posterior tibial (PTT):* Uses the groove in the medial malleo-lus as a pulley, continues through the tarsal tunnel to insert on the navicular, medial and middle cuneiforms, and the second through fourth metatarsal bases; acts as the principal inverter of the foot and maintains the longitudinal arch; *rupture usually occurs in women over 50 years of age and who have a clinical picture of acute painful flatfoot* that progressively worsens; patients with RA or previous flatfoot deformity are more prone to this disorder; patients with an accessory navicular ossifica-tion center may be predisposed to PTT injury; young athletes playing sports that require rapid changes in direction may also rupture the PTT; tears usually occur between the medial malle-olus and navicular and have *3 grades:* type I shows significant enlargement of the tendon, occasionally with vertical splits; type II shows attenuation of the tendon ($\frac{1}{3}$ to $\frac{1}{2}$ the size); type III shows a complete rupture with gap; there are three potential sources of misinterpretation; the PTT normally flattens out and appears bulbous with increased signal intensity near its insertion on the navicular, and should not be confused with a type I PTT injury at this site. *Rule of thumb: Except at the insertion, the normal PTT should not be greater than twice the diameter of the other posterior tendons.* There is normally

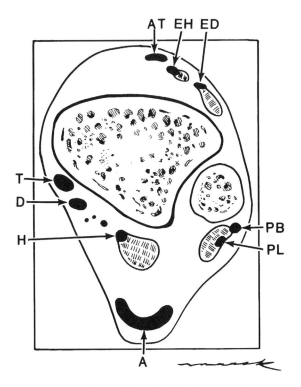

Fig. 3-44   Axial diagram through the tibiofibular joint, demonstrating the tendons of the ankle. A, Achilles; T, posterior tibial; D, flexor digitorum; H, flexor hallucis; PB, peroneal brevis; PL, peroneal longus; AT, anterior tibial; EH, extensor hallucis; ED, extensor digitorum longus/peroneus tertius.

a small amount of fluid in the tendon sheath that should not be mistaken for signs of tenosynovitis; the *"magic angle" effect* may cause normal tendons to have higher signal intensity on short echo TE sequences, the absence of morphologic abnormality and the absence of tendon signal on longer TE sequences should differentiate the magic angle effect from true PTT pathology.

b. Flexor digitorum longus: Uses the groove in the medial malleolus as a pulley, continues through the tarsal tunnel to insert on the fifth metatarsal; injury involving this tendon is rare.

c. *Flexor hallucis longus:* Is muscular further distally in the leg than the other flexor tendons; tendon passes posterior to flexor digitorum, passes beneath the sustentaculum tali of the calcaneus, using its groove as a pulley, and continues between the two sesamoids to insert on the base of the distal phalanx of the great toe; injury is uncommon except in *ballet dancers* due to repetitive push off from the forefoot; it may also be tethered against the tibia by a prominent os trigonum, leading to inflammation. One note of caution: In 20% of the population, there is contiguity between the ankle joint and the flexor hallusis tendon, allowing fluid in the tendon sheath to be a common finding; disproportionate fluid in the tendon sheath relative to the tibiotalar joint helps make a diagnosis of tenosynovitis.

2. Extensor tendons: In order from medial to lateral: anterior tibial, extensor hallucis longus, extensor digitorium longus, peroneus tertius (Tom, Harry, Dick, and Pete) (Fig 3-44); injuries are rare; the anterior tibial tendon injury occurs mostly in downhill runners and hikers, and rarely progresses to complete rupture.

3. Peroneal tendons: Peroneus brevis is located anterior to peroneus longus; both pass behind the lateral malleolus in a groove; peroneus brevis inserts on the fifth metatarsal base while the peroneus longus passes beneath the midfoot to insert on the base of the first metatarsal.
   a. Rupture, either partial or complete, is not common; seen more often in peroneus brevis; displacement of an os peroneum may suggest a ruptured peroneus longus tendon.
   b. Both peroneals are prone to stenosing tenosynovitis, especially if entrapped or impinged by calcaneal fracture fragments.
   c. Peroneals may sublux or dislocate due to avulsion of the overlying retinaculum (during forced plantar flexion), congenital absence or laxity of the retinaculum, or convexity or shallowness of the retromalleolar groove; axial MR while stressing the ankle in eversion and dorsiflexion may demonstrate the dislocated tendon.
   d. The magic angle effect during short echo TE sequences may cause increased signal intensity in the peroneals; as with the PTT, normal morphology and normal signal on long TE sequences should help avoid a misdiagnosis of tenosynovitis or partial tear.
   e. The peroneus brevis may normally be split by the peroneus longus, giving the appearance of injury.

4. *Achilles tendon:* Derived from the gastrocnemius and soleus muscles forming a thick tendon that inserts on the posterior calcaneus, with a prominent fat pad anterior to it.
   a. The tendon is *flat or concave* anteriorly and should be no more than 8 mm thick in its AP dimension.
   b. Achilles tendonitis is common in runners and jumping athletes;

tendon enlarges and may be edematous acutely, but signal intensity decreases once it becomes chronic.

   c. *Rupture:* Difficult clinical diagnosis since other structures may compensate; most injuries occur in *middle-aged males during running or jumping* athletic events, but may be seen in trained athletes as well; they are also seen in patients with weak tissues from systemic diseases such as RA, diabetes, renal disease, or steroid use. Injuries tend to occur *2 to 6 cm proximal to the calcaneal insertion* in a relatively avascular zone; acute partial tears usually have bright signal, either transverse or intrasubstance; as these become chronic, only thickening and rounding of the tendon may be seen; complete disruption shows retraction of the fibers.

   d. An intact plantaris tendon may mimic an intact fiber of the Achilles, but should be recognized as this normal variant by its location along the anteromedial margin of the Achilles tendon.

   e. An accessory soleus muscle may make the Achilles appear thickened; the muscle is recognized as this normal variant since it follows signal of muscle on all sequences.

   f. *Xanthomas* are common in the Achilles tendon in persons with hyperlipidemia; the low signal masses may have stippled high signal within; this may be difficult to differentiate from a partial Achilles tear or tendinitis.[53]

   g. The postsurgical Achilles may look thickened, retain high signal, and have cystic areas within it.

F. Soft tissue injuries of the ankle and foot: Ligaments.

   1. *Ligaments are more commonly injured than tendons;* the *lateral ligaments are more commonly injured than medial ligaments;* there are 3 major sets of ligaments.

   2. First-degree sprain: High signal around the ligament on T2.
Second-degree sprain: Partial discontinuity.
Third-degree sprain: Complete discontinuity.

   3. *Anterior and posterior tibiofibular ligaments* (Fig 3-45):

     a. *Most superior set of ankle ligaments, seen on axial views immediately above the ankle joint; at this level the fibula is convex or straight, so they should not be confused with the talofibular ligaments found more inferiorly where the fibula is concave.*

     b. Isolated tears of the tibiofibular ligaments are rare; usually associated with other ligamentous rupture.

     c. Nonvisualization need not mean there is a tear.

     d. *The posterior tibiofibular ligament may be seen in cross-section on sagittal images, giving the appearance of a loose body posterior to the talus at the level of the tibiotalar joint* (Fig 3-46).

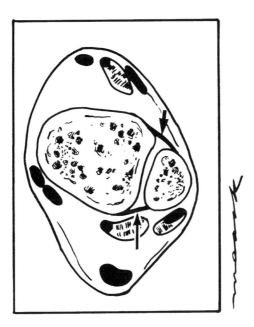

Fig. 3-45   Axial diagram immediately superior to the ankle joint, demonstrating the anterior and posterior tibiofibular ligaments (*short* and *long arrows,* respectively). Note that the fibular shape is convex at this level.

4. *Lateral collateral ligaments:* 3 structures:
   a. *Anterior talofibular ligament:* Extends from the anterior fibula to the lateral talar neck; this is *best seen in the axial plane, at the level where the medial aspect of the fibula is concave* (Fig 3-47); this is the *most frequently torn ankle ligament,* but is not clinically significant; however, it may become chronically enlarged and cause impingement, requiring resection.
   b. *Posterior talofibular ligament: Fan-shaped,* extending from the distal aspect of the lateral malleolar fossa to the lateral tubercle of the posterior talar process (Fig 3-47); because of the shape of these fibers, they may normally appear inhomogeneous; *they are seen at the same level on the axial image as the anterior talofibular ligament;* injury to the posterior talofibular ligament is rare unless the other two LCLs are ruptured as well; on sagittal images, this ligament may be seen in cross-section, giving the appearance of a loose body just posterior to the talus at the talocalcaneal joint (Fig 3-46).
   c. *Calcaneofibular ligament:* Extends from the tip of the lateral malleolus to the lateral aspect of the calcaneus (Fig 3-48); it

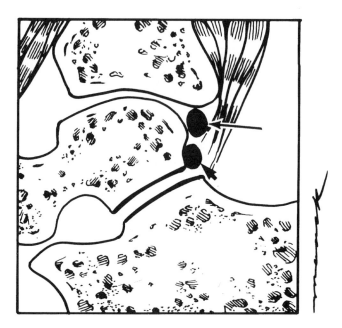

Fig. 3-46 Sagittal diagram demonstrating the posterior tibiofibular (*long arrow*) and posterior talofibular (*short arrow*) ligaments in cross-section, where they may simulate loose bodies.

is partially seen on either coronal or axial images, but is best seen on oblique axial images with the foot in plantar flexion; the calcaneofibular ligament is moderately frequently injured; if this ligament is injured, the anterior talofibular ligament is nearly always ruptured as well.

    5. *Medial collateral ligament* (deltoid): Five components; stronger than lateral collateral:
        a. *Always located deep to the flexor tendon.*
        b. Superficial ligaments (tibiocalcaneal, tibiospring, tibionavicular).
        c. Deep ligaments (anterior and posterior tibiotalar).
        d. The tibionavicular ligament is the weakest.
G. Soft tissue injuries of the ankle and foot: *Tarsal tunnel syndrome.*
    1. Analogous to carpal tunnel syndrome, with tingling, pain, and burning in the toes, sole, and medial foot.
    2. Tarsal tunnel is best seen on coronal or axial views (Fig 3-49) and consists of the *talus and calcaneus laterally and the flexor retinaculum medially, containing the flexor tendons as well as the*

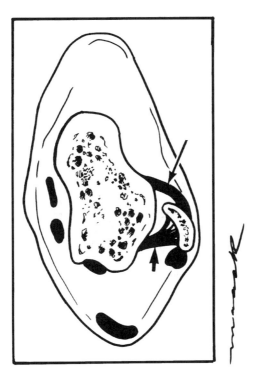

Fig. 3-47   Axial diagram demonstrating the anterior talofibular (*long arrow*) and posterior talofibular (*short arrow*) ligaments. Note that the fibular shape is concave on its medial aspect at the level you should expect to see these ligaments.

      posterior tibial nerve; pressure on the nerve causes the clinical syndrome.

  3. The tarsal tunnel has several septae, allowing minimal lesions to become symptomatic.

  4. Fifty percent of cases of tarsal tunnel syndrome will not have a morphologic abnormality.

  5. Abnormalities to search for include: neural tumors, ganglia, other masses, thickening of the flexor retinaculum, flexor tendon tenosynovitis, and hypertrophy of the abductor hallucis longus muscle.

H. Soft tissue injuries of the ankle and foot: *Sinus tarsi syndrome.*

  1. Tarsal sinus is a small opening between the posterior subtalar joint and the talocalcaneal navicular joint.

  2. Five ligaments are present (though only one or two may be seen distinctly on any one image), along with a small neurovascular bundle and joint capsule; all of these structures are surrounded by fat.

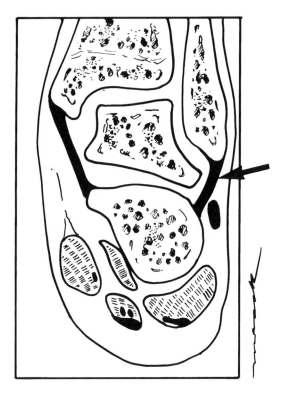

Fig. 3-48   Coronal diagram showing the calcaneofibular ligament (*arrow*), one of the LCLs.

   3. Clinical syndrome is caused by inflammation or hemorrhage at the site and gives lateral foot pain and instability of the hind-foot.
   4. *MR may show diffuse replacement of the fat by fibrosis or inflammatory change or fluid;* ligament tears may be subtle.
   5. Most patients have had prior LCL tears.
 I. Soft tissue injury of the ankle or foot: Accessory muscles.
   1. Eight percent of the population.
   2. Peroneus quartus (originates from the muscular portion of the peroneus brevis or from the fibula or peroneus longus and inserts on the peroneal tubercle of the calcaneus).
   3. Blood supply may be tenuous and patient may become symptomatic with exercise; may require fasciotomy if it leads to a compartment syndrome.
   4. May be a cause of tarsal tunnel syndrome.

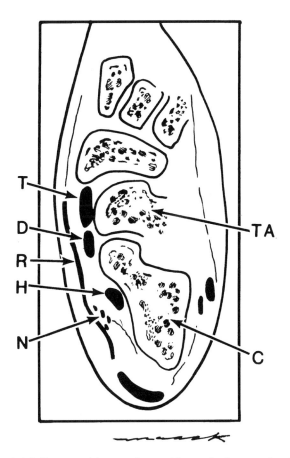

Fig. 3-49 Axial diagram of the tarsal tunnel located a few cuts in plantar direction from Fig 3-47. R, retinaculum; TA, talus; C, calcaneus; T, tibialis posterior tendon; D, flexor digitorum; H, flexor hallucis; N, posterior tibial nerve and associated vascular structures.

X. FOOT TRAUMA

Key Concepts

Calcaneal fracture is intra-articular if Boehler's angle is decreased. Calcaneal fractures are associated with lumbar spine fractures and are often bilateral. Tarsometatarsal (TMT) fracture-dislocations are very difficult to diagnose and require attention to precise anatomy at those joints. A child's stubbed toe may develop into a Salter 2 fracture and osteomyelitis.

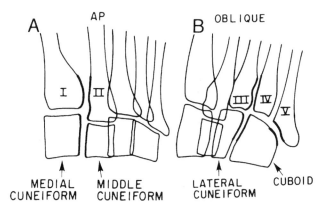

Fig. 3-50 Normal alignment of the tarsometatarsal joints, as outlined in the text. The first and second are evaluated on the AP film, while the third, fourth, and fifth are evaluated on the oblique film. The *bold lines* indicate the surfaces of the tarsometatarsals, which must align with one another on each view. The alignment must be precise, and the lateral film often appears normal even with severe derangement of these joints.

A. Anatomy.
　1. The calcaneus is tent-shaped on lateral. This is described by *Boehler's angle*, normally 28 to 48 degrees.
　2. The calcaneal apophysis and immature tarsal navicular normally appear dense and often fragmented. This is a normal variant rather than fracture or AVN.
　3. The articulations of the tarsals and metatarsals are very precise and must be observed carefully to rule out *midfoot (Lisfranc) fracture-dislocation* (Fig 3-50):
　　a. AP films: Lateral border of the first metatarsal aligns with the lateral border of the medial cuneiform; medial border of the second metatarsal aligns with the medial border of the middle cuneiform.
　　b. Oblique films: Lateral border of the third metatarsal aligns with the lateral border of the lateral cuneiform; the medial border of the fourth metatarsal aligns with the medial border of the cuboid; the base of the fifth metatarsal articulates with the cuboid but normally extends lateral to its lateral border.
　　c. The base of the second metatarsal is recessed between the medial and lateral cuneiform in a lock-and-key configuration.
　4. The apophysis of the base of the fifth metatarsal is longitudinally oriented and must not be mistaken for an avulsion fracture. It may also be normally bipartite.

5. The epiphysis of the proximal phalanx of the great toe may be bifid, simulating fracture.
6. Normal irregularities and excrescences may be seen along the shafts of all the phalanges.
7. Sesamoid bones may be bipartite or multipartite, simulating fracture.
8. Accessory ossicles are common and are not invariably bilateral. They are well-rounded and corticated, which helps differentiate them from fractures. The most common in the foot are the os peroneum (adjacent to the cuboid), os trigonum (on the lateral film, posterior to the talus), and os tibiale externum (on the AP film, adjacent to the navicular). Others are diagrammed in Keats' *Atlas of Normal Roentgen Variants That May Simulate Disease*.
9. The talocalcaneal joint has three different facets and appears least complicated when imaged by CT. It is completely described in Chapter 5 (Tarsal Coalition).

B. Trauma
1. Calcaneus: 75% intra-articular:
    a. Fractures sometimes are seen best on axial (Harris) view. CT is especially valuable if combined with reconstruction to evaluate fracture placement and, especially, involvement of the three calcaneal facets which articulate with the talus, forming the subtalar joint.
    b. Classified as intra- or extra-articular; a decreased Boehler's angle implies an intra-articular calcaneal fracture.
    c. Bilateral (10%).
    d. *Ten percent are associated with thoracolumbar fractures* (*Don Juan fractures*) since common mechanism is a fall from a height.
    e. *Stress fracture* may be seen only as a *vertical linear density* 10 to 14 days after onset of symptoms. These fractures are usually in the posterior portion of the calcaneus, and run superior-to-inferior (perpendicular to the major trabeculae of the calcaneus). In diabetics, one may see calcaneal insufficiency avulsion fracture (dubbed CIA), a fracture of the posterior tubercle of the calcaneus, avulsed by the Achilles tendon.
    f. *Extensor digitorum brevis avulsion:* An avulsion fracture of a small fragment from the anterolateral calcaneus; this fracture is easily overlooked and is best seen on an AP view of the ankle, with the fragment located adjacent to the calcaneus, 2 cm distal to the lateral malleous. It is also seen on an AP foot film, lateral to the anterior calcaneus.
    g. Heel pain syndrome may be due to plantar fasciitis, plantar

fascia rupture, tarsal tunnel syndrome, heel spur fracture, calcaneal stress fracture, or retrocalcaneal inflammatory arthritis.

2. Talus: 25% avulsion and chip; 75% neck and body:

   a. Other than chips and avulsions, the most common fracture is vertical neck; may be associated with talar dislocations.

   b. Very susceptible to AVN.

   c. Osteochondral fractures or osteochondritis dissecans may be seen on dome of talus either medially or laterally with an equal distribution. Lateral lesions are usually found in the midportion of the talar dome (from anterior to posterior), while medial lesions are usually found further posteriorly. They are most often seen in lax ankles. Osteochondritis dissecans is often bilateral. Stability of the osteochondral fragment may be evaluated by T2-weighted MR; high signal surrounding the fragment suggests lack of attachment; initial signal character is not useful.[54]

   d. Avulsion fractures from the talus are common on the superior, medial, lateral, and posterior parts of the talus; the most common is at the anterior superior surface of the neck of the talus, at the capsular attachment.

   e. Os trigonum syndrome: The os trigonum is an accessory ossicle, which has a synchrondrosis with the posterior lateral part of the talus. It may fuse with the talus, but 7% to 14% remain as a separate ossicle. Note that it may be difficult to differentiate the ossicle from an old un-united fracture of the lateral tubercle, which normally lies adjacent to the ossicle. Pain at the site can be caused by repetitive microtrauma and chronic inflammation. Forced plantar flexion of the foot may result in fracture of a fused trigonal process. Excessive dorsiflexion may fracture the adjacent lateral process of the posterior talus. The flexor hallucis longus tendon lies medial to the os trigonum; tenosynovitis may produce symptoms in the region. Posterior ankle impingement pain may be due to a posterior bony block caused by a large os trigonum or a large posterolateral process of the talus. Any of the abnormalities may cause localized pain typical of the os trigonum syndrome; careful imaging may reveal degenerative changes or fractures involving these structures.[55] On MR, a normal os trigonum will be seen as having a smooth but undulating synostosis; a fracture line is straight.

3. Navicular:

   a. Stress fractures are rare but tend to occur in joggers and basketball players, presenting with poorly localized pain along the medial arch of the foot. The fracture is usually in the sagittal plane at the junction of the middle and lateral thirds. If incomplete, the fracture is usually not seen on plain film. CT reconstruction or MR, performed tangential to the dorsal surface of the navicular (true axial and true coronal sections) make the diagnosis. Complications of a completed fracture include nonunion and AVN of the lateral fragment.

  b. Navicular avulsion fractures: Talonavicular capsule may avulse a dorsal fragment.

  c. Fractures of the navicular tuberosity (medially) must be different from the accessory ossicle, os tibial externum.

4. Lisfranc fracture-dislocation:

  a. Dorsal dislocation of TMT joints, usually associated with several chip and avulsion fractures.

  b. Precise study of these anatomic relationships on oblique and AP films may be required for diagnosis. Lateral films may appear normal.

  c. Classified as homolateral (usually lateral dislocation of metatarsals 2–5 or 1–5) or divergent (lateral dislocation of metatarsals 2–5 and medial subluxation of the first metatarsal). Early radiographic findings may be extremely subtle, with only slight widening and offset at the first and second metatarsals; with continued weight bearing, further separation occurs.

  d. Lisfranc fracture-dislocations are much more commonly a manifestation of a diabetic Charcot (neuropathic) joint than due to trauma; lateral film may appear normal.

5. Jones' fracture: Transverse fracture at the base of fifth metatarsal 1.5 to 2 cm distal to the tuberosity (also called dancer's fracture). The Jones' fracture is to be differentiated from the more proximal avulsion fracture; remember that the apophysis is oriented longitudinally and should not be mistaken for a fracture. More distal to the tuberosity, runners and basketball players may develop a stress fracture that is prone to delayed healing.

6. Metatarsal stress fracture (march fracture):

  a. Most common stress fracture.

  b. Second or third metatarsal most common.

  c. Nondisplaced and often not radiographically apparent until 7 to 10 days after injury, when fluffy callus formation or periosteal reaction is seen.

7. Stubbed great toe in a child:

  a. Nail bed of great toe is attached to periosteum at the level of the proximal metaphysis.

b. Stubbed great toe with a nail bed injury not infrequently results in a Salter 1 or 2 fracture and/or osteomyelitis.

XI. SPINE TRAUMA

Key Concepts

Cervical injuries may be extremely subtle, yet clinically devastating. Abnormal prevertebral soft tissues are usually an extremely reliable sign of significant injury if present, but may still appear normal postinjury. Numerous normal variants may suggest fracture. Each examination must be individualized.

Cervical Spine

A. Normal anatomy relevant to trauma.
  1. Lateral film: Initial film, to be cleared before further films are taken: *Must* see to top of T_1:
    a. Prevertebral soft tissues:
      (1) In adults:
        a Not more than 5 mm at C_3 and C_4.
        b Less than 22 mm at C_6.
      (2) In children:
        a Two-thirds the width of C_2 body at C_3 and C_4.
        b Not more than 14 mm at C_6.
    b. Cervical lordosis: Loss of the lordosis may represent muscle spasm; however, it is normally absent in 20% of patients in the neutral position. It is absent in 70% of normal patients if the chin is depressed only 1 inch; lordosis will, of course, be absent if the patient is on a back board or in a cervical collar.
    c. Four continuous curves describe the normal position of the bony elements (Fig 3-51)
      (1) Anterior vertebral body line.
      (2) Posterior vertebral body line; exception to this is in children, where there is often a physiologic offset of 2 to 3 mm of C_2 on C_3 or C_3 on C_4.
      (3) Spinal laminar line.
      (4) Posterior spinous process line.
    d. In the absence of disk disease, the distance between adjacent posterior vertebral bodies is uniform at all levels. A gap at one level suggests posterior ligamentous injury; this would be supported by an abnormal fanning of the spinous processes. Note that fanning of the spinous processes normally is not uniform: Normally it is greater for the proximal and distal

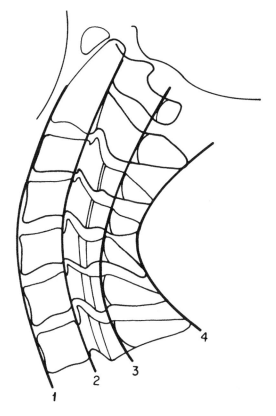

Fig. 3-51   Lateral cervical spine with four normal contiguous curves: *1,* anterior vertebral line; *2,* posterior vertebral line; *3,* spinal laminar line; *4,* posterior spinous line.

cervical elements than for the middle elements. Therefore, fanning of C_{3-5} spinous processes is indicative of posterior ligamentous injury (Fig 3-52,*A*).

e. The facets are bilateral. Since lateral films are usually not positioned perfectly, there is often overlap of the right and left facets at each level. This should be uniform at all levels in the absence of rotation. An abrupt change in amount of overlap indicates an abnormal rotation (Fig. 3-52,*B*). Occasionally, rotation from the lateral position is so significant that it is difficult to detect, since one set of facets is entirely superimposed over the vertebral bodies. To avoid missing this, be certain to see both sets of facets at each vertebral body level.

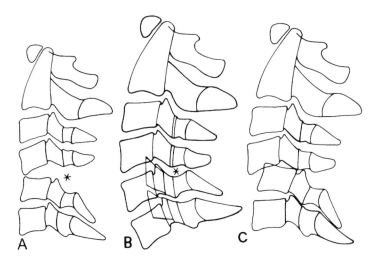

Fig. 3-52 **A,** Lateral cervical spine with fanning of spinous processes and a gap at the posterior vertebral body as well as spinous processes, indicating posterior ligamentous injury. **B,** Abnormal rotation of facets with an abrupt transition at C_{4-5}, indicating a rotational subluxation. **C,** Locked facets, with interruption of all four curves and total lack of contact between the articular surfaces of the facets at C_{4-5}.

    f. The inferior articular surface of the facet should be in full contact with the more distal element's superior facet articular surface. The absence of such full contact indicates a subluxed, perched, or locked facet (Fig. 3-52,*C*). A unilateral locked facet implies abnormal rotation as well.

    g. Odontoid process (dens) is normally tilted posteriorly on the body of C_2. If you do not see this tilt of the odontoid process, consider that there may be an occult fracture of the odontoid with anterior subluxation; check the spinolaminar line for confirmation.

    h. Atlantoaxial distance is measured at the base of the dens between the anterior cortex of the dens and the posterior cortex of the atlas' anterior arch. In adults, this distance is not more than 2.5 mm and does not change with flexion. In children, the distance may be as great as 5 mm and may change by 1 to 2 mm with flexion.

2. AP film: May provide a valuable clue to spinous process avulsion. The spinous processes should form a continuous line. In clay-shoveler's fracture, a "double" spinous process is caused by the

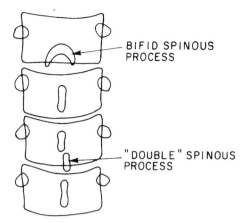

BIFID SPINOUS
PROCESS

"DOUBLE" SPINOUS
PROCESS

Fig. 3-53 AP cervical spine showing a normal bifid spinous process and an abnormal "double" spinous process, indicating a clay-shoveler's fracture. Note that facet joints are not seen on the AP because of their normal angulation.

slightly displaced fragment of the tip overlying the base of its process (see Fig 3-53).

3. Oblique film: Used to evaluate posterior elements for fracture and confirm normal overlap of facets. Often not a part of the trauma series.

4. Open-mouth film:
   a. Used to evaluate the odontoid process for fracture. Do not confuse the bottom of the incisors or the arch of the atlas with a fracture.
   b. Used also to evaluate the integrity of the ring of the atlas. In neutral position, there is exact alignment of C_1 on C_2 without offset of the facets (i.e., equal distance from the dens to the medial margin of each facet). With rotation, the atlas moves as a unit: the lateral facet of C_1 is offset laterally on one side of the dens and medially on the other. Bilateral lateral offset of the facets indicates a C_1 ring fracture in adults; in children, it may be a normal variant.

5. Other films to be tailored to the individual patient's needs:
   a. Lateral flexion-extension views:
      (1) If a fracture is not seen but there are other suggestions of ligamentous injury (usually abnormal gapping of the bodies posteriorly or fanning of the spinous processes on the lateral film), flexion-extension films will help evaluate the extent of the injury and the degree of stability.

(2) The patient is allowed to flex and extend alone, without force. A physician should supervise the filming, and the patient should be awake, cooperative, and neurologically intact.

(3) Watch for increase or reduction of the posterior splaying. Also evaluate facet subluxation as well as listhesis of the vertebral body.

b. Pillar views:

(1) AP with 20 to 30 degrees' caudad angulation.

(2) Used to profile the facets (they are normally angulated with respect to the AP film).

(3) Watch for facet compression or fracture. These are especially at risk in a hyperextension injury.

c. Tomograms/CT:

(1) Either may be useful in an individual situation: tailor to the problem.

(2) Tomograms require excellent technique and patient cooperation.

(3) CT may miss fractures in the axial plane (especially around C_1 and base of dens) if thin section with reconstruction is not utilized and must be interpreted with care since there is overlap of adjacent levels posteriorly. If there is a question bringing the patient to CT, at least sagittal reconstruction must be included.

B. Congenital anomalies and normal variants.

1. Fusion or lack-of-segmentation anomalies are common.

2. Occipitalization of the atlas: Lack of segmentation at atlanto-occipital junction; presents with atlantoaxial subluxation, simulating a traumatic disruption. There is also an abnormally large gap between the spinous processes of C_1 and C_2, with the atlas located unusually close to the occiput. The diagnosis is established by a flexion film, which demonstrates fixation of the atlas to the occiput. In addition, the odontoid often has a bizarre shape.

3. Absence or lack of fusion of ossification centers is especially confusing at C_1 and C_2:

a. Normal ossification of C_1: The body (occasionally bifid) and each of the neural arches (Fig 3-54); posterior arch defects are common in C_1. Also, the synchondrosis between the body and arch may fuse asymmetrically (usually by age 7 years).

b. Normal ossification of C_2 (Fig 3-55): Four ossification centers (one for each neural arch, the body [occasionally bifid], and the odontoid process). The body-neural arch synchondroses fuse asymmetrically between age 3 and 6; the body-odontoid

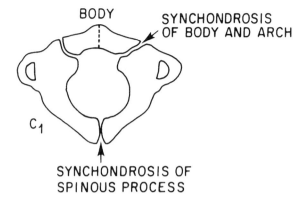

Fig. 3-54   Normal ossification centers of C_1, indicating sites at which lack of fusion may simulate a fracture.

    process synchondrosis also fuses between 3 and 6 years. A persistent lucent synchondrosis may remain into adult life, located well *below* the level of the apparent ''base'' of the odontoid. This is differentiated from an odontoid fracture, which usually occurs at the true base of odontoid.

    c. Os terminale: An ossification center at the superior tip of the odontoid process. Before it ossifies, the tip of the process is V-shaped. The os terminale normally fuses by age 12 (Fig 3-56,*A*) but may persist unfused, simulating a tip of odontoid fracture (Fig 3-56,*B*).

    d. Os odontoideum: In the presence of a hypoplastic odontoid, the os terminale becomes overgrown and is termed the os odontoideum. It is a large ossicle which is separated from the hypoplastic odontoid by a wide gap and which moves with the arch of the atlas. It may appear quite bizarre (Fig 3-52,*C*).

4. A bifid spinous process may project into the neural foramen on an oblique film, simulating a fracture.

5. A transverse process may be elongated, appearing as a bone fragment on the lateral film.

6. An enlarged uncinate process may simulate a vertebral body fracture on the lateral film. Confirm on the AP as DJD of the uncovertebral joint.

7. In a child, the ring apophysis (seen especially well anterosuperiorly on the lateral film) may simulate a chip or avulsion fracture. Before the ring apophysis is ossified, it appears as a corner notch in the vertebral body and may simulate anterior body wedging.

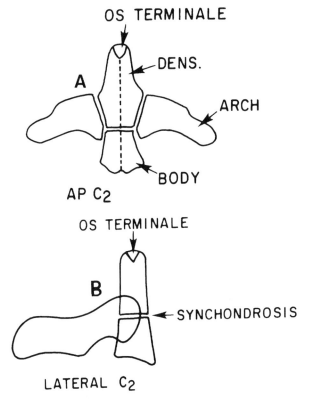

OS TERMINALE

DENS.

A

ARCH

BODY

AP C$_2$

OS TERMINALE

B

SYNCHONDROSIS

LATERAL C$_2$

Fig. 3-55 Normal ossification centers of C$_2$ (AP [**A**] and lateral [**B**]), indicating sites at which lack of fusion may simulate a fracture.

C. Injury pattern of the cervical spine.
   1. Occipital condyle fractures are more common than previously thought, and often require CT for diagnosis; they may involve the hypoglossal canal or jugular foramen, so clinical features of injury to cranial nerves IX to XII may be found.
   2. C$_1$ (atlas):
      a. Occipitovertebral dissociation: Normal occipitovertebral relationship is maintained by ligaments extending from the axis to the clivus; in patients with injuries resulting in severe facial trauma, trauma to this portion of the neck may also occur; a true dislocation is usually fatal and obvious on lateral film; subluxation is rare and may not have neurologic deficit or obvious plain film findings: Draw a line from the tip of the clivus, which is parallel to a line drawn along the posterior

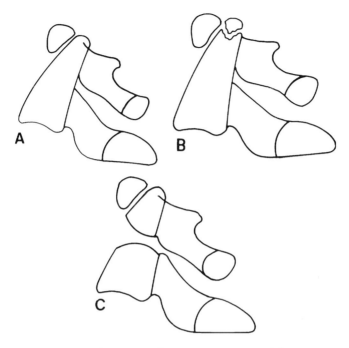

Fig. 3-56   Spectrum of os terminale variants: **A,** Normal fusion. **B,** A simple unfused os terminale. **C,** Os odontoideum, the result of a hypoplastic odontoid and overgrown os terminale.

body of C_2. If the distance between these two lines is less than 12 mm, then occipitovertebral subluxation is not likely.[56]

b. Bilateral vertical fracture through the neural arch is the most common fracture of the atlas; to be differentiated from congenital defects.

c. Jefferson's fracture: Vertical compression produces a burst fracture involving both anterior and posterior arches. It is stable, and usually the patient is neurologically intact unless there is also disruption of the transverse ligament. The latter may be seen or inferred by CT or MR.

d. Atlantoaxial rotatory displacement: A rotary locking of the facets, usually seen in childhood, presenting as torticollis. Most patients recover spontaneously:

(1) Open-mouth view: One lateral mass of C_1 appears wider and closer to the midline. The opposite is narrower and laterally offset. One of the facets may be obscured by overlapping. CT with reconstruction may be extremely helpful in diagnosing the condition.

(2) Lateral view: Posterior arches of the atlas fail to superimpose because of head tilt; may have wider atlas-dens space.

(3) The rotatory atlantoaxial dislocation described above is distinctly different from the rotatory atlantoaxial subluxation commonly seen in children after upper respiratory infection (URI), pharyngeal surgery, or minor trauma; these will resolve with conservative therapy; the more rare but serious rotatory atlantoaxial dislocation also usually occurs in children.

3. C_2(axis):

   a. Odontoid (dens) fracture: Usually through the base of the dens; if it has an oblique extension into the vertebral body anteriorly, it may not be seen on the open-mouth view; must be differentiated from congenital variants (see Section B, above); this is the most commonly missed cervical spine fracture (23%).[57]

   b. Hangman's fracture: Hyperextension injury resulting in bilateral neural arch fractures. The odontoid and its attachments are intact; nerve damage is uncommon owing to the width of the canal at this level. Type I (65%) involves the posterior part of the body of C_2 or any part of the ring without displacement or angulation, and the C_{2-3} disk is intact. If there is greater than 3 mm displacement of C_2 on C_3 or 15-degree angulation at this level, the C_{2-3} disk is likely disrupted, leading to a type II or III designation and implied instability.[57]

4. Flexion injuries:

   a. Anterior wedge: Relatively minor injury, not usually associated with posterior retropulsion of the body.

   b. Hyperflexion sprain-anterior subluxation: Posterior ligamentous complex disrupted; localized increased height of intervertebral disk space, associated with fanning of spinous processes and a local kyphotic angulation. These findings are accentuated on flexion films; may allow facet subluxation or locking. There is delayed instability in 20%.

   c. Unilateral locked facet: Due to flexion, distraction, and rotation; an abrupt change in amount of facet overlap on lateral film. Most common locations are C_{4-5} and C_{5-6}; 35% are associated with fracture (usually facet).

   d. Bilateral locked facet: Due to flexion with enough distraction for facets to become disarticulated; the vertebral body is displaced approximately 50% of the body length on the lateral film. Both lateral and oblique films show the "jumped," locked facets; high incidence of cord damage.

   e. Clay-shoveler's fracture: Avulsion of the spinous processes (usually C_6 or C_7) due to flexion; "double" process seen on AP. May occasionally be unstable.

   f. Teardrop burst fracture: Most severe flexion fracture compatible with life; 87% have neurologic changes, usually quadriplegia.[57] Coronal and sagittal comminuted vertebral body fractures with triangular fragment from the anteroinferior border of the body. The posterior body is displaced into the spinal canal with high probability of neural damage. Mechanism is combined flexion and compression (diving and motor vehicle accidents are most common).

5. Extension injuries (signs may be quite subtle): Stretch or tear the anterior longitudinal ligament, often interrupt the anterior annulus and avulse adjacent vertebral body endplates; may also disrupt the posterior longitudinal ligament, facet capsules, and other posterior support, leading to profound instability; despite these serious soft tissue disruptions, plain film findings may be extremely subtle:

   a. Prevertebral soft tissue swelling.

   b. Posterior body displacement.

   c. Widened intervertebral disk space, especially at the anterior portion of the bodies.

   d. Vacuum phenomenon at the anulus fibrosus (in the absence of degenerative disease) is highly suggestive of anterior soft tissue injury. Avulsion fracture from the anteroinferior margin, especially of C_2 or C_3. Facet (pillar) compression fracture may be unilateral and may require pillar views for diagnosis and results from hyperextension with rotation. May result in nerve root compression; not uncommonly, spinal cord injury occurs without fracture or dislocation.

   e. If mechanism, combined with or without any of the above extremely subtle plain film findings suggests hyperextension injury, MR should be performed to delineate the soft tissue injury and determine the likelihood of instability. The cord, any disk herniation, and epidural hematoma are directly visualized as well. Vertebral artery occlusions from facet fractures or instability may be seen as well.

   f. Less severe extension injuries include: Avulsion of the anterior arch of the atlas (horizontal), isolated fracture of the posterior arch of the atlas, extension teardrop (anterior inferior corner, usually in osteopenic patients), laminar fracture (including Hangman's).

6. Radiographic signs of instability:

   a. Spinous process fanning.

b. Widening of intervertebral disk space (in neutral, flexion, extension, or traction).

c. Horizontal displacement of one body on another more than 3.5 mm.

d. Angulation greater than 11 degrees.

e. Disruption of facets.

f. Severe injury, such as multiple fractures at one segment.

D. Cervical spine fractures in children.

1. Parameters for evaluation are different (see Section A, Normal and Abnormal Variants).

2. Sites of involvement tend to be different: Teenagers have cervical injuries similar in distribution to adults and need to be evaluated with the full adult series of films. Children under 12 years old involve mostly the atlanto-occipital and atlantoaxial regions, so greatest attention should be paid to this region.

E. Soft tissue injury in the cervical spine—diagnose by MR.

1. Acute disk herniation: Common with bilateral facet dislocation, hypertension injury, flexion-distraction injury, and flexion-compression injury.

2. Epidural hematoma: Less common, and may be delayed and accumulate slowly; MR signal depends on age of blood: acute (1 to 3 days) is low signal on T1 and T2 imaging, subacute is high signal on T1 and low signal on T2; may also be complex.

Thoracic Spine

A. Unusual site of fracture.

B. AP view: Watch interpediculate distance for abrupt widening suggestive of a burst fracture. There may be a paraspinous fullness secondary to hematoma. On chest films, this may simulate adenopathy or large vessel bleed.

C. Lateral view: Swimmer's view is necessary for upper spine. Vertebral body height should remain uniform over the length of the thoracic spine (except for a normal slight anterior wedging of T_{12}). Normal kyphosis is 20 to 40 degrees, measured from T_4 to T_{12}.

D. Thoracic spine fractures are generally stable because of support from the thoracic cage and the orientation of the facets. Instability is more likely with multiple rib fractures or a sternal fracture.

Lumbar Spine

A. Normal appearance:

1. On AP, interpediculate distance gradually widens from L_1 to L_5.

2. On lateral, disk spaces gradually increase in size from L_{1-2} to L_{4-5}; L_5 to S_1 may be slightly narrower.

3. Limbus vertebra is an unfused ring apophysis secondary to anterior disk herniation that may simulate a fracture.

B. Patterns of injury[58]:

    a. Sixty percent of thoracolumbar fractures are at T_{12}-L_2.

    b. Ninety percent are at T_{11}-L_4.

    c. Seventy-five percent are compression fractures (anterior wedging or depression of the superior end-plate) with intact posterior elements.

    d. Twenty percent are fracture-dislocations (involvement of posterior elements as well as body). These are burst fractures, requiring CT to evaluate for bony fragments in the spinal canal and to choose anterior or posterior surgical approach. The facets may be fractured, subluxed, perched, dislocated, or locked, and these situations are not always obvious on CT unless the anatomy is understood.[59] Facets are identified by their orientation with respect to the vertebral body (superior facets are directed posteromedially and inferior facets are directed anterolaterally) as well as the shape of the articular surface (superior facet articular surface is concave, inferior articular surface is flat or convex; Fig 3-57). Using these guidelines, facet dislocation (AP or lateral or superior with ''naked'' facets) will not be missed on CT; subluxation of facets can be seen well with sagittal reconstruction.

    e. Chance fracture: Transverse fracture through the posterior elements (spinous process, pedicles, facets, transverse processes); the vertebral body may or may not be fractured. Lap-type seat belts act as a fulcrum. The tensile stress in hyperflexion causes the usual transverse fracture; little to no vertebral body compression; abdominal injury is often associated.

C. Spondylolysis: A defect in the pars intra-articularis, seen on the AP and lateral films, but often seen best on the oblique film (fracture through the neck of the ''scotty dog'').

    1. Two thirds are at L_5.

    2. More common in males than females.

    3. More prevalent in whites than blacks.

    4. Usually diagnosed in second or third decade.

    5. Etiology uncertain, but many feel that it is a stress fracture (repeated normal trauma), perhaps aggravated by dysplasia or hypoplasia of the pars.

    6. May be unilateral or bilateral; if unilateral, hyperplasia and sclerosis of the contralateral facet may develop (simulating metastatic disease or osteoid osteoma); a congenitally absent pars may give a very similar appearance. If bilateral, associated spondylolisthesis may develop.

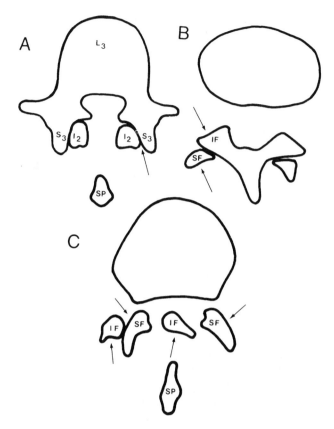

Fig. 3-57 CT appearance of facets in lumbar spine: **A,** Normal. **B,** Anterior lock. **C,** Lateral lock. SF, superior facet; IF, inferior facet; SP, spinous process; *arrows,* articular surface.

XII. NONACCIDENTAL TRAUMA (BATTERED CHILD SYNDROME)

Key Concepts

Typical fractures or combinations of injuries are suggestive. Watch especially for fractures at different stages of healing, metaphyseal fractures, and rib fractures. Periosteal reaction and growth disturbances are also suggestive.

A. Radiographic signs considered to be pathognomonic.
   1. Multiple fractures at different sites at different stages of healing (in the absence of metabolic or dysplastic disease).

2. Epiphyseal-metaphyseal fractures: Avulsion or bucket-handle fractures due to traction on the limb and avulsion of the metaphysis at the periosteal insertion (rare with accidental trauma in children under 5 years). Watch especially for such fractures at the medial portion of the proximal tibial metaphysis.

3. Rib fractures: Rare in accidental trauma owing to the plasticity of the thoracic cage. Fractures are usually posterior, at costovertebral junction. Watch also for callus formation at the costochondral junction, simulating a rachitic or scorbutic rosary.

B. Unfortunately, many cases are not typical; other areas to watch for:

1. Extremity fractures (long and short tubular bones) are most frequent focus of injury, long bones much more common than hands or feet.

2. Periosteal reaction without definite evidence of fractures. (Differential diagnosis is extensive, including physiologic reaction, Caffey's disease, infection, tumor, rickets, scurvy, hypervitaminosis A, prostaglandin administration, normal wavy radius.)

3. Skull fractures, usually linear, are common.

4. Pelvic fractures are rare, usually pubic rami.

5. Clavicle, usually midshaft.

6. Spine: Rare, usually thoracic and lumbar flexion injuries.

7. Growth disturbances or traumatic metaphyseal cupping.

8. Extraskeletal injuries: Subdural hematoma, visceral injury, usually associated with skeletal injury.

C. Bone scan:

1. May be useful for additional or confirmatory evidence in specific cases.

2. Epiphyseal-metaphyseal fractures are difficult to detect because of the normally increased activity in this region.

3. Especially sensitive for occult rib, spine, or diaphyseal fractures, particularly acutely.

D. Suggested plain films for screening of clinically suspected cases:

1. AP of extremities (including hands, feet, and pelvis) and AP thorax.

2. AP and lateral skull.

E. Epidemiologic considerations[60]:

1. Overall frequency of skeletal trauma associated with abuse is low (20% to 40%).

2. Incidence of skeletal injuries considered pathognomonic for abuse is low.

3. Most common sites of fracture are diaphyses of long bones and skull, but these are not, by themselves, diagnostic.

4. In abused children, skeletal trauma is most commonly seen in the

first 2 years of life. This is especially true of skull fractures (90% are in this age group). These data suggest that the efficacy of skeletal surveys is decreased in older children. A selective approach, rather than skeletal survey, may be indicated for them.

  5. Skeletal trauma is usually associated with clinical evidence of physical injury; it is much less commonly seen in conjunction with other forms of abuse (neglect or sexual).

  6. Yield is extremely low in skeletal survey of siblings of abused children in the absence of clinical evidence of physical trauma.

F. The pattern of inflicted injury in infants may be different than that in older children. One study of 31 infants (3 months average age) who died with inflicted skeletal injury showed rib fractures in 51%, fractures of long bones in 44% (89% of these were metaphyseal as opposed to the more common shaft fracture in older children), and skull fractures in 42% by histopathology. Only 58% of the fractures were seen on skeletal surveys, but 92% were seen with specimen radiography; even with children this young, most had fractures at multiple sites and of different ages.[61]

XIII. MYOSITIS OSSIFICANS

Key Concepts

The timing and zoning phenomenon of myositis is key to making the correct diagnosis. Without these considerations, osteosarcoma could be incorrectly diagnosed.

A. Juxtacortical myositis ossificans: Heterotopic formation of non-neoplastic bone and cartilage in soft tissue (usually muscle, but other soft tissue may be involved).

  1. Etiology: Usually traumatic, though the episode of trauma may be minor and not recalled.

  2. Sites: Anywhere, but most commonly, areas prone to trauma (e.g., thighs, elbows).

  3. Histologic evolution:

   a. Weeks 0 to 4: Pseudosarcomatous appearance of central zone suggests malignant neoplasm.

   b. Weeks 4 to 8: Centrifugal pattern of maturation: Periphery demarcated by initial immature osteoid formation, which organizes into mature bone about a cellular center (zone phenomenon).

4. Radiographic evolution:
   a. Weeks 0 to 2: soft tissue mass (clinically painful, warm, doughy).
   b. Weeks 3 to 4: Flocculated amorphous densities within the mass, with periosteal reaction in underlying bone. At this stage, it may be mistaken for an early osteosarcoma since the calcification looks like tumor bone. Occasionally, the mass may appear attached to underlying bone and may even elicit a periosteal reaction from the underlying bone, making it even more difficult to distinguish from tumor.
   c. Weeks 6 to 8: Sharp cortical bone surrounding a lacy pattern of new bone. Maturation proceeds centrifugally.
   d. Months 5 to 6: Maturity, with reduction in mass size. Often, a radiolucent zone separates the lesion from the underlying cortex.
5. The history and timing are crucial in supporting the early diagnosis of myositis ossificans. With good correlation of this information and radiographic findings, early and potentially confusing biopsies can be avoided.
6. Bone scans may be used serially to evaluate for maturation of myositis; surgical resection should not be considered prior to maturation, since it leads to a high rate of recurrence.
7. MR appearance of myositis ossificans relates to the age of the lesion, just as does the plain film. Early and intermediate lesions show a mass lesion isointense to muscle on T1, but high signal and very inhomogeneous on T2. Surrounding edema is prominent. Periosteal reaction and bone marrow edema may be seen if the myositis is located near bone. Mature lesions (over 2 months) are better defined. The center remains inhomogeneous, but approximates fat signal on T1 and T2 images, while the rim shows a ''halo'' of decreased signal on all sequences.[62] Thus, the zoning seen on plain film and histologically is also seen on MR.
   attached to bone resulting from trauma to the periosteum with hemorrhage beneath it.
B. Myositis ossificans associated with neurologic disorders or burns:
   1. Thirty-three percent to 49% of paraplegics show myositis in the paralyzed part, most commonly hips.
   2. Ossification in the muscles, tendons, and ligaments, not arising from the underlying bone.
C. Differential diagnoses of myositis:
   1. Parosteal osteosarcoma:
      a. Portions of the tumor may be separated from the underlying cortex by a radiolucent zone, but there is attachment; tends to

wrap around long bone; underlying marrow is usually involved, but not obviously until MR demonstrates it.

    b. Reversed zone phenomenon: More heavily calcified centrally, and the periphery is less dense and poorly circumscribed.

    c. Gradual increase in size.

2. Periosteal osteosarcoma: Usually appears more aggressive, often with scalloping of underlying cortex and amorphous tumor bone formation.

3. Juxtacortical chondroma: Scalloped underlying cortex, with juxtacortical calcific densities.

4. Osteochondroma: Arises from the underlying bone, with continuation of cortical and medullary bone. Should not be confused with myositis.

5. Tumoral calcinosis:

    a. Periarticular calcified soft tissue masses, usually around the hip, shoulder, and elbows that are entirely separate from the underlying bone, which is normal.

    b. Frequency higher among blacks; males and females affected in equal numbers.

    c. May progress to limit function, ulcerate, and undergo secondary infection.

    d. Very high recurrence rate after resection.

    e. Serum phosphate and erythrocyte sedimentation rate (ESR) are elevated; normal calcium.

    f. Etiology may be enhanced renal tubular phosphate resorption.

    g. May respond to a program of phosphate binding antacids and dietary phosphate and calcium deprivation.

6. Myositis ossificans progressiva:

    a. Hereditary mesodermal disorder characterized by progressive ossification of striated muscles, tendons, and ligaments.

    b. May be autosomal-dominant with a wide range of expressivity; many spontaneous mutations.

    c. Target tissue thought to be interstitial tissues, with muscle involvement secondary to pressure atrophy.

    d. Electromyogram (EMG) studies have shown abnormalities consistent with a myopathy.

    e. Pathologic abnormalities are similar to those of myositis ossificans.

    f. Most frequent presenting symptom is acute torticollis with a painful mass in the sternocleidomastoid muscle.

    g. Progresses to the shoulder girdle, upper arms, spine and pelvis, with bridging between adjacent bones and, eventually, severe restriction of motion.

h. High association of congenital digital anomalies: 75% show bilateral microdactyly of the first toes and/or synostosis of the phalanges; hallux valgus; thumbs less frequently involved.

i. Remissions and exacerbations frequently are precipitated by minor trauma.

j. Involvement of the insertions of fasciae, ligaments, and tendons produce "exostoses."

XIV. ORTHOPEDIC HARDWARE

Key Concepts

Femoral components of hip prostheses tend to loosen early, acetabular components late. Progression in signs of loosening is important to document. Subsidence of components may be subtle and is occasionally the only sign of failure. In knee prostheses, it is the tibial component that loosens most often and commonly shows no radiographic abnormalities, even though there is clinical failure. The patellar component fails more often than either the femoral or tibial, often through component or osseous failure rather than loosening.

A. Total hip arthroplasty: Whether device is cemented or uncemented (with or without porous coating for bony ingrowth) the principles of radiographic analysis are similar:

1. *Evaluation of placement*[63]:

a. *Lateral opening of the acetabulum* (measured by the angle of the cup to a line drawn between the ischial tuberosities) (Fig 3-58) is ideally 40 degrees ± 10 degrees. A wider opening angle increases the risk of dislocation. A decreased angle is stable in most positions, but not in abduction, so would be at risk for dislocation in a sexually active woman.

b. *Anteversion* of the acetabulum (evaluated on a groin lateral film) should be 10 to 15 degrees but may be as little as 0 degrees if compensated by an anteverted femoral component. Retroversion of the cup increases the probability of dislocation. Anteversion is only qualitatively evaluated on the groin lateral film.

c. Watch for *protrusio* acetabuli of the cup, especially in patients with RA, Paget's disease, or osteomalacia. The horizontal center of rotation is measured from the center of the head to a medial landmark such as the teardrop and compared with the opposite side. If the cup is not properly medialized (such as in a patient with OA), it is at risk for dislocation since the

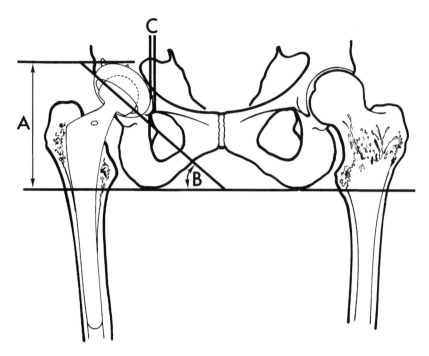

Fig. 3-58   Evaluation of total hip arthroplasty. The reference line for most of the evaluation is the transischial line. **A,** evaluates effective limb length; another way to evaluate this would be to compare the levels of the lesser trochanters with one another. **B,** measures the opening angle (lateral inclination) of the acetabular cup. **C,** is used to evaluate for either excessive or lack of medialization of the cup. (Reprinted with permission from Manaster BJ. *Total hip arthroplasty: Radiographic evaluation.* Radiographics 1996;16:645–660.)

iliopsoas tendon passes medial to the femoral head center of rotation and contraction would tend to force the head out.

d. Evaluate for *lengths of gluteus medius and* iliopsoas muscle groups and limb length; muscles are strongest at specific effective lengths. If they are overstretched, they may go into spasm, and if the space over which they contract is too short, they are ineffective. A side-to-side comparison of the position of the greater trochanters (insertion of gluteus) and lesser trochanters (insertion of the iliopsoas) should therefore be made. This comparison is frequently made with reference to the transischial line (Fig 3-58). Adjustments may be made in the length of the neck of the femoral prosthesis or by transplanting the greater tuberosity more distally to achieve the effective length.

e. *Position of femoral component:* Neutral to slight valgus (prosthesis resting against the lateral cortex proximally and against the medial cortex distally) is preferred to varus (which predisposes to loosening).

f. Inappropriate sizing, especially of a noncemented femoral component, may be problematic. These stems are chosen for optimal proximal canal fit, to maximize surface contact with the endosteal cortex.

g. Intraoperative fracture is extremely rare on the acetabular side; the femoral stem more commonly fractures the cortex, especially anteriorly. These fractures are often incomplete and difficult to see. Femoral fractures are significantly more common with the long-stemmed revision components than with the primary placements; fractures are more common among the primary press-fit prostheses than the smaller cemented components.

2. Evaluation for loosening:

a. Malpositioning (see above) promotes loosening.

b. If cement is used for femoral component fixation, it must be placed in areas of maximum stress—around the tip, on the lateral side of the distal stem, and on the medial side of the stem proximally.

c. A fracture in cement definitely indicates loosening.

d. Lucency at the bone–cement interface is suspicious for loosening, but not diagnostic. This is especially true at the superolateral aspect of the acetabular component, where a 2- to 3-mm lucency is common. *To be diagnostic of component loosening, lucency at the bone–cement interface must show progression over time.*

e. Extensive scalloped resorption around a femoral component (*massive osteolysis*) or lytic lesions developing in the acetabular region are indicative of particle disease. This destructive process results from particles of a specific size; the type of particle seems immaterial and may be bone, cement, metal, or polyethylene. The particles initiate a cascade of inflammatory reaction events, resulting in osteolysis. Watch particularly for particle disease related to polyethylene wear at the cup-femoral head interface. The wear is detected on an AP pelvis by a superior offset of the head within the cup (Fig 3-59). Be careful to detect this indication of polyethylene wear so as to avoid misinterpreting the osteolysis as loosening, infection, or even tumor.

f. Uncemented components often show a 1- to 2-mm lucency

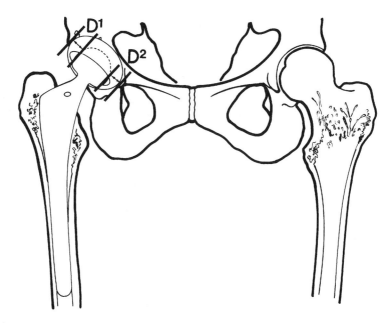

Fig. 3-59 Evaluation for polyethylene wear of the acetabular component. With polyethylene wear, the patient develops a superior offset of the head within the cup (D1 decreases relative to D2) since wear develops in the superior weight-bearing portion of the cup. (Reprinted with permission from Manaster BJ. *Total hip arthroplasty: Radiographic evaluation.* Radiographics 1996;16:645–660.)

around the component, with a very thin sclerotic margin. In our experience, unless this shows progression or evidence of toggling (windshield wiper sign) the lucency does not represent loosening.

g. Sclerosis at the tip of a femoral component alone does not suggest loosening in uncemented components. The cortex or endosteum may show bone formation as well; until such bone production "bridges" across the canal distal to the femoral stem, it is not considered indicative of *loosening, but should be watched for progression.*

h. *One of the most important signs of loosening is change in position of the component. Acetabular components tend to subside superiorly or tilt, and femoral components tend to subside inferiorly, with consequent shortening of the leg. Subsidence* may be extremely subtle, since the bone-component lucency may be obliterated by the change in component position.

Choose landmarks and use comparison films in order to detect subtle changes in position.

3. The pattern of loosening of cemented hip prostheses is interesting: Femoral components tend to loosen early, with a rapid rate, which then falls off to a slower rate after 5 years. On the other hand, the incidence of acetabular component loosening is low initially and shows a sharp increase after 5 years, so that acetabular loosening approaches, and in some series even surpasses, femoral component loosening. This observation has led to placement of "hybrid" prostheses, with cemented femoral components but uncemented cups.

4. Dislocation may be due to positional factors (placing the hip beyond the expected range of motion), soft tissue laxity (in multiply-operated hip revisions), soft tissue imbalance (abnormal reconstruction length or abductor length abnormalities), or component malposition (abnormal cup horizontal or anteversion or center of rotation).

5. Infection is suspected with the presence of periosteal reaction or large amounts of heterotopic ossification, but plain film findings are generally absent.

6. Bone scans show abnormal activity at the surgical site of the prosthesis, which decreases over a period of 9 months (longer in uncemented prostheses). Increasing activity over that period is abnormal. Loosening generally shows focal activity at the sites of greatest movement (especially the tip), whereas infection shows a more general increase in activity.

7. Arthrography is not reliable in detecting loosening (serial sequences of plain films are preferable). Specificity for loosening is especially low in noncemented prostheses: failure to demonstrate contrast tracking around components does not rule out loosening, while incomplete contrast tracking may not correctly diagnose loosening (solid fibrous union in porous coated prostheses may allow such tracking).

8. Revision arthroplasties are often uncemented, and bone graft is used liberally to fill defects (very large pieces such as femoral heads may be used).

   a. Lateral "windows" in the femoral shaft may be performed for cement extraction in revisions.

   b. Shafts commonly fracture from prosthesis and cement extraction, reaming of thinned bone, and reinsertion of femoral components (especially long-stemmed components that do not conform to normal anterior femoral bowing). The fractures are often subtle vertical ones. Cerclage wiring protects the revision.

c. As grafts compress or resorb, there is often significant change in position or orientation of components; several millimeters of subsidence is common and may be acceptable; stabilization should occur over about 12 months; serial films are crucial for evaluation.

9. *Endoprostheses* are utilized when there is no need for an acetabular replacement (e.g., in AVN or subcapital fractures). Either the older Austin Moore or Thompson prosthesis with a large head is used, or a bipolar (or Bateman) component (a cup that clamps on to the head of the femoral component; the femoral head can move within the cup, and the cup can move within the patient's normal acetabulum). In these bipolar prostheses, there is a large amount of movement expected at the outer cup with respect to the acetabulum; this outer cup must not be mistaken for a loose acetabular component.

B. Total knee arthroplasty[64]:

1. Normal placement:

a. Tibial component is placed 90 degrees ± 5 degrees to the long axis of the tibial shaft on the AP and ranges from 90 degrees to the long axis of the tibia to a slight posterior tilt on the lateral. Either through the tibial component placement, or through a differential polyethylene thickness, the normal 10-degree posterior tilt is retained.

b. Femoral component is placed in 5 degrees ± 5 degrees to the long axis of the femoral shaft on the lateral. Overall, there should be 4 to 7 degrees of valgus angulation of the knee.

c. Widened joint space on one side suggests soft tissue instability.

2. Evaluation of loosening:

a. As in the hip, watch for progressive lucency at bone–cement or bone–uncemented component interface.

b. Subsidence or other change in component position indicates loosening.

c. The tibial component is much more likely to loosen than is the femoral one. Early loosening is usually followed by tilting of the tibial component into a varus position with subsidence into the medial tibial plateau and collapse of the cancellous bone. Polyethylene wear, fragmentation, and dislocation may follow.

d. Loosening and/or infection in knee components is much more difficult to detect radiographically than in hip arthroplasties. Technical factors such as slight flexion, rotation, or change in centering can mask a lucency at the bone–component interface. To avoid those technical difficulties, fluoroscopic spot films of the tibial component–bone interface should be taken in order to evaluate for progressive lucency.

  e. In uncemented knee components it is common to see a nonprogressive 1- to 2-mm lucency at the tibial component–bone interface, which may have a sclerotic margin. It is speculated that the lucency may represent fibrous union. With porous-coated prostheses, there may even be loosened microspheres in this lucent region. As long as there is no progression, these findings are not likely to indicate loosening.

3. The femoral component rarely shows loosening. Uncemented femoral components frequently show the effect of stress shielding with bone resorption (but no sclerotic margin) at parts of the bone–prosthesis interface; distal femoral metaphyseal resorption may be widespread, appearing quite lucent, but this appears to bear no relationship to prosthesis failure. Buttressing may be seen at the site of stress (often the anterior cortex or posterior cortex or even streaming posteriorly from femoral prosthesis pegs).

4. Patellar complications occur most commonly (15%). They include:

  a. Subsidence: Common, and often stabilizes.
  b. Wear of polyethylene layer.
  c. Polyethylene may dissociate from the metal backing.
  d. Metal backing may disintegrate, leaving small metal particles lining the polyethylene and capsule (metalosis).
  e. Patellar dislocation.
  f. Surgical devascularization may result in patellar AVN or fracture.
  g. Patellar fracture may also result from stress raisers in the patellar component peg holes.

5. Particle disease may be initiated by wear debris, resulting in osteolysis.

6. Periprosthetic fracture: Usually insufficiency fractures in osteopenic patients (especially if there also was a tibial tubercle transfer).

C. Dynamic screws (Richard's screw is one common variety) for intertrochanteric fractures[65]:

1. Reduction may be stable and acceptable if it is anatomic or has had medial displacement of the shaft and impaction or valgus repositioning.

2. The screw fits within a coaxial sleeve in the femoral neck and is designed to ''telescope'' into its sleeve several centimeters to avoid cutting out of an osteoporotic femoral head if there is collapse or impaction at the fracture site.

3. The position of the screw head should be slightly inferior and

posterior to the middle of the femoral head and very close to the articular surface.

D. External fixators:
1. Used to maintain the length of a fractured limb in the presence of infection or severe comminution.
2. Rotation must be watched for carefully.
3. The Ilazarov fixator uses very thin (olive) wires, attached to the external frame, which is circular or semicircular. It was introduced for limb-lengthening procedures utilizing corticotomy rather than osteotomy, but is also used in posttraumatic stabilization.

E. Cerclage wires, Parham bands (older, wider, rarely used today), or cables may be placed around comminuted shaft fractures but may delay healing by stripping the periosteum and devascularizing the bone.

F. Intramedullary rod:
1. Watch for shaft shortening or telescoping if there is a butterfly fragment present. Interlocking nails prevent this complication.
2. Rotation should be watched for, especially if the fracture is beyond the isthmus (generally proximal or distal third of long bones), so that the rod does not occupy the entire canal of the fractured segments. Rotation may be controlled by placing interlocking nails or in rods.
3. Significant diastasis at the fracture site must be avoided. If there is diastasis or significant resorption at the fracture site such that nonunion is likely, the rod may be "dynamized" by removing the interlocking nails.

G. Swanson arthroplasties (MCP, MTP, IP joints):
1. Hinge is thinnest portion and, therefore, at risk for fracture.
2. Dislocation of the flange may occur, especially in diseases such as RA with soft tissue imbalance or contractures. Particle disease may result from and contribute to these complications.

H. Carpal implants:
1. Dislocation and rotation both are common.
2. Reactive synovitis and erosive changes may be seen. Particle disease may cause massive osteolysis.

I. Posterior spinal instrumentation: See Chapter 5, Section I, Scoliosis.

J. Anterior spinal instrumentation[66]:
1. In the cervical spine, complications arise from breakage or backing out of screws. Screws may be either cancellous or cortical; the latter must engage the posterior cortex of the vertebral body. Another complication is extrusion of the bone plug placed in the intervertebral disc space. The bone plug may disintegrate, collapse, and result in nonunion across the disk space.
2. In the lumbar spine, hardware failure most commonly involves

screw breakage. Longer fusions use Dwyer or Zilke fixation: A series of vertebral body screws attached to a cable or rod, respectively, placed on the convex site of a scoliosis.

K. Screws[65]:
1. Cortical screws: Threaded over their entire length; the threads are thinner and closer spaced than on cancellous screws; threads must traverse both cortices to assure stability.
2. Cancellous screws: Thin core with wide thread diameter to grip cancellous bone; may be either completely or partially threaded.
3. Herbert screws: Central portion is smooth, but both ends are threaded; the threads are at different pitches so that the fracture fragments that the screw traverses are compressed; most commonly seen in scaphoid fractures, but may be used elsewhere.

L. Plates[65]:
1. Straight plates: Flat metal strip with round holes.
2. Dynamic compression plate: Slightly concave plate with oval holes that allows compression of the fracture site as the screws are placed.
3. Tubular plates: Thin, with a concave inner surface that conforms to the bone surface and is easy to contour.
4. Reconstruction plates: Designed to allow bending and contouring; used most often in pelvic and distal humeral fractures.
5. T, L, or cobra plates have special contour to address particular fractures; blade plates have a portion that is intraosseous, usually crossing condyles.

REFERENCES

1. Heinke D, Erickson S, Chamoy L, Timins M: Ulnar collateral ligament of the thumb: MR findings in cadavers, volunteers, and patients with ligamentous injury (Gamekeeper's thumb). *AJR* 1994;163:1431–1434.
2. Fisher M, Rogers L, Hendrix R, et al: Carpometacarpal dislocations. *CRC Crit Rev Diagnostic Imaging* 1984;22:95.
3. Dunn A: Fractures and dislocations of the carpus. *Surg Clin North Am* 1972; 52:1513.
4. Gilula L: Carpal injuries: analytic approach and case exercises. *AJR* 1979; 133:503.
5. Yeager B, Dalinka M: Radiology of trauma to the wrist: dislocations, fracture dislocations, and instability patterns. *Skel Radiol* 1985;13:120–130.
6. Manaster B: Digital arthrography of the wrist. *AJR* 1986;147:563–566.
7. Manaster BJ: The clinical efficacy of triple-injection wrist arthrography. *Radiology* 1991;178:267–270.
8. Metz V, Mann F, Gilula L: Three compartment wrist arthrography: correlation of pain site with location of uni- and bidirectional communication. *AJR* 1993;160:819–822.

9. Dalinka M: MR imaging of the wrist. *AJR* 1995;164:1–9.

10. Smith O, Snearly W: Lunotriquetral interosseous ligament of the wrist: MR appearances in asymptomatic volunteers and arthrographically normal wrists. *Radiology* 1994;191:199–202.

11. Smith D: Scapholunate interosseous ligament of the wrist. MR appearances in asymptomatic volunteers and arthrographically normal wrists. *Radiology* 1994;192:217–221.

12. Oneson S, Scales L, Tinius M, Erickson S, Chamoy L: MR imaging interpretation of the Palmer classification of triangular fibrocartilage complex lesions. *Radiographics* 1996;16:97–106.

13. Mesgarzadeh M, Schneck C, Bonakdarpour A: Carpal tunnel: MR imaging. Part I: Normal anatomy. *Radiology* 1989;171:743–748.

14. Mesgarzadeh M, Schneck C, Bonadkdarpour A, Mitra A, Conaway D: Carpal tunnel: MR imaging. Part II: Carpal tunnel syndrome. *Radiology* 1989; 171:749–754.

15. Crowley D, Reckling F: Supracondylar fracture of the humerus of children. *Ann Fam Physician* 1972;5:113.

16. Patten R: Overuse syndromes and injuries involving the elbow: MR imaging findings. *AJR* 1995;164:1205–1211.

17. Ho C: Sports and occupational injuries of the elbow: MR imaging findings. *AJR* 1995;164:1465–1471.

18. Falchook F, Zlatkin M, Erbacher G, Moulton J, Bisset G, Murphy B: Rupture of the distal biceps tendon: evaluation with MR imaging. *Radiology* 1994; 190:659–663.

19. Coumas J, Waite R, Goss T, Ferrari D, Kanzaris P, Pappas A: CT and MR evaluation of the labral capsular ligamentous complex of the shoulder. *AJR* 1992;158:591–597.

20. Palmer W, Coslowitz P: Anterior shoulder instability: diagnostic criteria determined from prospective analysis of 121 MR arthrograms. *Radiology* 1995; 197:819–825.

21. Liou J, Wilson A, Totty W, Brown J: The normal shoulder: common variations that simulate pathologic conditions at MR imaging. *Radiology* 1993;186: 435–441.

22. Loredo R, Longo C, Salonen D, Yu J, Haghaigi P, Trudell D, Clapton P, Resnick D: Glenoid labrum: MR imaging with histologic correlation. *Radiology* 1995;196:33–41.

23. Tirman P, Feller J, Janzen D, Peterfy C, Bergman A: Association of glenoid labral cysts with labral tears and glenohumeral instability. Radiologic findings and clinical significance. *Radiology* 1994;190:653–658.

24. Reinus W, Shady K, Mirowitz S, Totty W: MR diagnosis of rotator cuff tears of the shoulder: value of using T2-weighted fat-saturated images. *AJR* 1995;164:1451–1455.

25. Neuman C, Holt R, Steinbach L, Jahnke A, Petersen S: MR imaging of the shoulder: appearance of the supraspinatus tendon in asymptomatic volunteers. *AJR* 1992;158:1281–1287.

26. Tirman P, Bost F, Steinbach L, Mall J, Peterfy C, Sampson T, Sheehan W,

Forbes J, Genant H: MR arthrographic depiction of tears of the rotator cuff: benefit of abduction and external rotation of the arm. *Radiology* 1994;192:851–856.

27. Haygood T, Langlotz C, Kneeland B, Iannatti J, Williams G, Dalinka M: Categorization of acromial shape: interobserver variability with MR imaging and conventional radiography. *AJR* 1994;162:1377–1382.

28. Peh W, Farmer T, Totty W: Acromial arch shape: assessment with MR imaging. *Radiology* 1995;195:501–505.

29. Tuite M, Toivonen D, Orwin J, Wright D: Acromial angle on radiographs of the shoulder: correlation with the impingement syndrome and rotator cuff tears. *AJR* 1995;165:609–613.

30. Tirman P, Bast F, Garvin G, Peterfy C, Mall J, Steinbach L, Feller J, Crues J: Posterosuperior glenoid impingement of the shoulder: findings at MR imaging and MR arthrography with arthroscopic correlation. *Radiology* 1994;193:431–436.

31. Erickson S, Fitzgerald S, Quinn S, Carrera G, Black K, Lawson T: Long bicipital tendon of the shoulder: normal anatomy and pathologic findings on MR imaging. *AJR* 1992;158:1091–1096.

32. Cartland J, Crues J, Stauffer A, Nottage W, Ryu R: MR imaging in the evaluation of SLAP injuries of the shoulder: findings in ten patients. *AJR* 1992; 159:787–792.

33. Fritz R, Helms C, Steinbach L, Genant H: Suprascapular nerve entrapment: evaluation with MR imaging. *Radiology* 1992;182:437–444.

34. Shankman S, Beltran J: MRI of the shoulder. *Current Problems in Diagnostic Radiology* 1995;24:201–228.

35. Gill K, Bucholy R: The role of CT scanning in the evaluation of major pelvic fractures. *J Bone Joint Surg Am* 1984;66A:34.

36. Resnik C, Stackhouse D, Shanmuganathan K, Young J: Diagnosis of pelvic fractures with acute pelvic trauma: efficacy of plain radiographs. *AJR* 1992;158:109–112.

37. Ben-Menachem Y, Coldwell D, Young J, Burgess A: Hemorrhage associated with pelvic fractures: causes, diagnosis, and emergent management. *AJR* 1991;157:1005–1014.

38. Affram P. An epidemiologic study of cervical and trochanteric fractures of the femur in an urban population. Analysis of 1664 cases with special reference to etiologic factors. *Acta Orthop Scand Suppl* 1964;64:11.

39. Schwappach J, Murphey M, Kokmayer S, Rosenthal H, Simmons M, Huntrakoon M: Subcapital fractures of the femoral neck: prevalence and cause of radiographic appearance simulating pathologic fractures. *AJR* 1994; 162:651–654.

40. Bayliss A, Davidson J: Traumatic osteonecrosis of the femoral head following intracapsular fracture. Incidence and earliest radiological features. *Clin Radiol* 1977;28:407.

41. Hodler J, Yu J, Goodwin D, Haghighi P, Trudall D, Resnick D: MR arthrography of the hip: improved imaging of the acetabular labrum with histologic correlation in cadavers. *AJR* 1995;165:887–891.

42. Allen W, Cope R: Coxa saltans: the snapping hip revisited. *J Amer Acad Orthop Surg* 1995;3:303–308.
43. Laurin C, Dussault R, Levesque H: The tangential x-ray investigation of the patellofemoral joint. *Clin Orthop* 1979;144:16.
44. Fisher S, Fox J, Del Pizzo W, et al: Accuracy of diagnoses from magnetic resonance imaging of the knee. *J Bone Joint Surg* 1991;73A(1):2–10.
45. Deutsch A, Mink J, Fox F, et al: Peripheral meniscal tears: MR findings after conservative treatment or arthroscopic repair. *Radiology* 1990;176: 485–488.
46. Deutsch A, Mink J, Fox J, et al: The postoperative knee. *Mag Reson Q* 1992; 8:23–54.
47. Applegate GR, Flannigan BD, Fox T, Del Pizzo W: MR diagnosis of recurrent tears of the knee: value of intraarticular contrast material. *AJR* 1993;161: 821–825.
48. Smith D, May D, Phillips P: MR imaging of the anterior cruciate ligament: frequency of discordant findings on sagittal-oblique images and correlations with arthroscopic findings. *AJR* 1996;166:411–413.
49. Manaster BJ. Imaging knee ligament reconstructions. *RSNA Categorical Course in Musculoskeleltal Radiology* 1993;211–218.
50. Mainwaring B, Daffner R, Reiner B. Pylon fractures of the ankle: a distinct clinical and radiographic entity. *Radiology* 1988;168:215–218.
51. Steinbach L, Tirmon P: MRI of the ankle. *The Radiologist* 1995;2:111–124.
52. Smith D: Imaging of sports injuries of the ankle and foot. *Operative Techniques in Sports Medicine* 1995;3:47–70.
53. Dussault R, Kaplan P, Roederer G: MR imaging of Achilles tendon in patients with familial hyperlipidemia. *AJR* 1995;164:403–407.
54. DeSmet A, Fisher D, Burnstein M, Graf B, Lange R: Value of MR imaging in staging osteochondral lesions of the talus (osteochondritis dessicans): results in 14 patients. *AJR* 1990;154:555–558.
55. Karasick D, Schweitzer M: The os trigonum syndrome: imaging features. *AJR* 1996;166:125–129.
56. Harris J, Carson G, Wagner L: Radiologic diagnosis of traumatic occipitovertebral dissociation: normal occipitovertebral relationships on lateral radiographs of supine subjects. *AJR* 1994;162:881–886.
57. El-Khoury G, Kathol M, Daniel W: Imaging of acute injuries of the cervical spine: value of plain radiography, CT and MR imaging. *AJR* 1995;164: 43–50.
58. Nicoll E: Fractures of the dorso-lumbar spine. *J Bone Joint Surg Br* 1949;31: 376.
59. Manaster BJ, Osborn AG: CT patterns of thoracolumbar facet dislocation. *AJR* 1987;148:335–340.
60. Merton D, Radkowski M, Leonidas J: The abused child: a radiological reappraisal. *Radiology* 1983;146:377–381.
61. Kleinman P, Marks S, Richmond J, Blackbourne B: Inflicted skeletal injury. A postmortem radiologic-histopathologic study in 31 infants. *AJR* 1995; 165:647–650.

62. Kransdorf M, Meis J, Jelinek J: Myositis ossificans: MR appearance with radiologic-pathologic correlation. *AJR* 1991;157:1243–1248.
63. Manaster BJ: Total hip arthroplasty: radiographic evaluation. *Radiographics* 1996;16:645–660.
64. Manaster BJ:. Total knee arthroplasty: postoperative radiologic findings. *AJR* 1995;165:899–904.
65. Slone R, Heare M, Vander Griend R, Montgomery W: Orthopedic fixation devices. *Radiographics* 1991;11:823–847.
66. Slone R, MacMillan M, Montgomery W, Heare M: Spinal fixation. Part 2. Fixation techniques and hardware for the thoracic and lumbosacral spine. *Radiographics* 1993;13:521–543.

BIBLIOGRAPHY

Berquist T: *MRI of the Musculoskeletal System,* 3rd ed. Philadelphia, Lippincott Raven, 1996.

Keats T: *An Atlas of Normal Roentgen Variants That May Simulate Disease.* Chicago, Year Book Medical Publishers, 1980.

Rang M: *Childrens' Fractures.* Philadelphia, JB Lippincott, 1974.

Rockwood C, Green D: *Fractures in Adults.* Philadelphia, JB Lippincott, 1984.

Rogers L: *Radiology of Skeletal Trauma,* vols. 1 and 2, 2nd ed. New York, Churchill Livingstone, 1992.

Stoller D: *Magnetic Resonance Imaging in Orthopedics and Sports Medicine.* Philadelphia, JB Lippincott, 1993.

4

Metabolic Bone Disease

I. OSTEOPOROSIS

Key Concepts

Abnormally decreased volume of bone which is, however, normal histologically and in its degree of mineralization; senile generalized osteoporosis, the most common form, contributes to significant morbidity, especially in older females; osteoporosis in childhood has a long and interesting differential diagnosis.

A. Definition: Any condition in which there is a reduction in the amount of bone tissue.
   1. This is a specific term and is not synonymous with osteopenia or deossification.
   2. Any bone tissue that is present is fully mineralized and normal histologically.
   3. Lab values are normal.
   4. Other major causes of osteopenia may be difficult to differentiate from osteoporosis.
      a. Osteomalacia: Looser's lines may be present; also, the trabeculae may appear smudged or indistinct.
      b. Hyperparathyroidism (HPTH): The presence of subperiosteal resorption, brown tumors, or end-plate sclerosis ("rugger jersey spine") is helpful.
      c. Multiple myeloma: Focal, punched-out lesions help make the diagnosis, but generalized myeloma may be indistinguishable from osteoporosis. One percent of patients with symptomatic osteopenia have multiple myeloma. Suspect myeloma in patients over age 50 with unexplained symptomatic osteopenia. Check for associated anemia, proteinuria, and increased erythrocyte sedimentation rate (ESR), as well as serum electrophoresis. Definitive diagnosis may require biopsy.

B. Etiologies and radiographic findings: Generalized osteoporosis.
   1. Senile (involutional) osteoporosis[1]:
     a. In women, loss of bone mass begins before menopause (perhaps even in the late childbearing years) and accelerates much more rapidly than in men. The time of onset and rate of acceleration determine the risk for fracture.
     b. Incidence is higher among women than men and among Caucasians and Asians than blacks. Gender, age, and race, thus, are prime factors.
     c. Modified by estrogens, calcium intake, weight (thin women store less estrogen), weight-bearing exercise, family history, amenorrhea (as in athletes or after oophorectomy), smoking, and heavy alcohol use. Major generalized risk factors are a low peak bone mass at skeletal maturity and accelerated postmenopausal bone loss.
     d. Thirty percent to 50% of women over 60 show evidence of significant bone loss.
     e. The process is usually irreversible, but the rate of bone loss may be altered by therapy.
     f. Etiology is unclear. Some studies favor a decrease in matrix formation, while others suggest increased osteoclast activity.
     g. Trabecular bone is resorbed faster than cortical bone.
     h. Most significant sites include the spine, femur (subcapital neck and intertrochanteric region), distal radius, and proximal humerus.
     i. Bone loss of 30% to 50% is required before it can reliably be detected by plain film.
     j. The spine shows the earliest radiographic signs: There is a loss of density due to resorption of the horizontal trabeculae. The vertical trabeculae appear more distinct and prominent. There is cortical thinning and only a relative increase in density of the end-plates (there is no significant subchondral sclerosis).
     k. Compression fractures are common and repair is slow. Fractures may be in the form of anterior wedging, biconcavity of the bodies, or true compression.
     l. The generalized osteoporosis is uniform and lacks cortical striation or tunneling (which indicate faster remodeling).
     m. In the femoral neck, the major stress-bearing trabeculae are accentuated.
     n. With fluoride therapy, trabecular accentuation and stress fractures occur.
   2. Hypercorticism (Cushing's disease or exogenous steroids) differs from osteoporosis in the following ways:

      a. Sclerotic (thickened) vertebral end-plates (callus from micro-fractures); abundant callus formation elsewhere as well.

      b. Aseptic necrosis, especially femoral and humeral heads, is a complication.

      c. Diaphyseal infarcts.

      d. Occasional Charcot-like joints.

  3. Homocystinuria: Young patient with scoliosis, osteoporosis, biconcave vertebrae, and arachnodactyly.

  4. Acromegaly: Should have typical hand findings of increased cartilage and soft tissues, bony excrescences, and spadelike tufts along with occasional osteoporosis.

  5. Ochronosis: See Chapter 2.

  6. Amyloidosis: See Chapter 2.

  7. Hyperthyroidism.

  8. Alcoholism: Direct effect on osteoblasts.

  9. Osteogenesis imperfecta: Discussed in a later chapter but characterized by diaphyseal fracture, bowing of long bones, and blue sclerae.

 10. Drug-related:

      a. Heparin (requires daily doses in excess of 15,000 units).

      b. Phenobarbital.

      c. Dilantin.

      d. Steroids.

      e. Smoking.

      f. Methotrexate.

      g. Aluminum-containing phosphate binders.

 11. Mastocytosis: See IX, below.

 12. Idiopathic juvenile osteoporosis: Acute onset in a previously healthy 8- to 12-year-old; osteoporosis with fracture and loss of height of vertebral bodies. Metaphyseal fractures are common; eventually stabilizes, but the osteoporosis remains; diagnosis of exclusion.

C. Localized osteoporosis:

  1. Disuse: May be uniform, spotty, or very aggressive-looking with cortical tunneling and metaphyseal bandlike lucencies.

  2. Reflex sympathetic dystrophy (Sudeck's atrophy):

      a. Soft tissue trophic changes (swollen, with hyperesthesia, then atrophic and contracted).

      b. Severe extremity involvement distal to the affected site: Rapid severe osteoporosis with a moth-eaten pattern, cortical tunneling, and lucent metaphyseal bands.

      c. Mediated by the sympathetic nervous system.

    d. Precipitating cause may not be identified but may be virtually any musculoskeletal, neurologic, or vascular condition.

3. Transient regional osteoporosis:
    a. Self-limited.
    b. Cartilage remains intact, differentiating it from septic arthritis.
    c. Two forms:
      (1) Migratory: Especially knee, ankle, and foot; male predominance; onset in fourth or fifth decade. Local pain, swelling, and osteoporosis; resolves within one year; recurs around other joints.
      (2) Transient osteoporosis of the hip: Described in a woman in the third trimester of pregnancy involving the left hip; in males, either hip may be involved; resolves within one year.
    d. MR may be indistinguishable from changes of edema in early avascular necrosis (AVN), with decreased signal intensity on T1 and increased signal intensity on T2, and without other distinguishing characteristics (see avascular necrosis).

D. Quantitative analysis of bone mass[2]: Identifying patients with low bone mass is only partially accurate when using risk factors alone, and generally inaccurate based on chest x-ray. Regarding the following methods, osteoporosis is present when the bone mineral is greater than two standard deviations below the mean of young adults of the same gender.

1. Quantitative computed tomography (QCT):
    a. Single-energy gives approximately 97% accuracy.
    b. Dual-energy not practical in most departments but may be more accurate.
    c. Radiation approximately 300 mR.
    d. Fat content in spine adversely affects accuracy, making this generally less accurate in elderly women.
    e. Positioning must be accurate for reproducible results and serial studies.
    f. Major advantage is that only the trabecular bone is imaged, which is thought to be the area of interest in bone mass studies.

2. Dual-photon absorptiometry (DPA): Transmission scanning with an isotope source (^{153}Gd):
    a. Accuracy similar to that of QCT.
    b. Significantly less radiation.
    c. Major disadvantage is that all the bone (cortical as well as trabecular) is imaged. Aortic calcification may also be a factor. It may also be difficult to distinguish a compression fracture, thus giving a false impression of increased bone mass due to impaction.

3. Dual-energy x-ray absorptiometry (DEXA):
   a. Bone mineral content is determined by measuring attenuation of x-rays passing through body tissues. Dual-energy x-ray source separates mineral mass from soft tissue mass.
   b. Accuracy is excellent, but as with DPA, aortic calcifications and degenerative osteophytes may give a falsely high reading.
   c. Very low radiation dose.
   d. Currently, the favored method of evaluation of bone density in the axial skeleton; dose is less than QCT and precision, resolution, and scan time are improved over DPA.
4. MR and broad-band ultrasound methodologies are being evaluated.

II. RICKETS/OSTEOMALACIA

Key Concepts

Lack of mineralization of normal osteoid. Rickets is characterized by a widened zone of provisional calcification and metaphyseal irregularity; osteomalacia is characterized by coarsened trabeculae and Looser's lines.

A. Definition:
   1. Lack of mineralization in osteoid that is otherwise normal. Rickets has the same metabolic process as osteomalacia, but is the childhood manifestation where the nonmineralized osteoid is deposited more rapidly in the growing portion of bone (epiphyseal plate—zone of provisional calcification) than in the already formed bones.
   2. Laboratory values (Fig 4-1):
      a. Serum: decreased Ca^{++} and HPO_4; elevated alkaline phosphatase.
      b. Urine: decreased Ca^{++} and HPO_4.
B. Radiographic signs:
   1. Generalized osteopenia due to decreased number of trabeculae seen in both osteomalacia and rickets.
   2. Coarsened trabeculae due to osteoid deposition on remaining trabeculae without adequate mineralization seen in both osteomalacia and rickets.
   3. Looser's lines: Wide transverse lucencies, often incomplete. Unmineralized osteoid is deposited during the repair process. Characteristic sites, often symmetric—pubic rami, ribs, axillary margins of scapulae, medial margins of proximal femurs, posterior margin of proximal ulna. Seen predominantly in adult osteomalacia.

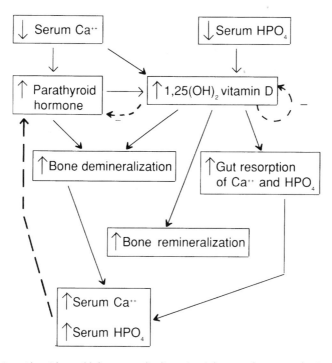

Fig. 4-1   Algorithm of laboratory findings in rickets and osteomalacia.

4. In rickets, changes predominate at sites of rapid growth: Proximal humerus, distal radius, distal femur, both ends of tibia. A cost-effective survey would, therefore, include anteroposterior (AP) view of knees, wrists, and ankles.

5. Rickets abnormalities are predominantly metaphyseal, with a widened lucent zone of provisional calcification consisting of unmineralized osteoid. With growth and continued weight-bearing on soft bone, the metaphyses become widened, irregular, and cupped. Occasionally, the epiphyses slip owing to normal weight-bearing stresses on an abnormally fragile epiphyseal plate.

6. Bearing weight may also produce bowing deformities of the long bones and vertebral end-plate depression.

C. Metabolism:

1. Vitamin D (cholecalciferol): A prohormone with two sources, it is produced endogenously in the skin (activated by ultraviolet light) and derived exogenously from dairy products and other food supplements.

2. Vitamin D undergoes two hydroxylations to become an active metabolite:
   a. In liver, 25 (OH) vitamin D.
   b. In kidney, 1,25 $(OH)_2$ vitamin D.
3. Vitamin D function:
   a. Maintains normal serum Ca^{++} and HPO_4.
   b. Maintains bone mineralization.
4. Effects of vitamin D on organ systems:
   a. Bone: Mobilizes Ca^{++} and HPO_4 by stimulating osteoclasts (requires parathyroid hormone [PTH]). By maintaining normal serum Ca^{++} and HPO_4, it maintains bone mineralization; also stimulates bone mineralization directly (independent of serum Ca^{++} levels).
   b. Gut: Stimulates increased resorption of Ca^{++} and HPO_4.
   c. Kidney: Stimulates tubular resorption of HPO_4.
   d. Parathyroid gland: Suppresses PTH (independent of serum Ca^{++} levels).
5. Regulation of vitamin D:
   a. Increased by low dietary intake of Ca^{++} (normally mediated by PTH, but may also regulate independently).
   b. Increased by hypophosphatemia (direct effect, not mediated by PTH).
   c. Decreased by vitamin D (self-regulator) directly as well as indirectly through decreased PTH.

D. Etiologies of osteomalacia and rickets (note that radiographically these cannot be differentiated reliably):
   1. Dietary calcium deprivation (rare in United States).
   2. GI malabsorption (due to surgery or various malabsorption syndromes).
   3. Liver abnormalities:
      a. Hepatocellular disease interferes with hydroxylation of the prohormone vitamin D.
      b. Biliary disease relates to malabsorption of vitamin D.
   4. Drug therapy: Phenobarbitol, Dilantin, Didronyl, Ifosamide.
   5. Renal osteodystrophy: Combination of osteomalacia (lack of second hydroxylation of vitamin D) and secondary HPTH (see Chapter 4, Section III).
   6. Renal tubular disorders:
      a. Also known as vitamin D-resistant (or refractory) rickets.
      b. Several syndromes with renal tubular defects, including cystinosis and X-linked hypophosphatemia (males with mild rachitic changes and only mild osteopenia).

      c. Rickets is due to renal tubular phosphate loss.

      d. The laboratory values are therefore different from classic rickets: decreased serum Ca^{++} and serum HPO_4, and elevated urine Ca^{++} and urine HPO_4.

  7. Tumor-associated rickets (also vitamin D refractory):

      a. Autosomal-dominant.

      b. Associated with small benign soft tissue or skeletal tumors (hemangioma, nonossifying fibroma, giant cell tumor).

      c. Possible tumor-related humoral substance causing decreased renal tubular phosphate resorption.

      d. Normocalcemic; decreased serum HPO_4; elevated urine HPO_4 and alkaline phosphatase.

      e. Responds to tumor resection.

  8. Neonatal rickets:

      a. Rickets normally is not seen radiographically before 6 months of age.

      b. May be seen in premature infants with low birth weight and long periods of parenteral nutrition.

      c. Due to rapid skeletal growth and possible insufficiency in dietary calcium, phosphate, and vitamin D.

      d. May be complicated by liver or kidney disease.

      e. Copper deficiency in premature infants mimics rickets.

E. Other etiologies that mimic rickets:

  1. Hypophosphatasia—spectrum of disease:

      a. Severely decreased alkaline phosphatase.

      b. Elevated phosphoethanolamine in blood and urine.

      c. Wide spectrum of disease.

      d. Severe: Victims die in infancy; ''tar babies''; no cranial mineralization (only face and base of skull); short bowed bones with severe fractures and deformities as well as ricketslike changes at metaphyses.

      e. Less severe: Osteopenic; looks like rickets at metaphyses, but there is craniostenosis and wormian bones; improves progressively.

      f. Least severe: Delay in fracture healing and mild bowing deformities.

  2. Metaphyseal chondrodysplasia (Schmid type):

      a. Abnormal endochondral bone formation.

      b. Normal serum values.

      c. Short bowed bones with widened growth plates; bony projections from the metaphysis into the growth plate.

      d. *Normal* mineralization and bone density.

3. Ifosamide: Chemotherapeutic agent used for sarcomas that may induce hypophosphatemic rickets.

III. HYPERPARATHYROIDISM (HPTH)

Key Concepts

Osteopenia or osteosclerosis; soft tissue and vascular calcification, several varieties of resorption, brown tumors, chondrocalcinosis. Though some manifestations are more prominent in primary than secondary HPTH, all may be found in either.

A. Laboratory values: Elevated serum Ca^{++} and alkaline phosphatase, decreased serum HPO_4; elevated urine HPO_4 and Ca^{++}.
B. Etiology:
    1. Primary HPTH: 90% due to adenoma.
    2. Secondary HPTH: Due to renal dysfunction; often see findings of rickets or osteomalacia as well.
C. Clinical findings:
    1. Nephrolithiasis.
    2. Gastric or duodenal ulcers.
    3. Weakness due to hypocalcemia.
    4. Bone pain and tenderness (10% to 25%).
D. Radiographic findings:
    1. Radiographically identifiable skeletal manifestations in 50%.
    2. For screening and serial studies, posteroanterior (PA) view of hand is most cost-effective.
        a. Predilection of many sites in the hand for manifestations of HPTH (subperiosteal resorption on radial side of digits, tuft resorption, soft tissue calcification, chondrocalcinosis of triangular fibrocartilage complex).
        b. Thin soft tissues and small bones, so bone detail is seen better.
        c. Fine detail extremity filming is performed routinely.
    3. Skeletal manifestations (Table 4-1):
        a. Generalized osteopenia; HPTH results in either excessive bone resorption or, occasionally, bone formation. There is a great variation in these activities, resulting in a spectrum of appearances, but generalized osteopenia is most common.
        b. Resorption; very common manifestation in both primary and secondary HPTH.
            (1) Subperiosteal resorption: Most common form, affects the radial aspect of phalanges (especially middle phalanx of

Table 4-1   Skeletal Manifestations of Primary and Secondary HPTH

Manifestations	Most Common in	
	Primary HPTH	**Secondary HPTH**
Generalized osteopenia	+	+
Resorption	+	+
Sclerosis		+
Brown tumor	+	
Chondrocalcinosis	+	
Soft tissue calcification		+
Vascular calcification		+

index and middle finger); also affects the tufts of fingers and margins of phalanges, giving marginal erosions; seen at medial proximal humeral, femoral, and tibial shaft.

(2) Endosteal resorption: Scalloped defects; usually not an isolated finding.

(3) Intracortical resorption: Linear striation and tunneling; not a specific finding (seen in any manifestation of rapid bone resorption).

(4) Trabecular resorption: Especially well seen in the diploe of the cranium, resulting in salt-and-pepper skull.

(5) Subchondral resorption: Results in collapse of subchondral surface and apparent widening and sclerosis of joint. Sacroiliac, acromioclavicular, temporomandibular joints and symphysis pubis are most common sites; must differentiate from sacroiliitis and other arthritides. Subchondral resorption is also seen in the tubular bones of the hand; with collapse, these appear very similar to erosions, though the latter are less well marginated.

(6) Subligamentous resorption: At sites of ligament origins, especially on pelvis, calcaneus, and distal clavical inferiorly.

c. Sclerosis: May be patchy or diffuse and is much more common in secondary than in primary disease. Mechanism is unclear, but PTH (as well as vitamin D) is known to stimulate osteoblastic activity. Bone formation may be more dramatic than bone resorption in some patients; this, combined with an element of subchondral resorption, collapse, and impaction, produces the rugger jersey appearance of dense vertebral end-plates seen most commonly in secondary HPTH.

    d. Brown tumors: Localized accumulations of osteoclasts producing expanded lytic lesions. Fibrous tissue and giant cells are also present. Radiographically and pathologically it may be difficult to differentiate from giant cell tumor. Usually other manifestations of HPTH are present as well, making the diagnosis. More common in primary than in secondary HPTH. May hyperossify after resection of the adenoma, giving the appearance of blastic metastases.

    e. Chondrocalcinosis: More common in primary than in secondary HPTH.

    f. Periarticular and soft tissue calcifications are more common in secondary than in primary disease. Vascular calcification may also be prominent. Large ''tumoral'' deposits most commonly are seen in dialysis patients.

IV. RENAL OSTEODYSTROPHY

Key Concepts

Chronic renal failure with a combination of bone abnormalities due to osteomalacia and secondary HPTH—and aluminum intoxication if the patient is on dialysis. The manifestations are highly individual depending on the predominant disease in each patient.

A. Definition:
    1. Bone disease seen in patients with chronic renal failure.
    2. Main features are osteomalacia or rickets, secondary HPTH and/or aluminum intoxication (if patient is on dialysis).
    3. In young patients, expressed mostly as rickets, with later changes of HPTH. More mature patients have more marked changes of HPTH.
    4. Secondary HPTH is due to renal failure which causes phosphate retention; phosphate retention causes a decreased serum calcium level, which in turn causes parathyroid hyperplasia. In renal failure, there is also decreased calcium resorption from the gut as well as skeletal resistance to PTH.
    5. Aluminum intoxication:
        a. Sources are aluminum salts in the dialysis fluid and aluminum hydroxide antacids administered to control hyperphosphatemia.
        b. Radiographic features are osteomalacia and stress fractures; resembles rickets in children.

      c. Clinical symptoms are bone pain, proximal muscle weakness; may be associated with dialysis encephalopathy.

      d. No response to vitamin D therapy.

      e. Distinctive histology: Osteomalacia with aluminum deposits at the interface of mineralized bone and osteoid.

B. Laboratory values: Serum Ca^{++} normal to decreased, serum phosphate and alkaline phosphatase elevated.

C. Radiographic features:

    1. *Rickets/osteomalacia:* Features osteopenia, widened zone of provisional calcification, and Looser's lines. *Slipped epiphyses* not uncommon in chronic disease.

    2. *Secondary HPTH: Resorption, osteosclerosis,* and *soft tissue and vascular calcifications* are prominent features. Chondrocalcinosis and brown tumors are less commonly seen. With severe chronic disease, *periosteal neostosis* may be seen, most commonly in the femurs, pubic rami, and metatarsals. There may be a lucent zone between the periosteal new bone and host bone. If present, neostosis helps distinguish secondary from primary HPTH.

    3. Abnormalities following dialysis:

      a. Changes of HPTH often resolve (depending on amount of calcium in the dialysis fluid and control of phosphate): reversal of resorption, healing brown tumors, resolution of vascular and soft tissue calcification.

      b. Effect on rickets/osteomalacia is controversial.

      c. Soft tissue calcification is common (50%) and may occur in large ''tumoral'' deposits.

      d. Osteomyelitis and septic arthritis (arteriovenous [AV] shunt is port of entry; patients often are chronically immunosuppressed).

      e. Aseptic necrosis: Due to steroid therapy as well as subchondral resorption and collapse.

      f. ''Dialysis cysts'' in phalanges and carpus; significance unknown.

      g. Shunt aneurysm.

      h. Aluminum intoxication: Osteomalacia and stress fractures.

      i. Carpal tunnel syndrome: Possibly related to altered hemodynamics at AV shunt.

      j. Spondyloarthropathy: Disc space narrowing, end-plate erosions and sclerosis, no osteophyte formation; looks like infection; biopsy should be taken since these patients are at risk for infection, but some material should also be evaluated for crystal deposition and amyloid.

V. HYPOPARATHYROIDISM

Key Concepts

Osteosclerosis or -porosis and soft tissue calcification are common to all varieties; pseudo- and pseudohypoparathyroidism also have a characteristic somatotype, shortened metacarpals or metatarsals, and small exostoses.

A. Definition: Deficiency in PTH production, usually secondary to excision or surgical trauma; rarely idiopathic; patient may have hypocalcemia and neuromuscular symptoms.
B. Radiographic abnormalities:
   1. *Osteosclerosis,* generalized or localized, is the most common finding.
   2. *Hypoplastic dentition.*
   3. *Subcutaneous calcification.*
   4. *Basal ganglia calcification.*
   5. Less common abnormalities:
      a. Osteoporosis.
      b. Premature closure of epiphyses.
      c. Enthesopathy and vertebral hyperostosis.
      d. Bandlike areas of increased density in metaphyses and endplates of vertebral bodies.
C. Pseudohypoparathyroidism:
   1. Etiology: End-organ resistance to PTH.
   2. Characteristic somatotype: Short, obese, brachydactyly.
   3. Has features similar to those of hypoparathyroidism:
      a. Hypocalcemia.
      b. *Osteosclerosis.*
      c. *Basal ganglia calcifications.*
      d. *Soft tissue calcifications.*
   4. Features that distinguish it from hypoparathyroidism.
      a. *Short metacarpals, metatarsals, and phalanges,* especially first, fourth, and fifth.
      b. Small *exostoses* projecting at right angles from the bone.
      c. Growth deformities, with wide bones and coned epiphyses.
D. Pseudopseudohypoparathyroidism:
   1. Normocalcemic form of pseudohypoparathyroidism with end-organ resistance to PTH.
   2. Somatotype identical to that of pseudohypoparathyroidism.
   3. Radiographic abnormalities identical to those of pseudohypoparathyroidism except that basal ganglia calcifications are rare.

VI. THYROID DISEASE

A. Juvenile hypothyroidism:
  1. *Delayed skeletal maturation,* may be severe.
  2. *Wormian bones.*
  3. Epiphyseal dysgenesis:
      a. *Stippled epiphyses* in infancy.
      b. *Fragmented epiphyses in childhood, especially the proximal femoral capital epiphysis.* This condition, which is called cretinoid epiphyses, may be misdiagnosed as Legg-Calvé-Perthes disease.
      c. *Coned epiphyses* may occur later.
  4. May have short vertebral bodies at the junction of the thoracic and lumbar spine, with anterior beaking and kyphosis (nonspecific).
  5. The diagnosis must be picked up in infancy, when it can be reversed in order to prevent mental retardation.
B. Hyperthyroidism:
  1. In children, accelerated skeletal maturation.
  2. In adults, *increased bone turnover and consequent osteoporosis,* with typical osteoporotic vertebral body pathologic fractures and kyphosis.
  3. *Myopathy* may simulate arthritis clinically.
C. *Thyroid Acropachy:* A rare complication following therapy for hyperthyroidism; the patient may be euthyroid, hypothyroid, even occasionally hyperthyroid.
  1. The *metacarpals and phalanges* are most commonly involved, *often asymmetrically;* other long bones involved only occasionally.
  2. Most common feature is a *dense feathery periosteal reaction.*
  3. *Soft tissue swelling.*
  4. *Clubbed fingers.*

VII. ACROMEGALY

A. Definition: *Excess of growth hormone* produces *proportional increase in size in the skeletally immature patient and tubular bone widening and acral growth in the skeletally mature patient.*
B. Radiographic abnormalities:
  1. *Soft tissue thickening, especially over the phalanges and in the heel pad.* (The distance from the calcaneus to the plantar aspect of the heel is normally less than 23 mm in males and 21.5 mm in females. The wide range of normal makes the question of heel pad thickness controversial.)
  2. *Enlarged sella,* often with destructive changes.
  3. *Prominent facial bones* and occipital protuberance, with *enlarged, excessively pneumatized sinuses.*

4. Increased vertebral body and disc height; posterior vertebral scalloping; exaggerated thoracic kyphosis.
5. *Hand and foot changes predominate over more proximal bones;* the bones are *wide,* with *spadelike tufts. Excresences at tendon attachments* along the phalanges are prominent. Overgrowth causes *cartilage widening,* and beaking osteophytes eventually develop into secondary degenerative joint disease (DJD).
6. There is also bony proliferation at the entheses.
7. Osteoporosis may be a late feature.

VIII. SCURVY (HYPOVITAMINOSIS C)

A. Definition: Lack of vitamin C results in *abnormal collagen formation;* hemorrhage is frequent, and bone production is decreased.
B. Radiographic abnormalities in children:
   1. Rarely seen before 6 months of age.
   2. *Subperiosteal hemorrhage* may cause spectacular elevation of the loosely attached periosteum in children, resulting in *extensive subperiosteal bone formation.*
   3. The abnormal bone production is most manifest at sites of rapid growth.
      a. Costochondral junction (*scorbutic rosary*).
      b. *Ends of long bones* (especially around the knee).
         (1) *Disorganized growth zone becomes densely calcified,* giving the *sclerotic epiphyseal rim* (Wimburger's sign) and the *dense metaphyseal line* (white line of Frankel).
         (2) More proximal metaphyseal lucent line.
         (3) With minor trauma, this brittle bone develops *metaphyseal corner fractures* (Pelkin's fracture).
         (4) *Generalized osteopenia.*
C. Radiographic abnormalities in adults: Nonspecific osteopenia and resultant pathologic fracture.

IX. MASTOCYTOSIS

A. Definition: *A proliferative disorder of mast cells* resulting in bone abnormalities as well as the clinical symptoms of flushing, nausea, vomiting, and skin lesions resembling urticaria pigmentosa.
B. Radiographic abnormalities: May show *either* osteoporosis or sclerosis.
   1. *Histamine release* from mast cells *results in osteoporosis,* usually generalized but occasionally focal.
   2. *Host reaction* to marrow infiltration *may result in bony sclerosis,* usually focal but occasionally diffuse.

X. GAUCHER'S DISEASE

Key Concepts

Storage disease: hepatosplenomegaly, femoral head avascular necrosis (AVN), osteoporosis, Erlenmeyer flask deformity of the knee.

A. Definition: Sphingolipid storage disorder, with accumulation in the reticuloendothelial system and marrow infiltration with Gaucher cells. Life span is normal in the usual form, but there are infantile and juvenile forms that produce mental retardation and early death.
B. Epidemiology:
   1. Familial; no gender predilection.
   2. Onset in childhood or young adulthood.
   3. Many patients are Ashkenazi Jews.
C. Radiographic abnormalities:
   1. *Erlenmeyer flask deformity* (expansion of the distal femur): Due to marrow infiltration, present in 40% to 50% of patients.
   2. *AVN*, especially of femoral head, present in 40% to 50% of patients.
   3. *Generalized osteoporosis* with fractures, especially of vertebral end-plates (H-shaped, as in sickle cell disease).
   4. Bone infarction with focal sclerosis and occasional bone-within-bone appearance.
   5. Occasional focal lytic ''cystic'' areas, simulating neoplasm.
   6. *Hepatosplenomegaly.*
   7. Increased susceptibility to osteomyelitis.
D. *Differential diagnoses for Erlenmeyer flask* deformity:
   1. *Anemias:* May appear very similar in that there may also be H-shaped vertebral end-plate collapse, AVN, and bony infarcts. Splenomegaly in Gaucher's should help differentiate.
   2. *Niemann-Pick disease:* Sphingomyelin accumulation with similar infiltrative bony findings (except AVN) as well as hepatosplenomegaly.
   3. *Pyle's disease:* A metaphyseal dysplasia that results in expanded metaphyses of tubular bones (especially about the knee) and normal diaphyses.

XI. MYELOFIBROSIS

A. Definition: *Fibrosis in areas of the skeleton normally involved in hematopoesis,* with subsequent compensatory hematopoesis in the fatty marrow of the large tubular bones. These latter sites, in turn, may become fibrotic.

B. Radiographic findings:
1. *Sclerotic bone marrow* (or patchy increased density with cortical thickening) in the hematopoetic bones (*vertebrae, pelvis, and ribs*) as well as long tubular bones.
2. Extramedullary hematopoiesis: Hepatosplenomegaly and paraspinous masses.
3. Occasional periosteal reaction secondary to bleeding associated with platelet deficiencies.
C. Differential diagnoses:
1. Mastocytosis, fluorosis, Paget's disease, metastases.
2. Splenomegaly and paraspinous masses help to differentiate.

XII. PAGET'S DISEASE OF BONE

Key Concepts

Skull, vertebral bodies, and pelvis most commonly affected; three sequential stages—lytic, mixed, sclerotic, affected bone enlarged; skeletal deformities, pathologic fracture, and occasional sarcomatous change; elevated alkaline phosphatase.

A. Definition: A disease of unknown etiology that causes abnormal remodeling of bone with *simultaneous osteoclast and osteoblast activity.* Thickened, disorganized, *fragile trabeculae* result.
B. Epidemiology:
1. *Males* more commonly affected than females.
2. *Rare before age 40 years.*
3. Most common in Great Britain, Australia, and the United States; rare in Asia.
C. Laboratory abnormalities:
1. *Elevated serum alkaline phosphatase* (due to bone formation).
2. Elevated serum and urinary hydroxyproline (due to bone resorption).
3. These values vary with the severity of the disease and are often normal initially.
D. Clinical signs:
1. Often asymptomatic.
2. Local pain, bowing of long bones, or pathologic fracture.
3. Enlarging bone, especially cranium.
4. Deafness (due to either middle ear ossicle involvement or cranial nerve compression).
5. Occasional spinal cord signs from platybasia or other compression.

6. Rare CHF secondary to high output from increased blood flow in involved bone.

E. Radiographic appearance: *three sequential stages* (though they may coexist):

1. *Lytic:* Initial destruction, usually geographic with a well-defined border (flame-shaped border in tubular bones).
2. *Mixed:* Intermediate stage, with cortical accretion and enlarging bones.
3. *Sclerotic:* Continued increase in both density and size.

F. Most common sites of involvement:

1. *Spine (75%* of patients): Lumbar most common; enlarged dense trabeculae, especially around the contours, give a *"picture frame" appearance.* If it is more uniformly dense, the increased body size helps differentiate it from metastasis or other etiology of an ivory vertebra. May develop compression fractures or spinal stenosis.
2. *Cranium (65%* of patients): Lytic phase, termed *osteoporosis circumscripta,* may start in either the frontal or occipital areas. Later, focal radiodense areas develop *("cotton wool"* appearance). *Basilar invagination in one third.* The cranium enlarges due to widening of the diploic space.
3. *Pelvis (70%* of patients): Initial finding is *cortical thickening* along the *ileopectineal line;* if unilateral involvement, the asymmetrical size increase becomes obvious. The softened bone develops a protrusio acetabuli deformity.
4. *Tubular bones (35%* of patients): *Lysis always begins in subarticular region,* advancing to diaphysis with a "flame" or "blade of grass" border. *Exception to this is the tibia, where the initial lysis may be diaphyseal.* Bone enlarges and bows.

G. Musculoskeletal complications:

1. *Stress fracture:* Horizontal lines on the convex (bowed) aspect of bone.
2. Osteoporosis if immobilized.
3. Neoplasm:
   a. Involved bone may degenerate to *sarcoma* (osteosarcoma more commonly than chondrosarcoma, malignant fibrous histiocytoma [MFH], or fibrosarcoma); a rare occurrence (probably less than 1% overall) but may be seen in 5% to 10% of patients with widespread disease. Paget's sarcoma should be suspected with unrelenting pain, a new rapid region of lysis or amorphous bone formation, focal cortical destruction, or soft tissue mass. MR may help differentiate underlying Paget's disease from a Paget's sarcoma. Uncomplicated Paget's disease usually shows

normal marrow signal.[3] This presumes the bone is not in the dense blastic stage. Paget's sarcoma is more likely to have both abnormal osseous signal and a soft tissue mass.

   b. *Giant cell tumors* (usually benign) involving the facial bones and cranium in 50% of cases.

   4. Osteoarthritis due to mechanical abnormalities.

XIII. DRUG- AND ENVIRONMENTALLY INDUCED ABNORMALITIES OF BONE

A. Drugs

   1. Coumadin: Embryopathy with stippled epiphyses.

   2. Heparin: Osteoporosis (dose-related).

   3. Dilantin and phenobarbital: Osteomalacia.

   4. Steroids: Osteoporosis, AVN.

   5. Lead: Widened metaphyses with dense bands, which may be multiple from several episodes of lead poisoning. A single dense metaphyseal line may be physiologic, but if one is present at the fibular metaphysis as well as other metaphyses around the knee, it is more likely to represent lead poisoning than physiologic findings.

   6. Bismuth: Same as lead.

   7. Vitamin A poisoning: Abnormalities appear only after 6 months of age. Periostitis of long bones (painful) is the first abnormality. An older child may have a growth disturbance and coned epiphyses.

   8. Vitamin D poisoning: Increased density and periostitis; prominent soft tissue calcifications. Osteoporosis also may be present.

   9. Fluorosis: Increased density, periostitis, ossification of ligaments (especially pelvic); stress fractures. Osteopenia and metaphyseal osteomalacia may also be seen.[4]

   10. Alcohol: Fetal alcohol syndrome (delayed development, among other findings); in adult, osteoporosis and AVN.

   11. Prostaglandins: Periostitis in infants.

SERUM LABORATORY VALUES IN METABOLIC BONE DISEASE

	Calcium*	Phosphate*	Alkaline Phosphatase*
Osteoporosis	nl	nl	nl
Osteomalacia/rickets	↓	↓	↑
Renal osteodystrophy (secondary HPTH)	nl to ↓	↑	↑
Hypophosphatasia	nl	nl	↓↓
Paget's disease	nl	nl	↑↑
Hypoparathyroidism	↓	↑	nl
Pseudohypoparathyroidism	↓	↑	nl
Pseudo-pseudohypoparathyroidism	nl	nl	nl

*nl = normal; ↑ = increased; ↓ = decreased.

B. Environmental causes:
   1. Polyvinyl chloride: Acro-osteolysis.
   2. Burns: Contractures, acro-osteolysis, heterotopic ossification.
   3. Frostbite: Acro-osteolysis (dense or resorbed distal phalangeal epiphyses in children); thumb often is spared.

REFERENCES

1. Riggs B, Melton L: Involutional osteoporosis. *N Engl J Med* 1986;314: 1676–1684.
2. Faulkner K, Glüer C, Majumdor S, Lang P, Engelke K, Genant H: Noninvasive measurements of bone mass, structure, and strength: current methods and experimental techniques. *AJR* 1991;157:1229–1237.
3. Mirra J, Briden E, Tehranzadeh J: Paget's disease of bone: review with emphasis on radiologic features. Parts I and II. *Skeletal Radiology* 1995;24:163–184.
4. Wang Y, Yin Y, Gilula L, Wilson A: Endemic fluorosis of the skeleton: radiographic features in 127 patients. *AJR* 1994;162:93–98.

BIBLIOGRAPHY

Resnick D, Niwayama G: *Diagnosis of Bone and Joint Disorders,* ed 2. Philadelphia, WB Saunders, 1988.
Jacobson H, Edeiken J (eds): *Syllabus—Metabolic and Endocrine Disorders Affecting the Skeleton.* Radiological Society of North America 67th Scientific Assembly, November, 1981.

5

Congenital Anomalies

The multitude of congenital syndromes is confusing. Furthermore, there is overlap in radiographic abnormalities among the syndromes. The more common congenital abnormalities are discussed briefly in this section; a practical approach to classifying dwarfs is also presented. An excellent reference for wider gamuts and less common syndromes is Taybi and Lachman *Radiology of Syndromes, Metabolic Disorders, and Skeletal Dysplasias,* ed 4 (St. Louis, Mosby, 1996). In this book, cross indexes reference the syndromes and give gamuts according to the nature of radiographic abnormalities as well as their sites.

In addition, many apparent abnormalities may be normal variants or, in children, a transitional state seen only at a certain age. The most complete reference for normal variants is Keats *An Atlas of Normal Roentgen Variants That May Simulate Disease,* ed 6 (St. Louis, Mosby, 1995). The best reference for different appearances of the skeleton through different periods of skeletal maturation is Keats and Smith *An Atlas of Normal Developmental Roentgen Anatomy* (Chicago, Year Book Medical Publishers, 1988).

I. SCOLIOSIS

> ### Key Concepts
>
> Must evaluate for intrinsic vertebral abnormalities, tumor, and neurofibromatosis. The latter disease may cause the spine to collapse rapidly, producing paraplegia. Posteroanterior (PA) views expose patients' breasts to less ionizing radiation than anteroposterior (AP) views.

A. Definition: Lateral deviation and rotation of the spine, often associated with thoracic hypokyphosis. Severe disease distorts the chest wall enough to restrict pulmonary and cardiovascular function, requiring correction. The cosmetic deformity may also be serious.
B. Etiology: Must be determined in each case of scoliosis since prognosis and treatment are highly dependent on etiology.

1. Idiopathic:
   a. By far the most common (85%).
   b. Thought to be related to defects in proprioception and vibratory sense.
   c. Girls are more often affected than boys (7:1) and their disease is more likely to progress and require treatment.
   d. Patterns may be thoracic (usually convex to the right), thoracolumbar, lumbar, or double major.
   e. Infantile idiopathic is uncommon, occurs more often in males, is usually thoracic and convex to the left, and is difficult to treat. Congenital forms must be ruled out.
   f. Juvenile (ages 3 to 10 years) and adolescent idiopathic scoliosis are much more common. Curves that are greater than 50 degrees or that show progression usually require surgical treatment. The curves are generally flexible (demonstrated by lateral bending films), and L_5 spondylolysis may be associated.
2. Congenital:
   a. Secondary to vertebral anomalies—hemivertebrae (failure of formation) or bars (failure of segmentation) causing unbalanced growth.
   b. May have associated tethered cord or diastematomyelia; magnetic resonance imaging (MRI) makes the diagnosis.
   c. Bracing is ineffectual, and progressing curves must be fused early.
3. Neuromuscular:
   a. Etiology may be spasticity, paralysis, arthrogryposis, or muscular dystrophy.
   b. The curves are long, single curves.
4. Diseases of collagen synthesis may all result in scoliosis:
   a. Marfan's syndrome—normal bone density.
   b. Ehlers-Danlos syndrome.
   c. Homocystinuria—decreased bone density.
5. Neurofibromatosis:
   a. Dysplastic vertebral bodies form a short, angular, usually high thoracic curve.
   b. Associated ribbon-shaped ribs and posterior vertebral body scalloping help make the diagnosis.
   c. These curves must be monitored carefully since they can collapse rapidly and produce paralysis.
6. Trauma: May require instrumentation if there is a burst fracture, especially in the lumbar spine.
7. Tumors:
   a. Osteoid osteoma is the most common tumor that causes scoliosis.

      b. The lesion may be lucent, but there is surrounding sclerosis. It is usually located in posterior elements.

      c. The scoliosis is long, with concavity on the side of the lesion. There is no rotational component.

      d. Bone scan may help locate an occult lesion, but precise localization within the posterior elements is best done by computed tomography (CT).

    8. Radiation therapy: If the entire vertebral body of a skeletally immature patient is not included in a radiation port, growth in the irradiated portion stops, with resultant scoliosis.

C. Filming:

    1. The initial film should be good quality AP erect films, in order to evaluate for intrinsic vertebral abnormalities.

    2. Subsequent films used only to evaluate progression should be high kVp and must be taken PA rather than AP, using gradient intensifying screens or filters. Gonad and breast shields should be utilized if possible. Collimation is essential. This approach reduces the dose to breast tissue to $\frac{1}{6}$ to $\frac{1}{10}$ that of AP films. The breast is the most radiation-sensitive tissue in adolescent females and should be protected.

D. Treatment:

    1. Bracing.

    2. Electrical stimulation.

    3. Posterior fusion: Rodding must be accompanied by sufficient graft for a fusion mass to form. For an excellent article describing the hardware used for posterior fixation, see Ref. 66 in Chapter 3.

      a. Harrington rods: Ratcheted portion is cephalad. Most common site of failure is at the junction of the ratcheted and smooth portion. The construct may also fail by the hooks ''popping'' off the laminae or pedicles; this may occur as early as immediately postop if the patient ''bucks'' while coming out of anesthesia. Superior and inferior hooks are different in size and shape. Either distraction or compression Harrington rods may be seen; those described above are the more common distraction type.

      b. Luque rods, ''U''s, or squares are another posterior system with a smooth rod that is secured either by sublaminar wiring (extremely secure but risks tearing dura during removal) or Wisconsin segmental spinal instruments (WSSI) wiring (through the thick portion of the spinous process, secured by buttons; almost as secure as sublaminar wiring and safer to place and remove). Luque rods are used most commonly in neuromuscular scolioses.

      c. Anterior rodding (Dwyer, Zielke, Dunn) rarely used for nontraumatic scoliosis. Anterior soft tissue release with bone grafting but combined with posterior rodding may be seen as therapy for a more severe and fixed scoliosis/kyphosis.

    d. Cotrel-Dubousset rodding: A complicated posterior rod system that reduces the scoliosis by correcting the rotatory deformity. This protects the thoracic kyphosis and also corrects the rib hump deformity of scoliosis. Multiple paired hooks are used, often connected by a crosslink; hooks may head either cephalad or caudad. May fail by the scored surface of the rod acting as a file and wearing down the screws which hold the hooks in place.

II. ARTHROGRYPOSIS MULTIPLEX CONGENITA

Key Concepts

Long scoliosis, multiple dislocations, and extremity deformities; atrophic soft tissues with webbed joints and ''dense'' capsules.

A. Etiology: The cause is disputed. Decrease in size and number of anterior horn cells; fibro-fatty changes in musculature are seen histologically.

B. Clinical features:
1. Apparent in utero or at birth.
2. Muscle wasting.
3. Symmetric contractures of appendicular joints.
4. Absence of normal skin creases.
5. Webbing of skin when joints are fixed in flexion.
6. Thickened articular capsules.
7. Intelligence usually normal.
8. Clubfoot, congenital dislocation of the hip (CDH), rudimentary or absent patella, club hand, flexed fingers, adducted thumbs.

C. Radiographic findings:
1. Atrophic musculature with relatively increased density of joint capsules.
2. Typical deformities:
    a. Fixed flexion deformities.
    b. Scoliosis (long, neuromuscular type).
    c. Hip subluxation/dislocation and hypoplastic pelvis
    d. Rudimentary or absent patellae.
    e. Clubfoot (or may have valgus deformities).
    f. Elbow dislocations.
    g. Club hand in ulnar deviation.
    h. Carpal fusion.
    i. Adducted thumb.

    3. Osteoporosis.

    4. Frequent fractures although bone is normal aside from being osteoporotic and gracile.

D. Distribution:

    1. Both upper and lower extremity disease: 50%.

    2. Upper extremity disease only: 40%.

    3. Lower extremity disease only: 10%.

III. NEUROFIBROMATOSIS

Key Concepts

A bone dysplasia with multiple manifestations; the kyphoscoliosis is the most significant since it may progress rapidly to collapse.

A. Skeletal involvement in 80% (90% if macrocranium is included).

B. Kyphoscoliosis in 50%:

    1. T_{3-7} most common.

    2. Short segment and angular.

    3. Need not be present at birth.

    4. Attributed to a primary mesodermal dysplasia.

    5. May be rapidly progressive, causing paraplegia.

C. Posterocentral vertebral body scalloping with erosion of pedicles:

    1. May be progressive.

    2. Usually due to dural ectasia, with or without the presence of neurofibromas.

D. Loosely attached periosteum is easily stripped causing large calcified subperiostal hemorrhage or poor callus response and pseudarthrosis.

E. Bowing and pseudarthrosis of the tibia, most commonly at the junction of the middle and distal thirds; an abnormally formed, deficient, gracile fibula with pencil-pointing of the segments is often seen, with or without a tibial pseudarthrosis. Osseous dysplasia is very commonly seen in the tibia, and may be manifest as bowing with or without incomplete fractures on the convex cortex.

F. Irregular, notched, scalloped, twisted, ribbon-like ribs are usually due to the primary bone dysplasia, but occasionally there is a neighboring intercostal neurofibroma.

G. Localized gigantism (occasionally dwarfism).

H. "Cystic" lesions are controversial:

    1. May relate to deossification of bone, reaction to subperiosteal hemorrhage, or local erosion rather than replacement by tumor.

    2. Biopsy of some large, expanded lesions has proven them to be nonossifying fibromas.

   3. Multiple nonossifying fibromas (NOF) are uncommon; if present, consider neurofibromatosis as an underlying etiology; the lesions are not neurofibromas but NOF.
 I. Small exostoses may arise adjacent to a soft tissue neurofibroma.
 J. Local erosion due to a soft tissue neurofibroma.
 K. Skull:
   1. Deficient or absent sphenoid wing.
   2. Hypoplasia of posterosuperior orbital wall with herniation into posterior orbit and exophthalmos.
   3. Cranial defects, most commonly at the left lambdoid suture, sometimes accompanied by an ipsilateral hypoplastic mastoid, are due to underlying mesodermal dysplasia rather than neurofibromatous tissue.
   4. Enlargement of cranial foramina, especially optic and internal auditory canals, due to neuromas or gliomas.
   5. Macrocranium in 75%.
 L. Neurofibromas often, but not invariably, demonstrate a "target sign" on MR T2 imaging, with low signal centrally surrounded by high signal tissue (a more detailed discussion of neurofibroma is found in the tumor section).

IV. MARFAN'S SYNDROME

Key Concepts

Connective tissue abnormality with ocular (bilateral ectopic lenses), cardiovascular (ascending aortic dissection, valvular insufficiency), and musculoskeletal (arachnodactyly, kyphoscoliosis, posterior vertebral body scalloping) abnormalities.

 A. Definition: Familial (usually autosomal-dominant) *connective tissue disorder* in which the primary defect is unknown. Patients are tall and thin, with *disproportionately long extremities, especially distally (arachnodactyly)*.
 B. Epidemiology: No race or gender preponderance.
 C. Nonmusculoskeletal features:
   1. Ocular: Ectopic lenses.
   2. Cardiovascular: Cystic medial necrosis of the ascending aorta or pulmonary artery predisposes to dissection and rupture. Aortic and mitral valve insufficiency also occur.
 D. Musculoskeletal features:
   1. *Arachnodactyly.*

2. *Kyphoscoliosis* in a pattern similar to that of idiopathic scoliosis but occurring earlier.
3. *Posterior scalloping of vertebral bodies* (secondary to dural ectasia).
4. *Spondylolysis,* especially of L$_5$, often with high-grade spondylolisthesis.
5. *Pectus excavatum.*
6. *Normal bone density:* This feature is important in differentiating Marfan's syndrome from homocystinuria (arachnodactyly with osteoporosis).
7. Deformities may occur secondary to hypermobility (pes planus, genu recurvatum, patella alta), as can dislocations.
8. Hypermobility may lead to premature osteoarthritis, but otherwise the joints are normal.

V. HOMOCYSTINURIA

Key Concepts

Familial connective tissue disorder with ocular (lens dislocation) and skeletal abnormalities resembling Marfan's syndrome (disproportionately long extremities, scoliosis, joint laxity). Major differences are the frequent thrombotic episodes and osteoporosis found in homocystinuria.

A. Definition: A *familial* (autosomal-recessive) disease resulting from deficiency of the enzyme cystathionine synthetase. There is an associated *defect in collagen* synthesis, which affects multiple organ systems.
B. Epidemiology: More common in patients of Northern European extraction.
C. Nonmusculoskeletal features:
  1. *Mental retardation* and seizures.
  2. Frequent, often life-threatening, *thrombotic episodes* (venous and arterial) secondary to abnormal platelet aggregation.
  3. *Lens dislocation,* often bilateral.
  4. Cystic medial necrosis in all elastic arteries, but dissections are rare (unlike Marfan's).
D. Musculoskeletal features:
  1. *Arachnodactyly* (as in Marfan's).
  2. *Scoliosis.*
  3. AP diameter of vertebral bodies may be increased, with *posterior scalloping.*
  4. Pectus excavatum.
  5. *Osteoporosis* is an important feature that is constant in homocysti-

nuria but not seen in Marfan's; end-plate biconcavity and *vertebral compression fractures are common.*

6. Joint laxity occurs, as in Marfan's, but *flexion contractures* are more common.

VI. EHLERS-DANLOS SYNDROME

Key Concepts

Familial connective tissue disorder with many features similar to those of Marfan's syndrome (arachnodactyly, kyphoscoliosis, posterior vertebral scalloping, spondylolysis). Subcutaneous calcifications and the history of skin hyperelasticity help make the correct diagnosis.

A. Definition: Familial (usually autosomal-dominant) spectrum of connective tissue diseases characterized by hyperelasticity of the skin, laxity of the joints, and a bleeding disorder, affecting multiple systems; there is an associated defect in collagen synthesis.
B. Epidemiology: Usually patients are Caucasians of European origin; males are affected predominantly.
C. Nonmusculoskeletal features:
  1. *Thin, hyperelastic skin.*
  2. *Fragile vessel walls predispose patient to bleeding and dissecting aneurysms.*
D. Musculoskeletal features:
  1. No primary osseous abnormality.
  2. *Ligamentous laxity allows subclinical trauma to joints, as well as dislocations. Early osteoarthritis results.*
  3. *Kyphoscoliosis and other deformities* (genu recurvatum and pes planus are the most common).
  4. *Posterior vertebral scalloping.*
  5. *Arachnodactyly.*
  6. *Spondylolysis.*
  7. *Subcutaneous calcification,* most often *in forearms and shins,* result from fat necrosis and hematomas. Calcifications look like phleboliths.

VII. OSTEOGENESIS IMPERFECTA

Key Concepts

Spectrum of connective tissue diseases with both congenital and late forms. Blue sclerae, osteoporosis, wormian bones, and multiple fractures are the most common abnormalities.

A. Definition: A congenital connective tissue abnormality (both osteoid and collagen are abnormal) which is manifested in a wide clinical spectrum. This spectrum has been divided into three main groups but there is overlap among them.
B. Epidemiology: No race or sex predilection.
C. Features common to all three groups:
    1. *Blue sclerae.*
    2. Severe *osteoporosis* and resultant multiple *fractures.*
    3. *Elevated alkaline phosphatase* secondary to multiple fractures.
    4. *Exuberant callus formation* and fracture healing (though often with deformity).
    5. *Wormian bones* in the skull.
    6. Dental abnormalities.
    7. Thin skin.
    8. Joint laxity.
    9. Otosclerosis.
    10. Platelet abnormalities and vascular structural abnormalities resulting in bleeds.
    11. Platybasia, wedge deformities of the vertebral bodies, and kyphoscoliosis.
D. Three major groups:
    1. *Osteogenesis imperfecta congenita.*
      a. *Autosomal-recessive disorder.*
      b. *Long bones are short, thick, and bowed* (resembling dwarfism).
      c. *Multiple fractures at birth* (usually acquired in utero).
      d. Large skull.
      e. Infants are stillborn or die very early.
      f. Rare survivors may develop cystic metaphyses.
    2. *Osteogenesis imperfecta tarda 1.*
      a. *Autosomal-dominant* disorder.
      b. *Long bones are thin and of normal length.*
      c. *May have fractures at birth but not prenatally.*
      d. Fracture rate decreases at puberty.
    3. *Osteogenesis imperfecta tarda 2:* Similar in appearance to osteogenesis imperfecta tarda 1 but with *fewer fractures* and *later onset.*

VIII. SCLEROSING DYSPLASIAS

Key Concepts

Spectrum of diseases with various patterns of increased osseous density. Some are asymptomatic; others cause brittle bones that develop pathologic fractures.

A. Definition: A *spectrum of diseases* resulting from a *failure of osteoclasts to resorb bone* during remodeling. This failure may occur at sites of either endochondral or intramembranous ossification.
B. Individual diseases in the spectrum:
   1. *Osteopetrosis* (Albers-Schonberg disease):
     a. *Sclerotic, fragile long bones with frequent transverse fractures.*
     b. Transverse dense metaphyseal bands are common.
     c. May have *bone-within-a-bone* appearance.
     d. Metaphyseal flaring is secondary to abnormal remodeling.
     e. Infantile autosomal-recessive form is severe and often fatal; adult form, which may be recessive or dominant, is more benign.
     f. Patient is anemic and subject to infection.
     g. Sclerosis and lack of remodeling of surrounding bone cause cranial nerve damage (blindness and deafness).
   2. *Pyknodysostosis:*
     a. Similar to osteopetrosis with *sclerotic long bones that sustain transverse pathologic fractures.*
     b. Additional features are *wormian bones, hypoplastic angle of the jaw, and acro-osteolysis.*
   3. *Osteopoikilosis: Multiple bone islands located in the epiphysis and metaphysis.*
   4. Osteopathia striata (Voorhoeve's disease): Linear striations in the metaphyses.
   5. Progressive diaphyseal dysplasia (Camurate-Engelmann disease):
     a. Symmetrically thickened cortex with sparing of the metaphyses and epiphyses.
     b. Both the endosteum and periosteum are involved, narrowing the medullary cavity.
   6. Ribbing disease: Asymmetric, painful cortical thickening.
   7. Melorheostosis:
     a. A wavy hyperostosis ("dripping candle wax") that is endosteal as well as periosteal, involving only one side of the bone.
     b. Lower extremities more commonly affected than other sites.
     c. Unilateral predisposition, tendency to involve multiple bones in the same way; tarsals may be involved as well.

IX. CONGENITAL DISLOCATED HIP (CDH) DEVELOPMENTAL DYSPLASIA OF THE HIP (DDH)

Key Concepts

Lateral and superior migration of the femoral head, often associated with acetabular dysplasia and hypoplasia of the femoral head ossification center.

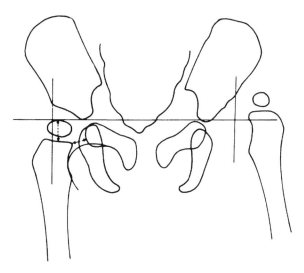

Fig. 5-1 *Left* CDH; normal right hip. Hilgenreiner's line (line through triradiate cartilages) serves as a reference. The left hip shows both lateral and superior displacement (as measured from the teardrop and Hilgenreiner's line, respectively) and is, therefore, dislocated. Shenton's line (shown on the normal right side outlining the obturator foramen and femoral neck) would be distorted on the abnormal left side.

A. Definition: Perinatal relaxation of the capsule of the hip joint allows dislocation of the hip. Acetabular deficiency, femoral head and neck deformity, and contractures of periarticular muscles are secondary features.

B. Epidemiology:
   1. *Caucasians* have the highest incidence.
   2. Incidence greater in *females* than males 5:1.
   3. Breech delivery and oligohydramnios are predisposing factors.
   4. Very common in neonatal period, but 75% to 95% of newborns with clinical signs of CDH revert to normal after a few weeks.
   5. Incidence after neonatal period 1:1000.

C. Radiographic signs:
   1. *Films prior to 6 weeks of age have a high false-negative rate.* Early films may, however, be useful in ruling out other etiologies of leg shortening (such as proximal focal femoral deficiency).
   2. *Primary radiographic signs[1] of CDH* (Fig 5-1):
      a. Draw *Hilgenreiner's line* (through triradiate cartilages), then *Perkin's line* (from the anterior inferior iliac spine perpendicular to Hilgenreiner's line); *normally the femoral head ossifica-*

tion center is located in the inner lower quadrant formed by these lines.

    b. Measure horizontal distance from teardrop to metaphysis and compare to normal side; a difference of 2 mm or more indicates *lateral subluxation* of the hip.

    c. Measure vertical distance from Hilgenreiner's line to metaphysis; a difference of 2 mm or more indicates superior subluxation of the hip. *If the hip is displaced both laterally and superiorly, it is considered dislocated.*

    d. *Shenton's line* (following the curve from the obturator foramen extended to the femoral neck) may be helpful.

  2. *Secondary radiographic signs of CDH:*

    a. *Acetabular dysplasia:* Present when the angle described by Hilgenreiner's line and the acetabular roof is greater than 30 degrees. This ''shallow acetabulum'' is rarely present initially but develops because of inadequate stress by the malpositioned femoral head; often reconstitutes normally after reduction of the hip dislocation.

    b. Excessive *anteversion* of the femoral head. The 30 degrees' anteversion of the head at birth normally decreases to 10 degrees by the time of skeletal maturity. This process often fails to occur in CDH.

    c. Delayed ossification of the proximal femoral epiphysis is often present but nonspecific. Normal femoral heads may show asymmetric ossification.

D. Complications of CDH:

  1. Avascular necrosis (AVN) secondary to manipulation; tenotomy and traction may reduce the risk.

  2. Development of pseudoacetabulae in the iliac wings and associated mechanical problems.

  3. Secondary osteoarthritis occurs surprisingly late, generally in the fifth or sixth decade.

E. *Ultrasound,* in experienced hands is extremely accurate.[2]

F. *Arthrography* is employed in patients with persistent and unexplained CDH, primarily to demonstrate sources of mechanical obstruction to a successful reduction such as:

  1. *Inverted limbus* ''*thorn*'' (superior acetabular labrum).

  2. *Pulvinar* (intracapsular soft tissue).

  3. *Elongated ligamentum teres* and *hourglass constriction* of the joint capsule.

  4. Tight *iliopsoas* muscle.

G. CT or MRI is occasionally useful in further defining abnormal bone relationships, especially deficiency in the posterior rim of the acetabulum. Hip reduction post casting is easily evaluated by CT. A minimal number of 4-mm axial cuts (2 to 3) through the affected femoral head will determine its location relative to the acetabulum. If this is performed at a 30-mAs technique, dose is minimal to the infant.[3]

H. Treatment of CDH: All aimed at improving femoral head coverage by the acetabulum, to promote normal growth and development of both head and acetabulum[4]:

1. Closed reduction.
2. Skeletal traction.
3. Adductor tenotomy and iliopsoas release.
4. Open reduction for mechanical obstruction.
5. Varus rotational osteotomy of the femoral subtrochanteric region (results in increased femoral head coverage by the acetabulum).
6. Pemberton acetabuloplasty: An osteotomy extending from the anterior inferior iliac spine to the tri-radiate cartilage, using the latter as a hinge. An opening wedge is placed. This reconstructive osteotomy for the skeletally immature patient affords coverage of the femoral head and allows congruent growth of the femoral head and acetabulum.
7. Salter opening wedge osteotomy: A reconstructive osteotomy that is less difficult to perform than the Pemberton. The osteotomy extends from the anterior inferior iliac spine straight across to the sacrosciatic notch. An opening wedge is placed, using the symphysis pubis as a hinge. As with the Pemberton operation, the acetabular roof is shifted anterolaterally to cover the femoral head.
8. Triple innominate (triple Steele) osteotomy: A reconstructive procedure for the skeletally mature patient. Osteotomies are performed across the iliac neck, ischium, and superior pubic ramus, leaving a free-floating acetabulum, which is rotated so that femoral head coverage is attained and secured with hardware at the iliac neck osteotomy site.
9. Chiari medial displacement: This is not a reconstructive, but a salvage procedure for older patients. An intra-articular osteotomy is extended across the superior acetabulum. The inferior portion of the osteotomy as well as the femoral head are displaced medially, thus attaining the goal of femoral head coverage.

X. PROXIMAL FEMORAL FOCAL DEFICIENCY

A. Definition: A spectrum of abnormalities involving agenesis of all or part of the proximal femur. The entity usually is an isolated abnormality and unilateral.

B. Radiographic abnormalities:
   1. Short, displaced femur.

2. Normal distal femur.
3. Proximal femoral abnormality ranges from complete absence to a large gap between the diaphysis and capital femoral epiphysis, to pseudarthrosis at the femoral neck, to a varus deformity. Imaging procedures seek to classify the abnormality early so that prognosis and treatment may be established. In younger patients, where apparently absent structures may in fact be cartilaginous, magnetic resonance (MR) or MR arthrography may demonstrate nonossified structures.
4. Major differential diagnosis is infantile coxa vara.

XI. INFANTILE COXA VARA

A. Definition: Development of coxa vara (neck-to-shaft angle of less than 120 degrees) in infancy, often related to walking. Etiology is unknown, and the abnormality may be progressive; 25% are bilateral. Leg-length discrepancy and limp develop.
B. Differential diagnosis:
   1. Proximal femoral focal deficiency, mild.
   2. Renal osteodystrophy and rickets.
   3. Coxa vara in cleidocranial dysostosis.
   4. Slipped capital femoral epiphysis. At so young an age, it is more likely due to infection. An idiopathic variety is seen in adolescents.

XII. PRIMARY PROTRUSIO OF THE ACETABULUM (OTTO'S DISEASE)

A. Definition: Protrusio acetabuli without any recognized etiology and no other radiographic abnormality; perhaps due to abnormal acetabular remodeling; usually bilateral and more common in women; often familial; secondary osteoarthritis is common.
B. Differential diagnosis:
   1. Arthritides with axial migration—rheumatoid arthritis (RA), rheumatoid variants, 20% of degenerative joint disease (DJD).
   2. Diseases that soften bone, leading to protrusio, such as osteomalacia or Paget's disease of bone.

XIII. PSEUDARTHROSIS

A. Definition: Interruption in the diaphysis of a long bone, usually with tapering ends and mobility at the site of pseudoarthrosis.
B. Pseudarthrosis is most common in the tibia, followed by the fibula and clavicle; may be congenital or may develop in infancy.
C. May be an isolated phenomenon or related to neurofibromatosis or fibrous dysplasia.

D. If it develops in an infant, there is anterior bowing first, then pathologic fracture, then tapering of the bones at the fracture site.

XIV. CONGENITAL FOOT ANOMALIES

Key Concepts

Most foot anomalies can be described using the following parameters: hindfoot equinus or calcaneus, hindfoot varus or valgus, forefoot varus or valgus. Clubfoot consists of hindfoot equinus, hindfoot varus, and forefoot varus. Congenital vertical talus deformity consists of hindfoot equinus, hindfoot valgus, forefoot valgus, and talonavicular dislocation. All of these parameters should be evaluated *only on weight-bearing films.*

A. Terminology[5,6]:
  1. *Cavus:* Raised longitudinal arch of the foot (literally, *hollow*).
  2. *Planus:* Flattened longitudinal arch of the foot.
  3. *Equinus:* Fixed plantar flexion of the hindfoot.
  4. *Calcaneus:* Fixed dorsiflexion of the hindfoot.
  5. *Varus (adductus):* Inverted (hindfoot or forefoot).
  6. *Valgus (abductus):* Everted (hindfoot or forefoot).
  7. *Supination of the forefoot:* Inward rotation of forefoot on hindfoot (sole faces inward).
  8. *Pronation of the forefoot:* Excessive outward rotation of forefoot on hindfoot.
B. Most valuable measurements are *all made on weight-bearing films.*
  1. *Hindfoot equinus or calcaneus:*
      a. Normal on the lateral film: The calcaneus is normally dorsiflexed. The angle between the longitudinal axis of the tibia and the calcaneus (measured along the base) ranges between 60 and 90 degrees (Fig 5-2,*A*).
      b. *Hindfoot equinus: Plantar* flexion of the calcaneus such that the calcaneotibial angle is greater than 90 degrees (Fig 5-2,*B*); seen in clubfoot and congenital vertical talus).
      c. *Hindfoot* calcaneus: Excessively dorsiflexed calcaneus such that the calcaneotibial angle is less than 60 degrees (Fig 5-2,*C*); seen in cavus and spastic deformities.
      d. Another method of evaluating the dorsi- or plantar flexion of the calcaneus is "calcaneal pitch": on a lateral view a line drawn along the anterior and posterior prominence on the inferior border of the calcaneus should slant upward from the horizontal surface by 20 to 30 degrees.
  2. *Hindfoot varus or valgus:* Talus is the point of reference since it

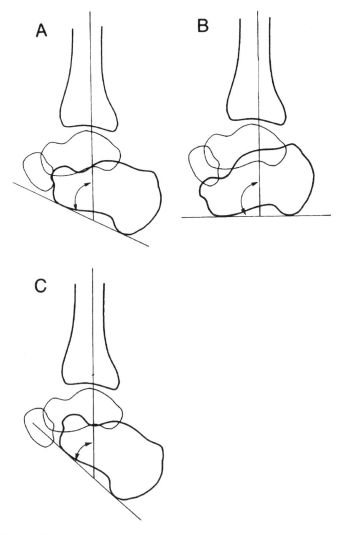

Fig. 5-2 **A,** Normal hindfoot with the tibiocalcaneal angle measuring between 60 and 90 degrees. **B,** Hindfoot equinus (angle greater than 90 degrees). **C,** Hindfoot calcaneus (angle less than 60 degrees).

is assumed to be fixed relative to the lower leg; calcaneus rotates around it.

a. *Normal:*

    (1) *Lateral:* Talocalcaneal (TC), or Kite's, angle 25 to 45 degrees (50 degrees in newborns; Fig 5-3,*A*).

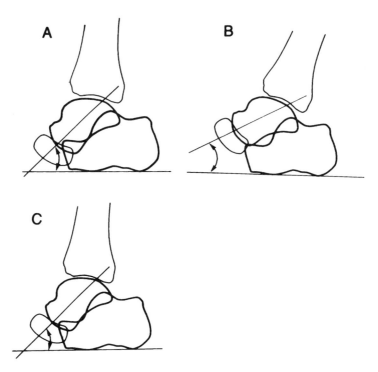

Fig. 5-3   Lateral view: **A,** Normal hindfoot with the lateral talocalcaneal (TC) angle measuring 25 to 50 degrees. **B,** Hindfoot varus with a decreased lateral TC angle. **C,** Hindfoot valgus with an increased lateral TC angle.

    (2) *AP:* TC angle 15 to 40 degrees (30 to 50 degrees in newborns). The midtalar line passes through or slightly medial to the base of the first metatarsal (MT). The midcalcaneal line passes through the base of the fourth MT (Fig 5-4,*A*).

  b. *Hindfoot varus:* With fixed talus, the calcaneus can adduct. Hindfoot varus is seen in clubfoot and some paralytic deformities.

    (1) *Lateral: Decreased TC angle* (less than 25 degrees), with the talus and calcaneus, approaching parallelism (Fig 5-3,*B*).

    (2) *AP: Decreased TC angle* (less than 15 degrees) (Fig 5-4,*B*). The talus points lateral to the first MT because the entire foot swings medially.

  c. *Hindfoot valgus:* With fixed talus, the calcaneus can abduct. Hindfoot valgus is seen in congenital vertical talus, flexible flatfoot deformity, and neurologic deformities.

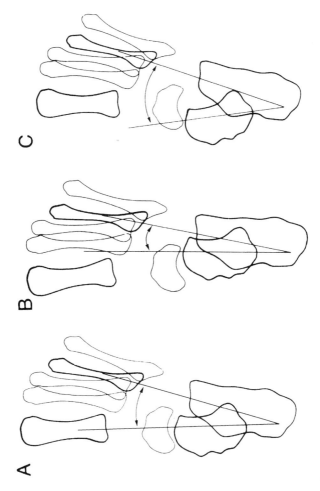

Fig. 5-4 AP view: **A,** Normal hindfoot with a TC angle of 15 to 40 degrees. **B,** Varus hindfoot with a decreased TC angle. **C,** Valgus hindfoot with an increased TC angle.

(1) *Lateral: Increased TC angle* (greater than 45 degrees, or, in newborns, 50 degrees) (Fig 5-3,*C*).

(2) AP: Increased TC angle (Fig 5-4,*C*). The talus points medial to the first MT because the calcaneus (and, therefore, the entire foot) swings laterally.

d. Residents seem to have a terrible time remembering whether the TC angle is increased or decreased in varus or valgus. First, remember that the TC angle is usually increased on *both* AP and lateral films, or decreased on *both* AP and lateral films. One radiologist gives the hint that hindfoot *valgus* has an *increased angle* as well as an *increased number of letters* relative to hindfoot varus.[7]

3. *Forefoot varus or valgus:*

a. *Normal:*

(1) AP: MTs converge proximally with slight overlap at the bases (Fig 5-5,*A*).

(2) Lateral: Fifth MT is in most plantar position, with other MTs superimposed (Fig 5-6,*A*).

b. Forefoot varus (inverted, often supinated). Forefoot varus is seen in clubfoot.

(1) AP: Forefoot is narrowed, with increased convergence at bases (Fig 5-5,*B*).

(2) Lateral: Ladderlike arrangement, with first MT most dorsal and fifth MT most plantar (Fig 5-6,*B*)

c. *Forefoot valgus* (everted, often pronated). Forefoot valgus is seen in congenital vertical talus, flexible flatfoot, and spastic deformities.

(1) AP: Forefoot is broadened with decreased overlap at bases (Fig 5-5,*C*).

(2) Lateral: May see ladderlike arrangement, but first MT is in most plantar position (Fig 5-6,*C*).

C. Common foot deformities:

1. Clubfoot (talipes equinovarus):

a. Incidence: 1 in 1000 births.

b. Ratio of males to females affected: 2 to 3:1.

c. Etiology unclear. Possible contributing factors are:

(1) Defective connective tissue with ligamentous laxity.

(2) Muscle imbalance.

(3) Intrauterine position deformity.

(4) Persistence of an early normal fetal relationship.

d. Radiographic findings (Fig 5-7):

(1) Hindfoot equinus.

(2) Hindfoot varus.

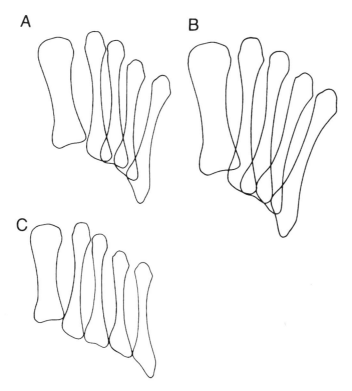

Fig. 5-5 AP view: **A,** Normal forefoot with mild MT convergence at bases. **B,** Forefoot varus with increased MT convergence. **C,** Forefoot valgus with decreased convergence.

      (3) Forefoot varus (more or less, depending on severity of deformity).

2. Congenital vertical talus (rocker-bottom foot). The talus is in extreme plantar flexion with dorsal dislocation of the navicular, locking the talus into plantar flexion.

  a. Rigid flat foot.

  b. May occur in isolation or as part of a variety of syndromes, frequently associated with myelomeningocele.

  c. Radiographic findings (Fig 5-8):

    (1) *Lateral:*

      a Abnormal talus with *dislocated navicular.*

      b Valgus hindfoot.

      c Equinus.

      d Forefoot dorsiflexed and valgus.

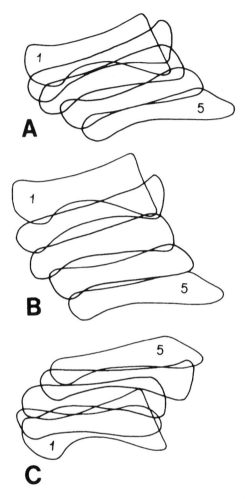

Fig. 5-6   Lateral view: **A,** Normal forefoot with MT superimposition (but fifth in plantar position). **B,** Forefoot varus with ladder configuration of MTs and 5th in plantar position. **C,** Forefoot valgus with MT superimposition (first MT in plantar position).

      (2) *AP:*
         a Severe hindfoot valgus.
         b Forefoot normal to valgus.
   3. Flexible flatfoot deformity (pes planovalgus):
     a. Affects 4% of population.
     b. Hereditary influence.

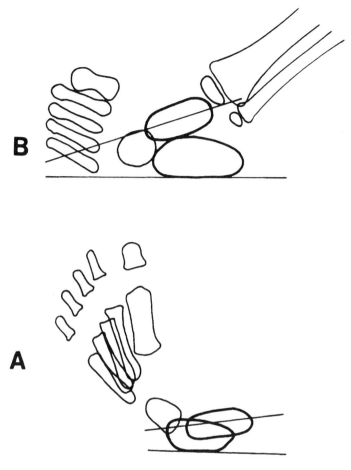

Fig. 5-7   Clubfoot deformity: hindfoot equinus, hindfoot varus, forefoot varus.
A, AP. **B,** Lateral.

    c. Etiology may be lax ligaments that allow the calcaneus to rotate into a valgus position. The talus becomes more vertical, but the navicular follows it.

    d. Radiographic findings: (Note: It is flexible: *non–weight-bearing films are normal.*)

      (1) AP:

        a Hindfoot and forefoot valgus.

        b Forefoot valgus with flattened midtarsal arch.

      (2) Lateral:

        a Hindfoot and forefoot valgus.

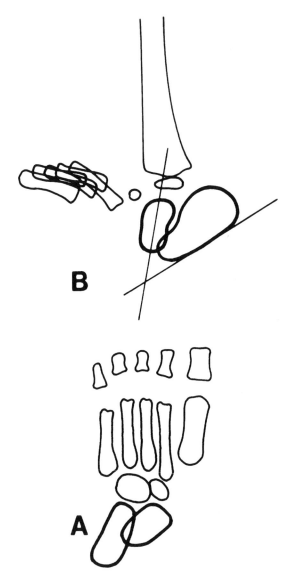

Fig. 5-8   Congenital vertical talus: hindfoot equinus, hindfoot valgus with dislocated talonavicular joint, forefoot valgus. **A,** AP. **B,** Lateral.

       b May superficially resemble congenital vertical talus, but the talonavicular joint is not dislocated and there is no equinus.

  4. Pes cavus: High arched foot (calcaneus) with compensatory plantar flexion of the forefoot.

    a. Etiology:

      (1) Upper motor neuron lesions (Friedreich's ataxia).

      (2) Lower motor neuron lesions (poliomyelitis).

      (3) Vascular ischemia as in Volkmann's contracture.

      (4) Muscular dystrophy of the peroneal type (Charcot-Marie-Tooth disease).

  5. Metatarsus adductus:

    a. Most common structural abnormality of the foot seen in infancy.

    b. Ten times as common as clubfoot.

    c. Usually bilateral.

    d. Etiology unknown.

    e. More common in females.

    f. Radiographic findings:

      (1) *Forefoot adductus and in varus.*

      (2) *Hindfoot normal* to moderate valgus.

      (3) No equinus (dorsiflexion normal).

D. MR studies show that early ossification in the talar, calcaneus, and navicular bones does not begin in the center of their cartilaginous anlages. The orientations of the long axis of the ossification center is slightly different from the cartilaginous anlage. Part of the change in alignment seen on radiographs with growth is due to the ossification proceeding eccentrically in the cartilage rather than a true change in alignment.[8]

XV. TARSAL COALITION (PERONEAL SPASTIC FLATFOOT)

Key Concepts

    May be the etiology of painful flatfoot in young males. Secondary changes of sclerosis and beaking are seen on lateral film. Coalition seen on oblique (calcaneonavicular) or Harris (TC) views; CT is extremely useful.

A. Epidemiology:

  1. Occurs in 1% of population.

  2. May be familial, but with great variability.

  3. May be congenital (vast majority) or secondary to infection, trauma, arthritis disorders, or surgery.

4. May be a part of various syndromes: hereditary symphalangism, Aperts' acrocephalosyndactyly, hand-foot-uterus.
5. Congenital probably due to a failure of segmentation in the fetus. (Coalitions are seen in fetuses.)
6. Calcaneonavicular more common than TC, more common than talonavicular, more common than calcaneocuboid.
7. Males more commonly affected.
8. Bilateral 25%.

B. Signs and symptoms:
 1. Symptoms generally first occur in the second or third decade.
 2. Physical examination findings: Limited subtalar motion, pes planus, shortening with persistent or intermittent spasm of the peroneal muscles.

C. Radiographic findings:
 1. Coalition may be fibrous, cartilaginous, or osseous, so may not demonstrate bony bridging in all cases. In the absence of a bony bridge, close approximation of the bones with cortical irregularity or sclerosis suggests fibrous or cartilaginous bridging.
 2. Calcaneonavicular coalition.
    a. Symptoms are less severe than in a TC coalition.
    b. Secondary radiographic signs are less marked.
    c. Talar "beaking" uncommon.
    d. Best seen on 45-degree medial oblique (Fig 5-9).
 3. Talocalcaneal coalition.
    a. Talocalcaneal joint has three facets: Posterior (lateral), middle (medial), and anterior. The coalition usually occurs at the middle facet between the talus and sustentaculum tali. Ankylosis of the posterior or anterior facets is far less common.
    b. The TC coalition is never seen on routine AP, lateral, and oblique films of the foot; initial diagnosis depends on secondary radiographic signs:
       (1) Talar beaking on lateral film: Dorsal subluxation of the navicular is produced by subtalar rigidity, which leads to elevation of periosteum, which leads to subperiosteal proliferation and bony excrescence. Talar beaking is not pathognomonic; it is also seen in RA, diffuse idiopathic skeletal hyperostosis (DISH), and acromegaly.
       (2) Narrowing of the posterior subtalar joint on lateral film, representing DJD due to calcaneal eversion.
       (3) Ball-and-socket ankle seen on AP ankle (provides inversion-eversion function that is restricted at the TC joint).
    c. Comparison views may be necessary to evaluate for asymmetry

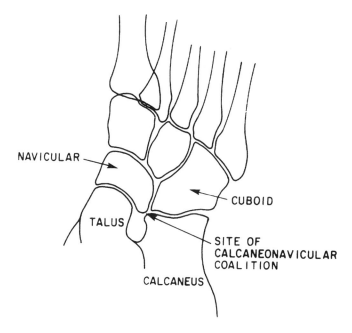

Fig. 5-9 Medial oblique view showing site of calcaneonavicular coalition.

of the undersurface of the talar neck or broadening of the lateral process of the talus.
d. Harris-Beath view (tangential calcaneus) required but may give a false-positive or -negative impression if patient is positioned incorrectly (Fig 5-10).
D. Special techniques:
1. Bone scan may be useful as a screening device. In positive cases, the subtalar joint as well as talar beak show increased uptake.
2. Tomography: Lateral, complex motion; four sections. Where W equals the heel width:
a. W–1 cm demonstrates the medial facet.
b. W–1.5 cm and W–2 cm demonstrate the anterior facet.
c. W/2 demonstrates the posterior facet.
3. CT: Easily demonstrates the three facets of the subtalar joint with both feet viewed symmetrically in the same exam (Fig 5-11). Gantry either is not angled or is angled away from the knees. If mistakenly angled toward the knees, a false-positive impression may result.
4. Arthrography: Rarely performed today but can conclusively demonstrate a coalition whether it is osseous, cartilaginous, or fibrous.

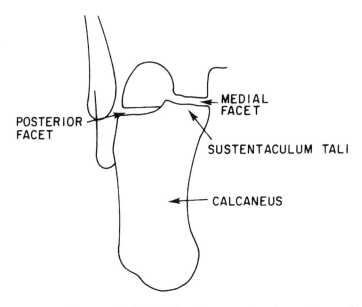

Fig. 5-10 Harris-Beath view of subtalar joint, demonstrating the position and medial facet. The latter is the most likely site of a TC coalition.

XVI. CLEIDOCRANIAL DYSOSTOSIS

A. Definition: Autosomal-dominant abnormality with retarded development of the membranous bones.

B. Radiographic abnormalities:
  1. *Delayed cranial suture closure;* platybasia.
  2. *Wormian bones.*
  3. Partial or total *absence of the clavicle,* usually bilateral. Pseudoarthroses may be present.
  4. Ossification of the pubis absent or delayed. Valgus or varus deformities of the femoral neck.
  5. Various other epiphyseal or metaphyseal abnormalities may be present.

XVII. OSTEO-ONYCHODYSOSTOSIS (NAIL-PATELLA SYNDROME, OR FONG'S DISEASE)

A. Definition: Autosomal-dominant disorder characterized by multiple bone abnormalities, dysplastic fingernails, and renal disease.

B. Radiographic abnormalities:
  1. Absent patella.
  2. Posterior iliac horns are pathognomonic.

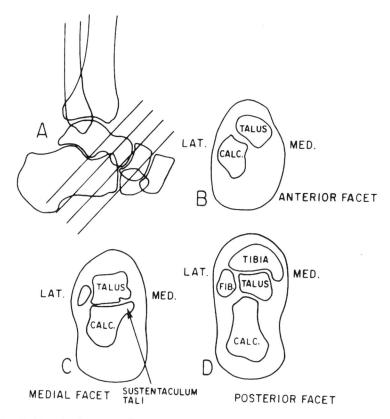

Fig. 5-11   CT for TC coalition: **A,** Position of cuts. **B,** Anterior facet. **C,** Medial facet. **D,** Posterior facet.

3. Hypoplastic capitellum and radial head dislocation.
4. Hypoplastic lateral femoral condyle and resultant genu valgum.

XVIII. CAUDAL REGRESSION SYNDROME (SACRAL AGENESIS)

A. Definition: Spectrum of abnormalities ranging from agenesis of part of the sacrum to agenesis of the sacrum, lumbar spine, and lower part of the thoracic spine. Twenty percent of patients are infants of diabetic mothers.

XIX. MADELUNG'S DEFORMITY

A. Definition: Bowing of the distal radius in an ulnar and volar direction. The ulna is therefore relatively long and is often dorsally dislocated.

The deformity results in a narrowed carpal angle. Madelung's deformity may be seen:
1. As an isolated finding.
2. In dyschondro-osteosis dwarfism.
3. In Turner's syndrome.
4. As a deformity after radial fracture.
B. More common in women than men.

XX. CHROMOSOME DISORDERS

A. Down's syndrome (trisomy 21):
1. Flared iliac wings with flattened acetabular roofs.
2. Clinodactyly.
3. Eleven ribs.
4. Microcephaly.
5. Atlantoaxial instability.
B. Trisomy 18:
1. Adducted thumb and other finger and toe deformities.
2. "Rocker-bottom" feet.
3. Sternal aplasia or hypoplasia.
4. Hypoplastic ribs and clavicles.
C. Turner's syndrome (deletion of one X chromosome):
1. Short stature.
2. Osteoporosis.
3. Short metacarpals, especially the fourth.
4. Madelung's deformity.
5. Flattening of the medial tibial plateau with overgrowth of the medial femoral condyle.
6. Cubitus valgus.

XXI. DWARFISM by PAULA SHULTZ, M.D.

Key Concepts

Differentiation of dwarfism is important for prognosis and genetic counseling. A standard set of films and an algorithm is presented that we have found useful in diagnosing different types of dwarfism.

Current research is revealing the modes of inheritance, life expectancy, and expected quality of life of the various dwarfs. Correct classification, based in large part on the radiographic findings, must be made to insure appropriate genetic counseling as well as appropriate transmission of information to parents regarding their child's life expectations and limitations.

Volumes have been written on the subject of dwarfism. The classifications and subclassifications change constantly as knowledge increases. The numerous synonyms and eponyms in use for clinical entities add to the confusion. The latest generally accepted classification was established by the European Society for Pediatric Radiology and the National Foundation March of Dimes; it is titled *International Nomenclature of Constitutional Diseases of Bones.* In this section, the eleven most common dwarfism complexes are described. This is followed by a simplified approach to classifying the different types of dwarfs.[9–15]

Selected Major Dwarf Syndromes

Achondroplasia

A. Synonyms: Chondrodysplasia, chondrodystrophia fetalis, chondrodystrophic dwarfism.
B. Inheritance: Autosomal-dominant (most cases, however, are new mutants).
C. Age of manifestation: Birth.
D. Main clinical features:
   1. Short-limbed dwarfism with proximal segments of limbs shorter than distal (rhizomelic).
   2. Macrocrania, with or without hydrocephalus; characteristic facies with small maxillary area, prominent, bulging brow, and depressed nasal bridge; normal intelligence.
   3. Lumbar kyphosis in infancy progressing to lumbar lordosis in childhood and adulthood; occasional scoliosis; normal to relatively long trunk.
   4. Prominent buttocks and abdomen.
   5. Limitation of elbow extension; trident hand with relatively short fingers; genu varum.
   6. Possible neurologic symptoms due to relative spinal stenosis resulting from the narrowed interpedicular distance.
E. Major radiographic features:
   1. *Large calvaria with small area of facial bones* in comparison to vault; short base of skull and reduced size of the foramen magnum.
   2. *Decrease in the interpediculate distance from upper to lower lumbar spine;* short pedicles; *posterior scalloping of vertebral bodies;* occipitalization of C_1.
   3. *Squared iliac wings with horizontal acetabular roofs;* narrow greater sciatic notch; narrowed pelvic inlet.
   4. *Shortened and thickened tubular bones with flared metaphyses and normal epiphyses.*
   5. "Trident" hands in about 50% of cases.

F. Progression and prognosis: Normal life span; complications occurring include hydrocephalus, nerve root irritation, and paraparesis and paraplegia.
G. Differential diagnosis: Other forms of short-limbed dwarfism:
   1. Hypochondroplasia: Similar but milder changes; normal skull.
   2. Pseudoachondroplasia: Normal skull; epiphyseal abnormality.
   3. Thanatophoric dwarfism (infancy): Lethal condition; smaller thorax, more severe changes.

Hypochondroplasia
A. Synonyms: Chondrohypoplasia.
B. Inheritance: Autosomal-dominant; is distinct from achondroplasia and not a variation or manifestation of a single mutant gene.
C. Age of manifestation: Early childhood.
D. Main clinical features:
   1. Small stature with disproportionately short extremities.
   2. Slightly increased lumbar lordosis with mildly protuberant abdomen; kyphosis is not a feature.
   3. Limitation of elbow extension.
   4. Mild generalized joint laxity.
E. *Major radiographic features:*
   1. *Normal skull.*
   2. *Mild narrowing or lack of widening of the interpedicular distances from upper to lower lumbar spine.*
   3. Tubular bones short and thickened with *mild rhizomelic predominance.*
   4. *Large capital femoral epiphysis with short, broad femoral neck;* prominent femoral trochanters.
   5. Often *increased length of fibula.*
F. *Progression and prognosis:* Normal life span. Caesarean section for delivery is necessary because of the small pelvis.
G. *Differential diagnosis:*
   1. Achondroplasia: Skull involvement is present; has greater disproportion of limb length (rhizomelic); trident hand deformity present in about 50% of cases, more prominent narrowing of interpediculate distance.
   2. Metaphyseal chondrodysplasia, Schmid type: Pronounced coxa vara; growth plate line is vertical and irregular; no vertebral abnormalities.
   3. Dyschondrosteosis: Madelung-type deformity present.

Pseudoachondroplasia
A. Synonyms: Pseudoachondroplastic type of spondyloepiphyseal dysplasia.

B. Inheritance: Probably heterogeneous; some are autosomal-dominant, others recessive.
C. Age of manifestation: Second to fourth year of life.
D. Main clinical features:
    1. Normal face and head.
    2. Short-limbed dwarfism but no rhizomelic predominance.
    3. Marked joint laxity at all joints except elbow.
    4. Short, stubby hands and feet.
E. Major radiographic features:
    1. *Grossly abnormal epiphyses* with irregular calcification.
    2. Normal skull.
    3. *Variable deformities of the vertebrae* on the lateral view ranging from near normal to persistent oval shape to anterior beaking and platyspondyly; may have irregular ossification at the end-plates of the vertebral bodies.
F. Progression and prognosis: Normal life expectancy; early disability from osteoarthritis.
G. Differential diagnosis:
    1. Achondroplasia: Head is large with frontal bossing and depression of bridge of nose; epiphyses are normal.
    2. Multiple epiphyseal dysplasia: Vertebral anomalies are not present.

Thanatophoric Dwarfism
A. Synonyms: Severe achondroplasia.
B. Inheritance: Unknown; autosomal-recessive has been suggested.
C. Age of manifestation: At birth or in utero.
D. Main clinical features:
    1. Death in early infancy.
    2. Disproportionate dwarfism with marked rhizomelic tubular bone shortening.
    3. Relatively normal trunk length, narrow thorax, protuberant abdomen.
    4. Large head with frontal bossing, protruding eyes, and depressed nasal bridge.
E. Major radiographic features:
    1. *Cloverleaf deformity of skull* may be present; short skull base.
    2. *Platyspondyly* with notchlike ossification defects of the central portion of the upper and lower vertebral end-plates causing an H or U configuration. *Trunk length is normal due to widened disc spaces.*
    3. *Lumbar interpedicular distance fails to widen caudally;* narrowing is greatest in midlumbar area.
    4. *Short ribs* with consequent narrow thorax in AP and lateral views.

5. Decreased height and horizontal inferior margins of the iliac bones with small sacrosciatic notch.
6. *Marked rhizomelic tubular bone shortening with curving and irregular metaphyseal flaring; "telephone receiver-shaped" femurs.*

F. Progression and prognosis: Death within first few days of life due to respiratory distress and cardiac failure.
G. Differential diagnosis:
  1. Achondroplasia: Fails to show the marked flattening of the vertebral bodies, widened intervertebral spaces, or the irregular flaring of the metaphyses.
  2. Achondrogenesis: Lacks the telephone receiver-shaped femur; no narrowing of sacrosciatic notch; lacks ossification of lower vertebral bodies, iliac, and sacrum.
  3. Metatropic dwarf: Decreased trunk length.

Achondrogenesis (Types I and II)

A. Synonyms: None.
B. Inheritance: Autosomal-recessive.
C. Age of manifestation: At birth or in utero.
D. Main clinical features:
  1. Incompatible with life.
  2. Extremely short limbs, protuberant abdomen, disproportionately large head.
  3. Hydropic, edematous appearance.
E. Major radiographic features:
  1. Poorly mineralized skull.
  2. *Ossification of spine absent or severely retarded more caudally than cranially in spine.*
  3. Absent ossification of talus and calcaneus.
  4. *Barrel-shaped thorax with short, horizontal ribs* with multiple fractures.
  5. Very *small, broadened long bones* with concave ends and longitudinally projecting spines or spikes.
  6. *Type II is less severe* with more complete ossification and no evidence of rib fracture.
F. Progression and prognosis: Patients are stillborn or die in neonatal period.
G. Differential diagnosis: All lethal forms of dwarfism. Thanatophoric dwarfs demonstrate markedly bowed femurs; ossification of vertebral bodies, sacrum, and pubic and ischial bones is present.

Asphyxiating Thoracic Dysplasia

A. Synonyms: Asphyxiating thoracic dystrophy, Jeune syndrome, thoracic-pelvic-phalangeal dystrophy, infantile thoracic dystrophy.

B. Inheritance: Autosomal-recessive.

C. Age of manifestation: Usually birth.

D. Main clinical features:
1. Respiratory difficulties due to small thoracic cage.
2. Short extremities at birth, usually acromelic but sometimes rhizomelic.
3. Renal disease, progressive with age.

E. Major radiographic features:
1. *Normal skull and spine.*
2. *Small thoracic cage with short, horizontal ribs;* with time this becomes normal.
3. *Sometimes flared ilia;* spurlike downward projections at the medial and lateral aspects of the acetabular roof; normalization of the pelvis with age.
4. Short middle and distal phalanges with some coned epiphyses and premature fusion of epiphyses.
5. *Disproportionately (usually acromelic) short extremities with metaphyseal irregularities.*

F. Progression and prognosis: If the patient survives the respiratory difficulties in the first year of life, there may be no further complications. Renal failure may develop in later childhood or adult life.

G. Differential diagnosis:
1. Chondroectodermal dysplasia: Hair and teeth abnormalities.
2. Thanotophoric dwarfism: Very short long tubular bones with characteristic bowing of the femurs.
3. Achondroplasia: Thoracic cage is only mildly reduced in size, if at all; middle and distal phalanges are normal.

Chondroectodermal Dysplasia

A. Synonyms: Ellis-van Creveld syndrome; ectodermal dysplasia; chondrodystrophy with ectodermal defects; mesoectodermal dysplasia.

B. Inheritance: Autosomal-recessive.

C. Age of manifestation: Birth.

D. Main clinical features:
1. Disproportionate dwarfism with short limbs, particularly in the distal portions.
2. Polydactyly of the hand and often of the feet; extranumerary digit is on the ulnar aspect.
3. Sparse hair and disordered eruption or absence of teeth due to ectodermal dysplasia; hypoplastic nails.
4. Long, narrow thorax.
5. Congenital heart disease.

E. Major radiographic features:
1. *Normal skull and spine.*

2. *Short ribs and long narrow thorax in infancy,* progressing to normal as child grows.
3. *Long bones are markedly short,* particularly the distal segments.
4. *Polydactyly* with or without fusion of metacarpals and/or phalanges.
5. In infancy, dysplasia of the pelvis with small iliac bones and, sometimes, a downward-directed spike in the region of the triradiate cartilage. This, too, progresses to normal with age.
6. *Fusion of capitate and hamate;* coned epiphyses of middle and distal phalanges.
7. *Proximal tibial epiphyses hypoplastic and displaced medially.* Defect of the lateral tibia causes severe genu valgum.

F. Progression and prognosis: Prognosis is related to the congenital heart defect with infant mortality estimated to exceed 50%. Also, the long, narrow thorax produces pulmonary insufficiency. Some disability may result from the genu valgum.

G. Differential diagnosis:
1. Asphyxiating thoracic dystrophy in neonatal period; hypoplastic nails are associated, and polydactyly is inconstant.
2. Later, other forms of short-limbed dwarfism, but upper tibial deformity and fused capitate and hamate should distinguish chondroectodermal dysplasia.

Diastrophic Dwarfism (Dysplasia)

A. Synonyms: None.
B. Inheritance: Autosomal-recessive.
C. Age of manifestation: Birth.
D. Main clinical features:
1. Small stature, short extremities; clubfoot and hitchhiker's thumb.
2. *Contractures of many joints.*
3. Cystic swelling of external ear.
E. Major radiographic features:
1. *Normal skull.*
2. *Appearance of spine variable:* Spectrum ranges from flattening to some increase in height, but may be normal. Posterior scalloping may be present.
3. Short clubbed long bones; epiphyses may be flattened and stippled.
4. *Severe talipes equinovarus* with short, thick MTs.
5. *Short first metacarpal with abnormal origin of thumb.*
6. Scoliosis.
F. Progression and prognosis: Perinatal mortality is increased, but those who survive past infancy can expect a normal life span. Moderate to severe restriction of physical activity due to combination of severe clubfoot deformity and scoliosis. Osteoarthritis is inevitable.

G. Differential diagnosis:
   1. Arthrogryposis multiplex: Marked decrease in muscle mass; lack of characteristic skeletal changes in hands and feet.
   2. Achondroplasia: Skull will be affected; contractures are not a feature and epiphyses are normal.

Chondrodysplasia Calcificans Punctata

A. Synonyms: Chondrodysplasia punctata, Conradi's disease, congenital stippled epiphysis, Conradi-Hunerman disease, chondropathia calcificans, chondropathia punctata, chondroangiopathia punctata, dysplasia epiphysealis congenita, punctate epiphyseal dysplasia.
B. Inheritance: Two types, both autosomal-dominant and autosomal-recessive.
C. Age at manifestation: Birth or early infancy.
D. Main clinical features:
   1. Congenital short-limbs, short stature; may be asymmetric (dominant type) or disproportionate short stature of the rhizomelic type (recessive type).
   2. Flat face with depressed bridge of nose.
   3. Ichthyosiform skin changes; joint contractures; cataracts.
   4. Associated anomalies include congenital heart disease (dominant type).
E. Major radiographic features:
   1. Dominant type (Conradi):
      a. Infancy:
         (1) *Stippling of epiphyses,* primarily at the ends of long bones, carpal, and tarsal regions.
         (2) *Unilateral, less frequently bilateral, shortening of the long tubular bones.*
         (3) Coronal cleft vertebral bodies; scoliosis may be present.
      b. Childhood and adulthood:
         (1) *Assymmetric, less frequently symmetric, shortening of the long tubular bones* and metacarpal bones.
         (2) *Epiphyseal dysplasia or irregularity* in places where previous stippling was located.
   2. Recessive type:
      a. *Severe symmetric shortening and metaphyseal splaying and calcific stippling of the ends of humeri and/or femurs.*
      b. *Dorsal and ventral ossification centers of vertebral bodies, which are separated by radiolucent bars of cartilage.*
F. *Progression and prognosis:*
   1. Dominant type: If severely affected, patients may be stillborn or die within the first week of life. After the first week, life expectancy

and intellectual development are normal. Complications arise from cataracts, joint contractures, and other orthopedic problems.

2. Recessive type: Prognosis is extremely poor. Failure to thrive, severe retardation in psychomotor development and death in infancy from repeated infection are demonstrated.

G. *Differential diagnosis:*
  1. Dominant type:
     a. Recessive type: Coronal clefts in vertebral bodies and symmetric shortening of the limbs.
     b. Zellurger's syndrome: Associated clinical, cytologic, and biochemical findings differentiate it.
     c. Epiphyseal dysplasia.
  2. Recessive type:
     a. Dominant type: Vertebral bodies lack coronal clefts; more often asymmetric.
     b. Epiphyseal dysplasia.

Dyschondrosteosis

A. Synonyms: Leri-Weill disease, Madelung's deformity with short forearms.
B. Inheritance: Autosomal-dominant with female preponderance.
C. Age of manifestation: Later childhood.
D. Main clinical features:
  1. Short-limbed, short stature associated with forearm, tibia, and fibular shortening.
  2. Dorsal dislocation of distal ulna with short, bowed radius.
  3. Limitation of motion at the elbow and wrist.
E. Major radiographic features:
  1. *Normal skull, spine, thorax,* shoulder girdle/humerus, *pelvic girdle,* and *femur.*
  2. *Dorsal dislocation of ulna at wrist* and sometimes at elbow.
  3. *Shortening of radius with bowing* and increase in distance between distal radioulnar articulation.
  4. *Pyramidal appearance of the carpus with the lunate at the apex,* fitting between the radius and ulna.
F. Progression and prognosis: Normal life expectancy. Some limitation of wrist motion, occasionally accompanied by pain.
G. Differential diagnosis:
  1. Other mesomelic dwarfs: Madelung's deformity is not present.
  2. Turner's syndrome: Clinical manifestations should easily differentiate.

Spondyloepiphyseal Dysplasia Congenita
A. Synonyms: None.
B. Inheritance: Autosomal-dominant with considerable variability of expression; may be sporadic.
C. Age of manifestation: Birth.
D. Main clinical features:
  1. Markedly reduced stature with short trunk.
  2. Pectus carinatum.
  3. Gross coxa vara.
  4. Decreased muscle tone and waddling gait.
  5. Myopia and retinal detachment.
  6. Occasionally clubfoot and/or cleft palate.
E. Major radiographic features:
  1. *Flattening of vertebral bodies* with shortening of the trunk; *hypoplasia of the odontoid.*
  2. *Small ilium* with irregular acetabula with horizontal roofs; *delayed ossification of pubic rami.*
  3. Capital femoral epiphyses, if present, are small and deformed with delayed presentation.
  4. *Limb epiphyses vary from normal to severely fragmented. Metaphyses also may be disordered and irregular.*
  5. *Shortening of the long bones.*
  6. Scoliosis.
F. Progression and prognosis:
  1. Premature osteoarthritis in affected joints is inevitable.
  2. Scoliosis is probable, and paraplegia has occurred.
G. Differential diagnosis:
  1. Morquio's disease: Clinically similar but radiographically dissimilar.
  2. Other forms of spondyloepiphyseal dysplasias: Most have less severe coxa vara, lack the delayed ossification of the pelvis and proximal femur, and do not demonstrate major changes in hands and feet.

Approach to Radiographic Classification of Dwarfism

Radiographic evaluation should be performed as early in life as possible since many of the typical findings become less apparent as the patient matures. A specific set of radiographs should be obtained in all evaluations and should include the following:
A. Lateral skull.
B. AP and lateral of the thoracolumbosacral spine.
C. Chest (shoulders must be included).
D. AP pelvis and hips.

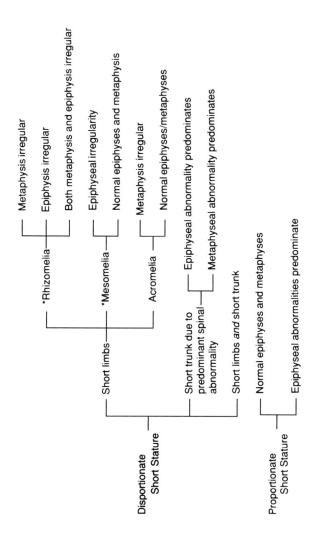

Fig. 5-12 Flow chart for characterization of most types of dwarfism. Asterisk indicates conditions for which tables of limb ratios are available for subtle or questionably abnormal cases.

Table 5-1   Group 1: Disproportionate Short Stature

A. Short-limbed, normal trunk
1. *Rhizomelia* (proximal limbs more affected)
   a. Metaphysis irregular or abnormal
      (1) Achondroplasia
         a Macrocrania with short skull base and small foramen magnum
         b Decreasing interpedicular width from upper to lower lumbar spine
         c Squared iliac wings with narrow sacrosciatic notch
      (2) Hypochondroplasia
         a Normal skull
         b Mildly decreasing interpediculate distances from upper to lower lumbar spine
         c Often increased length of fibulas
      (3) Achondrogenesis
         a Lack of ossification of lower lumbar and sacral spine
         b Disproportionately large head
         c Marked micromelia
      (4) Thanatophoric dwarfism
         a Marked shortening, curving of tubular bones with metaphyseal flaring
         b Platyspondyly; H- or U-shaped vertebrae
         c Narrow thorax both AP and lateral views due to rib shortening
   b. Epiphysis irregular or abnormal
      (1) Chondrodysplasia calcificans punctata (recessive)
         a Symmetric rhizomelic shortening of extremities
         b Coronal clefts of vertebral bodies
         c Calcific stippling ends of humeri and/or femurs
   c. Both epiphyses and metaphyses are abnormal
      (1) Pseudoachondroplasia
         a Normal face and head
         b Grossly abnormal epiphyses
         c Variable deformities of vertebrae

E. AP upper extremity (one side only).
F. AP lower extremity (one side only).
G. AP hand/wrist (one side only).

Initially one should determine what feature constitutes the most striking abnormality. Fig 5-12 is a flow chart that should allow a physician to accurately characterize most dwarfs. Tables 5-1 through 5-6 give the most likely diagnoses once the flow chart has been consulted. Each of these tables lists only the three most common radiographic abnormalities. Because of this limitation and the fact that most dwarfism syndromes have a spectrum of involvement that may or may not include the most common

Table 5-2   Group 1: Disproportionate Short Stature

A. Short-limbed, normal trunk
   2. *Mesomelia*
      a. Epiphyses irregular or abnormal
         (1) Chondroectodermal dysplasia
            a Short-limbed dwarfism most pronounced distally
            b Postaxial polydactyly
            c Fusion of capitate and hamate
      b. Normal epiphyses and metaphyses
         (1) Dyschondrosteosis
            a Normal skull, spine, thorax
            b Dorsal dislocation of ulna at wrist with Madelung's deformity
            c Pyramidal appearance of the carpus with the lunate at the apex

radiographic findings, one may also have to refer back to the more complete descriptions or use the excellent references listed at the end of this chapter for further clarification. In difficult cases starting over on the flow chart with the second most striking abnormality may prove more helpful in reaching the correct diagnosis.

You will note that several types of dwarfs appear in more than one table. The explanation is threefold. First, for many types, there is a wide spectrum of findings with certain of the findings present in one individual and not in another. Second, the age at evaluation will affect the abnormality most predominant at presentation because with growth, certain characteristic abnormalities either resolve or become more dominant. Third, as more is learned about dwarfs with individual characteristic manifestations, more

Table 5-3   Group 1: Disproportionate Short Stature

A. Short-limbed, normal trunk
   3. *Acromelia*
      a. Normal metaphyses and epiphyses
         (1) Acrodysostosis
            a Short stature predominantly distal, with peripheral dysostoses
            b Occasional brachycephaly and thickening of vault and base
            c Nasal hypoplasia
      b. Irregular or abnormal metaphyses
         (1) Asphyxiating thoracic dysplasia
             a Small thorax with short, horizontal ribs
            b Short limbs with acromelic predominance and metaphyseal irregularity
            c Short middle and distal phalanges; coned epiphyses

Table 5-4   Group 1: Disproportionate Short Stature

B. Short trunk and major spinal involvement
  1. Epiphyseal abnormalities predominate
     a. Spondyloepiphyseal dysplasia
        (1) Platyspondyly with hypoplastic odontoid
        (2) Shortening of long bones with epiphyseal, and less often metaphyseal, abnormality
        (3) Coxa vara
     b. Chondrodysplasia calcificans punctata (dominant type)
        (1) Asymmetric shortening of limbs
        (2) Scoliosis with irregular deformities of vertebral bodies
        (3) Calcific deposits in and around epiphyses and other cartilaginous areas
  2. Metaphyseal abnormalities predominate
     a. Spondylometaphyseal dysplasia
        (1) Platyspondyly with mild irregularity of end-plates
        (2) Metaphyseal irregularities with almost normal epiphyses

Table 5-5   Group 1: Disproportionate Short Stature

C. Short limbs and short trunk: All listed have both metaphyseal *and* epiphyseal abnormalities, so this focus will not help to differentiate
  1. Diastrophic dysplasia (dwarf)
     a. Severe talipes equinovarus with short, thick MTs
     b. Short first metacarpals with abnormal origins of thumbs
     c. Scoliosis
  2. Pseudoachondroplasia
     a. Normal face and head
     b. Variable deformities of the vertebrae
     c. Grossly abnormal epiphyses
  3. Kniest's disease
     a. Large cranium; hypoplasia of odontoid; flat face with depressed nasal bridge
     b. Severe platyspondyly
     c. Flared metaphyses; large, irregular, punctate epiphyses
  4. Metatropic dwarfism
     a. Kyphoscoliosis
     b. Striking platyspondyly
     c. Diaphyseal constriction and widely flaring metaphyses

Table 5-6   Group 2: Proportionate Short Stature

A. Normal epiphyses and metaphyses
　　1. Systemic diseases/metabolic abnormalities (most are addressed in other chapters)
　　　　a. Pituitary dwarfism
　　　　b. Renal osteodystrophy
　　　　c. Gonadal dysgenesis
　　　　d. Cardiopulmonary disease
　　　　e. Regional enteritis
　　　　f. "Hepatic" dwarf (biliary atresia or cirrhosis)
　　　　g. Hematologic abnormality (severe anemias)
　　　　h. Mucopolysaccharidosis
　　　　i. Mucolipidosis
　　　　j. Other storage diseases
　　　　k. Malnutrition
B. Predominant epiphyseal abnormalities
　　1. Multiple epiphyseal dysplasia
　　　　a. Irregularity of end-plates in lower dorsal spine
　　　　b. Pair of joints almost always symmetrically involved; fragmented ossification centers
　　　　c. Capital femoral epiphysis almost always involved
　　2. Chondrodysplasia punctata dominant (Conradi-Hünermann)
　　　　a. Stippled epiphyses
　　　　b. Mild shortening to normal limb length; if abnormal, usually asymmetric
　　　　c. Irregular deformities of the vertebral bodies
　　3. Hypothyroidism
　　　　a. Broad provisional zones of calcification
　　　　b. Retarded skeletal and skull maturation
　　　　c. Stippled epiphyses, especially femoral capital epiphyses, which has been termed "cretinoid" and resembles Legg-Calve-Perthes disease
C. Predominant metaphyseal abnormalities
　　1. Metaphyseal chondrodysplasias
　　　　a. Vertebral bodies may retain their oval shape
　　　　b. Limb metaphyses expanded and irregular; may be coned
　　　　c. Femoral metaphyses (proximal) demonstrate medial beaking, irregularity and widening; develops coxa vara
　　2. Spondylometaphyseal dysplasia
　　　　a. Universal platyspondyly; mild irregularity of the end-plates
　　　　b. Almost normal epiphyses; metaphyseal irregularities
　　　　c. Marked coxa vara may develop

distinct entities are described. In the earlier literature, some of these same entities would have been considered together, so there is some disagreement among the resources regarding some of the characteristic findings.

Finally, good luck! Although the task of classifying a dwarf is tedious and often quite frustrating, the final diagnosis is very important to the patient and his or her family—for genetic counseling and a better understanding of life's expectations and limitations.

XXII. MUCOPOLYSACCHARIDOSES

A. Definition: *Spectrum* of hereditary diseases characterized by a distinctive dwarfism pattern and distinguished in part by clinical presentation and largely by the difference in type of mucopolysaccharide excreted in the urine; all but Morquio's patients are *mentally retarded.*

B. *Radiographic findings common to all the mucopolysaccharidoses:*
   1. *Macrocephaly,* with a *J-shaped sella.*
   2. *Ribs are oar shaped* (i.e., narrow at costovertebral junction, then broad).
   3. Lateral view of the thoracolumbar spine is distinctive. There is *a focal kyphosis at the thoracolumbar junction, with an L_1 or L_2 body that is distinctly small, retrolisthesed, and oval in shape with a central anterior beak.*
   4. *AP pelvis demonstrates constricted iliac necks and flared iliac wings.*
   5. *Long bones are shortened,* often with wide metaphyses and diaphyses.
   6. PA view of hands demonstrates *short wide metacarpals, with constricted proximal ends.* The overall appearance is that of a *fan-shaped configuration of the metacarpals.*

C. *Morquio's* syndrome: Treated separately since these patients are *not mentally retarded.* In addition to the osseous abnormalities seen in other mucopolysaccharidoses, they have the following distinctive osseous findings:
   1. *Severe platyspondyly* with anterior beaking of the vertebral bodies.
   2. *Hypoplastic odontoid.*
   3. *Atlantoaxial instability.*
   4. Compression and fragmentation of the femoral capital epiphyses.
   5. Restricted chest wall motion secondary to sternal buckling.

REFERENCES

1. Gold R, Amstutz, H: Surgical procedures for congenital dislocation of the hip. *Radiol Clin North Am* 1975;13:123–137.
2. Morin C, Horcke H, MacEwan G: The infant hip: real-time US assessment of acetabular development. *Radiology* 1985;157:673–677.

3. Eggli K, King S, Boal D, Quirogue T: Low-dose CT of developmental dysplasia of the hip after reduction: diagnostic accuracy and dosimetry. *AJR* 1994;163:1441–1443.

4. Hubbard A, Dormans J: Evaluation of developmental dysplasias, Perthes disease and neuromuscular dysplasia of the hip in children before and after surgery: an imaging update. *AJR* 1995;164:1067–1073.

5. Ozonoff M: *Pediatric orthopedic radiology.* Philadelphia, WB Saunders, 1979.

6. Freiberger R, Hersh A, Harrison M: Roentgen examination of the deformed foot. *Semin Roentgenol* 1970;5:341–353.

7. Koleoyne R, Rych S, Gloeb H: Radiological measurement of congenital and acquired foot deformities. *Applied Radiology* 1993(December volume): 35–41.

8. Hubbard A, Meyer J, Davidson R, Mahboubi S, Hartz M: Relationship between the ossification center and cartilaginous anlage in the normal hindfoot in children: study with imaging. *AJR* 1993;161:849–853.

9. Bailey JA II: *Disproportionate short stature—Diagnosis and Management.* Philadelphia, WB Saunders, 1973.

10. Felson B (ed): Dwarfs and other little people: a roentgen guide. *Semin Roentgenol* 1973;8

11. Greenfield GB: *Radiology of bone diseases,* ed 4. Philadelphia, JB Lippincott, 1986.

12. Spranger JW, Langer LO Jr, Wiedemann HR: *Bone dysplasias: an atlas of constitutional disorders of skeletal development.* Philadelphia, WB Saunders, 1974.

13. Robinow M, Chumlea WC: Standards for limb bone length ratios in children. *Radiology* 1982;143:433–436.

14. Tabyi H. *Radiology of syndromes and metabolic disorders,* ed 2. Chicago, Year Book Medical Publishers, 1983.

15. Wynne-Davis R, Hall CM, Apley AG: *Atlas of skeletal dysplasias.* New York, Churchill Livingstone, 1985.

6

Miscellaneous, Including Hematologic Disorders and Infection

I. HEMATOLOGIC DISORDERS

A. Hemophilia

> **Key Concepts**
>
> Males only are affected; hemarthroses may appear dense; deformities and contractures; arthropathy in knees, elbows, ankles; pseudotumor in femur, pelvis.

A. Definition: A bleeding disorder due to a clotting factor deficiency that results in hemarthroses, deformities, and arthropathy.
B. Epidemiology: The 2 most common varieties are inherited through an X-linked recessive pattern and are, therefore, found only in *males:*
 1. *Hemophilia A (factor VIII).*
 2. *Hemophilia B (factor IX; Christmas disease).*
 3. *von Willebrand's disease* is due to a combined factor VIII deficiency and platelet abnormality and is found in *males or females.*
C. Radiographic abnormalities:
 1. *Hemarthroses:*
  a. Often lead to *flexion contractures* and arthropathy.
  b. May involve multiple joints, but often *asymmetric.*
  c. Joints most commonly involved are *knee, elbow, ankle,* hip, shoulder (in descending order of occurrence).
 2. Arthropathy: Follows multiple episodes of hemarthroses.
  a. *Effusions appear dense* radiographically due to *hemosiderin deposits* in hypertrophied synovium. This hypertrophic synovium is low signal on T1 and intermediate signal on T2 MR imaging.
  b. The synovial inflammation causes *hyperemia,* which in turn causes *osteoporosis, epiphyseal overgrowth* (seen as *flared, enlarged joints,* with gracile diaphyses), and *early epiphyseal fusion* (and resultant short bones).

    c. *Cartilage degeneration, erosions,* and *subarticular cysts* are seen uniformly throughout the joint.

    d. *Secondary degenerative joint disease (DJD)* eventually develops.

    e. Distinctive findings in the *knee* include *widening of the intercondylar notch* and *squaring of the inferior pole of the patella,* but they are not pathognomonic since juvenile rheumatoid arthritis (JRA) may have the same appearance.

    f. Distinctive findings in the *elbow* include an *enlarged radial head* and *enlarged trochlear notch.*

    g. Distinctive findings in the ankle include a nonspecific tibiotalar slant.

3. Pseudotumor:

    a. Due to an *intraosseous, subperiosteal, or soft tissue bleed.*

    b. Occurs most commonly in the *femur, pelvis,* and tibia.

    c. Most commonly appears as *extrinsic and/or intrinsic scalloping and pressure erosion.* The *area of destruction may be extremely large,* but the *margins are generally sclerotic and sharp.*

    d. There *may be a large soft tissue mass,* depending on the site of origin of the bleed. The mass has a hypointense rim on magnetic resonance (MR) due to fibrous structure as well as hemosiderin deposits. The central signal will vary according to the age of the blood and clot contained therein. Usually, many different combinations of signal intensities are seen, reflecting the process of remote and recurrent bleeding as well as clot organization.[1]

    e. *Periosteal reaction* may be extensive.

    f. The size and extent of destruction may simulate neoplasm, but sclerotic margins with both extrinsic and intrinsic scalloping suggest the correct diagnosis.

B. Anemias

Key Concepts

Sickle cell—dactylitis, avascular necrosis (AVN), infarcts, infections; thalassemia—more severe marrow hyperplasia with squared phalanges and "hair-on-end" appearance on skull.

A. Definition: The congenital anemias represent abnormalities in one of the chains comprising hemoglobin that affects the shape and/or function of hemoglobin.

B. Radiographic abnormalities: The following skeletal abnormalities may be found in each of the anemias, but each may be more predictably seen with one in particular:

1. *Marrow hyperplasia* due to long-term anemia: *Osteopenia,* but *coarsened trabeculae, widening of tubular bones and mandible, widened diploic spaces* in the skull.

2. *Infarction* due to vascular occlusion: *Dactylitis* (hand-foot syndrome) due to infarcts in the small tubular bones of the hands and feet, where hematopoietic marrow is persistent and digits are unprotected from *vasoconstriction due to ambient cold. Periosteal reaction and soft tissue swelling occur,* and the entity is *often confused with osteomyelitis.*

   a. *Diaphyseal infarcts:* Patchy sclerosis or serpiginous calcified density with occasional periosteal reaction.

   b. *Vertebral body end-plate infarcts:* Pattern is different, depending on type of anemia (see C, below).

   c. *AVN:* Especially femoral and humeral heads; often bilateral.

3. Predilection for *osteomyelitis,* often indistinguishable from infarction. *Staphylococcus* is the most common organism, but *Salmonella* osteomyelitis is seen much more often in the anemias than in the normal population.

C. Features of the various anemias:

   1. *Sickle cell (Hb SS):*

      a. Found in 1% of North American blacks.

      b. *Dactylitis* is very common (10% to 20% of children with sickle cell disease).

      c. *AVN* is extremely common.

      d. Necrosis of *vertebral body* end-plates is described as *H-shaped* and is due to the distribution of small vessel arcades in which the sickled cells "sludge."

      e. Other radiographic findings include *renal papillary necrosis, cholelithiasis, splenic infarction, cardiomegaly,* and *pulmonary infarction.*

   2. Sickle cell trait (Hb AS): Very few musculoskeletal findings, only an occasional bone infarct.

   3. Sickle cell hemoglobin C (Hb SC): Marrow hyperplasia of the skull and avascular necrosis predominate; splenomegaly.

   4. *Thalassemia* (Cooley's anemia):

      a. Thalassemia major manifests early, and death usually occurs by young adulthood.

      b. *Marrow hyperplasia* is spectacular, with dense striations in a very widened diploic space (hair-on-end); obliteration of paranasal sinuses; Erlenmeyer flask deformity; squared phalanges.

      c. AVN much less common than in sickle cell disease.

5. Sickle cell thalassemia: Ranges from asymptomatic to typical sickle cell manifestations (infarcts overshadow hyperplastic marrow changes).

II. MARROW

Key Concepts

Conversion of red to yellow marrow occurs normally during growth and development, and has a predictable pattern; a neonate has almost entirely red marrow; distribution of red marrow differs in each skeletal site and changes with age at different rates at the different sites.

A. Generally, progressive conversion to fatty marrow occurs from the peripheral (appendicular) toward the central (axial) skeleton.
1. Terminal phalanges convert first.
2. In long bones, conversion begins in the diaphysis and progresses to the distal ends.
3. Conversion to fatty marrow is mostly complete by age 25, when red marrow remains only in the axial skeleton and proximal humeri and proximal femurs (except the proximal epiphyses, which are fatty).
4. Women often retain residual spotty red marrow in the femurs, likely related to the demands of menstruation.
5. With further aging beyond age 25, there is a slower continuation of the fatty conversion process; by the eighth decade, the pedicles and posterior elements have fatty marrow.
B. Fatty marrow is quite labile and reconverts with any stress for hematopoiesis.
1. Reconversion begins in the spine and flat bones and can be spotty or complete, especially in the femurs and humeri (including the proximal humeral epiphysis) and is often seen incidentally in MR exams.[2,3,4]
2. Conditions in which one sees marrow reconversion include anemias (hemolytic, chronic disease, chronic blood loss), smoking,[5] hypoventilation hypoxia, poorly compensated heart disease, AIDS, "sports anemia" (marathon runners).[6]
3. Pathologic processes mimicking reconversion: Polycythemia vera, osteomyelitis, hemochromatosis, amyloidosis, Gaucher's, lymphoma, myelofibrosis, myeloma, metastases.
4. One hint for differentiating infiltrative marrow pathology from hematopoietic marrow in the spine on MR: at T1-weighted SE imaging, marrow signal alteration that is less than skeletal muscle or

normal disk, should not be attributed to hematopoietic marrow alone; exceptions to this include TR weighting that is greater than 700 ms (not a true T1), infants, and patients with profound anemia (sickle cell, bone marrow transplant, and transfused AIDS patients).

C. Evaluation of marrow after treatment can be extremely complex.
   1. Some chemotherapeutic agents may stimulate red marrow conversion.
   2. Even after irradiation of osseous tumor by therapy, marrow may retain abnormal signal of tumor for an undetermined amount of time.
   3. After bone marrow transplant, marrow regeneration in vertebral bodies appears to have a T1-weighted MR pattern showing a peripheral zone of intermediate signal intensity and central zone of bright signal intensity, with the peripheral zone relating to regenerating hematopoietic cells.[7]
   4. After radiation, normal bone containing hematopoietic marrow (spine and pelvis in adults) shows cell death and conversion to fatty marrow as early as 8 days post-treatment and complete replacement by 8 weeks.[8]

III. INFECTION

Key Concepts

Osteomyelitis may appear extremely aggressive, simulating neoplasm. Soft tissue planes often are obliterated. Osteomyelitis in infants may involve the epiphyses. It is metaphyseal in children; radiographic changes lag behind clinical findings. Septic joints must be proven emergently by aspiration.

A. *Organisms:*
   1. Overall, *Staphylococcus aureus* is by far the most common organism.
   2. In *neonates, group B Streptococcus* is more common.
   3. *Drug abusers* have increased incidence of *Pseudomonas* and *Serratia* osteomyelitis compared to the rest of the population; even in this group, *Staphylococcus* is still the most common organism.
   4. *Sickle cell* patients have an increased incidence of *Salmonella* osteomyelitis, but *Staphylococcus* is most common in this group as well.
   5. Tuberculosis and syphilis, which are of radiographic interest as separate entities, are discussed in F1 and F2 below.
B. Osteomyelitis: *Routes of involvement.*
   1. *Direct penetrating wound.*

2. *Contiguous spread* from soft tissue to periosteum and subsequent bone involvement. Some areas are particularly at risk:
   a. Metacarpals and phalanges (as well as metacarpophalangeal [MCP] and proximal interphalangeal [PIP] joints) from a human bite (most often from punching an adversary in the mouth).
   b. A felon (infection in the terminal pulp of the digit) may progress to osteomyelitis of the tuft.
   c. In the hand, soft tissue infection may spread along tendon sheaths and fascial planes, so the site of bone involvement may be distant from an initial injury.
   d. Decubiti in bedridden or paraplegic patients often result in osteomyelitis, especially of the sacrum and ischial tuberosities.
   e. Ulcers on the feet of diabetics are discussed in F3, below.
   f. A stubbed toe with a nail bed injury may result in osteomyelitis of the distal phalanx of the hallux since the periosteum is immediately adjacent to the nail bed.

3. *Hematogenous spread:* As is the case with bone tumors, site of bone involvement (both site within the bone and the individual bone) is a major determinant in making the diagnosis of hematogenous osteomyelitis. The site of involvement is strongly influenced by vascular anatomy.
   a. *Infant* (neonate to 12 months): Some metaphyseal vessels penetrate the epiphyseal plate to anastomose with epiphyseal vessels. *Metaphyseal infections,* therefore, *not uncommonly involve the epiphysis and joint* in this age group, *resulting in slipped epiphyses and growth deformity.* It is not uncommon to have *multifocal* sites of involvement in infants, often clinically benign, radiographically simulating metastatic neuroblastoma or an aggressive histiocytosis.
   b. *Child: Terminal vessels* occur as loops with sluggish blood flow *in the metaphyses* and do not cross into the epiphyses. This, combined with a relative *lack of phagocytes* in the metaphyseal region, *leads to the metaphyses being the most common site of infection in the child. Epiphyseal and joint involvement are uncommon, but MR examination often demonstrates extension of infection from the metaphysis into the epiphysis, which may not be suspected from plain film evaluation.* The *tubular bones of the lower extremities* are the most common sites (65% to 75% of childhood osteomyelitis occurs in the metaphyses of the femur or tibia).
   c. *Adult:* With closure of the epiphyseal plate, the terminal metaphyseal vessels anastomose with epiphyseal vessels. Thus *joint involvement secondary to osteomyelitis is more common.* The *spine*

and small bones are more commonly involved than tubular bones.

C. Osteomyelitis: Radiographic appearance varies depending on the clinical course of the infection.

  1. *Acute osteomyelitis:*

     a. Radiographic change lags behind onset of infection by 1 to 2 weeks. *First sign* is *blurring* or *obliteration of soft tissue fat planes.* This may be an important differential point since fat planes are often retained but displaced by soft tissue tumor.

     b. Soft tissue changes are followed by *intramedullary destruction,* often in an extremely subtle permeative pattern that may appear only as a focal decrease in density. If this permeative pattern is serpiginous, it assures the diagnosis of osteomyelitis.

     c. This is followed by *cortical destruction, endosteal scalloping,* and *periosteal reaction* (expected by 2 weeks).

     d. These initial bone changes appear highly aggressive and may be difficult to differentiate from tumor. Knowing the time course of the disease may be helpful since an acute osteomyelitis may cause destructive changes more rapidly than does tumor.

     e. Eventually, a *sequestrum and involucrum* may develop. A sequestrum is necrotic bone isolated from living bone by granulation tissue; it appears relatively dense because it has no blood supply while the surrounding bone is hyperemic and loses its mineralization. A sequestrum may harbor bacteria, leading to chronic osteomyelitis. An involucrum develops secondary to lifting of the periosteum by the abscess and subsequent reactive new bone formation and is living normal bone that envelopes the sequestrum. Involucrum formation is more common in children than adults since the periosteum is relatively loosely attached at the metaphysis, allowing easier periosteal elevation to initiate the formation of the host bone reaction.

  2. Subacute osteomyelitis: *Brodie's abscess.*

     a. Usually found in the *metaphysis of a child.*

     b. A lucent focus of osteomyelitis *sharply delineated* by a *sclerotic margin.*

     c. Therefore, appears much less aggressive than acute osteomyelitis.

     d. Clinically it is also less distinctive, often without fever or elevated sedimentation rate.

     e. The diagnosis may therefore be difficult, with the *differential* including *eosinophilic granuloma* and other benign metaphyseal lesions.

     f. *Occasionally,* a Brodie's abscess is *cortically based, eliciting more sclerosis* and periosteal reaction. The *differential* diagnosis in this situation may include *osteoid osteoma and subacute stress fracture.*

3. *Chronic osteomyelitis:*
   a. *More host reaction,* often with thickened cortices and variable sites of lucency and density; *may have sequestra* present.
   b. *Plain film appearance may not change* for a period of several years, *yet may reactivate.*
   c. Evaluate by watching for change in osteolysis or development of periosteal reaction. If no radiographic change is seen in a patient who clinically suggests reactivation of chronic osteomyelitis, *nuclear medicine studies* are indicated (see D4, below).

D. Osteomyelitis: Diagnostic difficulties.
   1. Differentiation of osteomyelitis from aggressive lytic tumor may be difficult since the nature of destructive pattern or periosteal reaction is not pathognomonic. Soft tissue characteristics may be useful.
   2. Patients on partial antibiotic therapy may have delayed radiographic changes.
   3. Diagnosing infection in total knee arthroplasties (TKAs) is notoriously difficult since radiographic change is seldom seen. The physician should be very cautious about diagnosing absence of infection in TKA.
   4. Other modalities may be useful in the diagnosis of osteomyelitis and should be tailored to the individual needs of the case.
      a. Tomography may be useful in identifying sequestra for surgical resection.
      b. CT findings usually mirror those of the plain film: Destructive bone changes, sometimes with serpiginous tracking, are seen. Soft tissue fat planes are obliterated. Soft tissue abnormality often involves several muscle groups and is less discrete than many soft tissue tumor masses. Contrast enhancement is usually nonuniform and often forms a swirling pattern through the soft tissue mass, with an enhancing rim.
      c. Radionuclide studies:
         (1) 99mTc-MDP bone scans: In adults, highly sensitive in detecting early occult osteomyelitis; in children, perfectly symmetric position for side-to-side comparison, as well as pinhole collimators allow differentiation of metaphyseal osteomyelitis from the normal increased uptake in the metaphyseal-epiphyseal growth centers. Specificity is not as good as sensitivity in bone scans, but a 3- or 4-phase technique (perfusion, blood pool, bone uptake, and, sometimes, 24-hour images) increase the specificity. Increasing lesion-

to-background ratios make osteomyelitis more likely than cellulitis.

(2) Both ^{67}Ga and ^{111}In white blood cell (WBC) imaging improve specificity (75% to 85%)[9,10] but at the cost of delaying the diagnosis.

d. MR[11]:

(1) Osteomyelitis: STIR and T1 MR imaging are highly sensitive, as is T1 with contrast; specificity is more limited.

(2) Soft tissue abscesses: Contrast-enhanced T1 imaging is highly sensitive for abscesses, showing rim enhancement around low signal fluid; the contrast enhances conspicuity between the abscess and surrounding edema; the appearance is not specific: ruptured popliteal cyst, phlegmon, posttraumatic seroma, and necrotic tumors may give the same rim-enhancing appearance.

E. Complications of osteomyelitis.

1. Chronic osteomyelitis with exacerbations.

2. Slipped epiphyses and deformity.

3. Joint involvement and eventual osteoarthritis.

4. Amyloid deposit in chronic active lesion;

5. Squamous cell carcinoma developing in a chronic draining sinus tract, usually 10 to 20 years following development of chronic osteomyelitis.

F. Special cases of osteomyelitis.

1. *Tuberculosis* (TB):

a. Tends to have a *slower course* and *less host reaction* than pyogenic osteomyelitis. In this appearance, it is similar to many fungal infections.

b. TB dactylitis (*spina ventosa*) is an unusual manifestation seen in the tubular bones of the hands and feet, usually in children; may be multifocal. Radiographic characteristics are soft tissue swelling with periostitis followed by expansion of the bone. Differential diagnosis includes JRA, sickle cell dactylitis, and other infections.

2. *Syphilis* osteomyelitis.

a. *Congenital:* Initially demonstrates *metaphyseal irregularity* and a widened zone of provisional calcification, occasionally resulting in slipped epiphyses. May progress to invade the diaphysis and elicit *periosteal reaction.* Congenital syphilis is in the extensive differential for infants with periosteal reaction, including nonaccidental trauma, tumor, other infections, and metabolic diseases.

b. *Acquired* (not distinguishable from reactivated congenital syphilis): This chronic osteomyelitis elicits a periostitis and endosteal reaction which result in an *enlarged, bowed bone with mixed lytic and sclerotic areas.* In the tibia, the bow is anterior and is called a *saber shin* deformity. This differs from Paget's disease of the tibia since syphilis is diaphyseal and rarely involves the subarticular region of the bone. Flat bones and cranium may also be involved in syphilis osteomyelitis.

   c. Another manifestation of syphilis is neuropathic joints, especially knees (see Chapter 3).

3. Osteomyelitis in the diabetic foot.
   a. Ulcerations and underlying osteopenia make the diagnosis of acute osteomyelitis difficult since early findings of osteomyelitis consist of soft tissue abnormality and decreased bone density. Therefore, there is heavy reliance on periosteal reaction, cortical destruction, and progression on serial films.
   b. Diabetics also often have neuropathic joints (most commonly the talonavicular and tarsometatarsal joints). This process results in cortical destruction, fragmentation, loss of cartilage, and effusion—findings that, in other joints, are suggestive of infection.
   c. Radionuclide studies or MR with contrast may be very useful.

4. *Pin tract osteomyelitis.*
   a. Suspect with an enlarging lucency adjacent to a pin and associated periosteal reaction.
   b. If a lucency about the pin is due only to motion of the pin, the lucency is usually uniform and well-marginated.
   c. A *ring sequestrum* (a dense ring of sclerotic bone surrounded by irregular lucent destruction) is diagnostic of osteomyelitis in a pin tract.

G. *Septic arthritis.*
   1. Radiographic signs in bacterial septic arthritis:
      a. *Joint effusion* is first sign.
      b. Hyperemia leads to *osteoporosis.*
      c. Cartilage destruction with *decreasing joint space.*
      d. *Bone erosion* and destruction follow rapidly.
      e. Osteomyelitis may develop via contiguous spread.
      f. *Sclerotic* host *reaction.*
      g. Ankylosis may occur eventually.
   2. *TB* and *fungal septic arthritis.*
      a. *Little* or no host bone *reaction.*
      b. *Cartilage destruction* is much *slower.*
      c. *Slow progression of erosions,* often without other abnormalities.
      d. Hip and knee are most common areas of involvement, followed by wrist and elbow.
   3. Radionuclide studies may be helpful, but joint aspiration more

quickly assures the diagnosis. Note that a prior aspiration, with or without the use of radiographic contrast material, does not alter bone scan results.[12]

H. Special considerations in diagnosing septic arthritis.
  1. *Hip in childhood:*
     a. Common site of septic arthritis since the hematogenous focus of infection in the metaphysis is within the hip joint capsule.
     b. Soft tissue signs of effusion (bulging psoas, gluteal, and obturator internus fat planes) are of limited usefulness since they may be false-positive with any pelvic rotation or flexion or rotation of the hip.
     c. Inducing an *air arthrogram* with traction on the hip rules out an effusion.
     d. *Increased teardrop* distance is more reliable evidence of hip effusion.
     e. *Hip aspiration* may require injection of 5 to 10 ml nonbacteriostatic saline and reaspiration. A small amount of contrast material confirms needle position in joint.
     f. *Differential diagnosis* of septic arthritis in the juvenile hip is extensive, including *transient synovitis, hemarthrosis* due to trauma or hemophilia, *JRA* and *early Legg-Calvé-Perthe's disease.*
  2. *Arthroplasties:*
     a. Infection is difficult to differentiate from simple loosening. Lucency at the prosthesis or cement-bone interface is seen in either case.
     b. *Periosteal reaction* and *heterotopic bone* formation are more suggestive of an infected arthroplasty.
     c. Aspiration with culture should be a part of all arthrograms of prosthetic joints.
  3. *Sacroiliac (SI) joint* septic arthritis:
     a. Radiographic feature is *widening* of the SI joint with *indistinct cortices.* (Note that wide SI joints are normal in adolescents.)
     b. Overlying bowel gas and the overlapped configuration of the joint may make plain film diagnosis difficult.
     c. *CT* may be particularly useful since it demonstrates the widened joint, cortical erosions, and a soft tissue mass or psoas abscess. The differentiation of nonseptic arthritides or other causes of unilateral SI joint abnormalities is much easier with CT or MR images.
  4. *Sternoclavicular* septic arthritis:
     a. The major differential diagnosis of a mass at the sternoclavicular junction is dislocation and septic arthritis (often in drug users).

    b. *CT* limited to a few axial images through the joint will very clearly define erosion involving both sides of the joint and a soft tissue mass, easily differentiating septic arthritis from dislocation.

I. *Infection of the spine.*

  1. Pertinent anatomy: *Veins of Batson* provide communication between the pelvic and thoracolumbar venous systems; thus, genitourinary (GU) infections are a frequent source of spine infection.

  2. Despite the frequent GU source, *Staphylococcus aureus* is still the most common infecting organism.

  3. Radiographic appearance:

    a. The infection starts in the subchondral portion of the body, then extends to the disk and adjacent vertebral end-plate.

    b. Radiographic changes are relatively late (2 to 8 weeks).

    c. Pathognomonic appearance therefore is two *adjacent end-plate abnormalities* (irregularity and loss of cortex) *with decrease in height of the corresponding disk.* A paravertebral mass or displaced psoas may be seen, especially by CT or MR. Later, a sclerotic host reaction may evolve.

  4. *TB of the spine (Pott's disease):*

    a. Usually there is pulmonary TB.

    b. Tends to involve the *thoracolumbar junction* and, late in the disease, may cause an acute *angular kyphosis* (gibbus).

    c. Features that favor the diagnosis include *slow progression,* with *preservation of disk height* and lack of sclerotic response.

    d. May develop a *calcified psoas abscess.*

  5. *Discitis:*

    a. A less significant, often *self-limited,* disk infection in *skeletally immature* patients.

    b. Probably a direct hematogenous infection of the disk.

    c. Present with back pain, low-grade fever, elevated sedimentation rate; often there is a preexisting minor infection (e.g., upper respiratory).

    d. Radiographic changes are delayed but include *decrease in disk height, end-plate irregularities,* and *eburnation.* Paravertebral *soft tissue mass is minimal.*

    e. Bone scan demonstrates abnormality earlier than plain film.

    f. *Organisms are often not cultured,* either from blood culture or percutaneous biopsy. When proven, it is usually *Staphylococcus aureus.* At some institutions, these patients are treated empirically for *Staphylococcus* infection.

  6. *Discogenic sclerosis* (idiopathic segmental sclerosis):

    a. A *degenerative change that may mimic a disk space infection.*

b. Degenerative disk leads to *decreased disk height.* Occasionally disk height is not decreased. Adjacent vertebral end-plates are smooth (except in the presence of a Schmorl's node—intravertebral disk herniation) *but sclerotic;* end-plate *sclerosis is often triangular in shape and may be limited to the anterior aspect of the upper involved vertebral body.*

c. No progression (and even occasional resolution) with time.

J. AIDS: Musculoskeletal[13]:

1. Lymphoma.
2. Kaposi sarcoma—bone or soft tissue.
3. Bacillary angiomatosis—multifocal bacterial infection that may produce osteolytic lesions with mass and periosteal reaction.
4. Low signal marrow—anemia of chronic disease.
5. Arthritis—especially psoriatic and Reiter's.
6. Infection—common or opportunistic.
7. Myositis—either septic or aseptic; contrast MR should differentiate.
8. Secondary hypertrophic osteoarthropathy.

IV. SARCOIDOSIS

Key Concepts

Lytic lesions with lacy trabeculae (usually in phalanges) or focal sclerotic lesions. Generally, if bone lesions are present, lung and skin abnormalities are as well.

A. Definition: A systemic granulomatous disorder; osseous involvement 1% to 15%.[14] If bone lesions are present, skin lesions usually are also (90%). Lung abnormalities (hilar adenopathy, pulmonary infiltrates, fibrosis, and apical bullous disease) are also usually present (80% to 90%). Nodular liver disease with hepatosplenomegaly may be present, as may ocular abnormalities (uveitis, iritis).

B. Epidemiology:
1. Young adults.
2. No sex predominance.
3. Blacks affected much more frequently than Caucasians or Asians.

C. Osseous manifestations: There are several very different appearances:
1. Generalized osteopenia.
2. Lytic lesions with lacy trabeculae, usually in middle or distal phalanges.
3. Sclerosis of tufts may occur.
4. Focal or generalized sclerosis.

5. Polyarticular arthralgias, usually without radiographic abnormalities but occasionally with nonspecific erosive arthritic changes.
D. Differential diagnoses:
   1. For lytic phalangeal lesions:
      a. Enchondroma.
      b. Brown tumor.
      c. Tuberous sclerosis.
   2. For lytic or sclerotic lesions at other sites:
      a. Paget's disease.
      b. Metastases.
      c. Myelofibrosis.
      d. Mastocytosis
E. Muscular sarcoidosis[15] is common, but rarely symptomatic:
   1. Early myosotic type is controlled by steroids and is negative on MR.
   2. Chronic myopathic type shows nonspecific atrophy on MR.
   3. Nodular type (palpable mass) is least common; on MR may have a central low signal on T1 as well as T2 due to fibrous scar, surrounded by nonspecific low signal on T1 and high signal on T2.

V. RADIATION-INDUCED ABNORMALITIES*

A. Growth disorders: Depends on site of radiation:
   1. Epiphyseal fusion and limb-length discrepancy.
   2. Scoliosis (if entire vertebral body is not included in the field).
   3. Iliac wing hypoplasia.
B. Radiation osteonecrosis:
   1. May appear aggressive (simulating tumor).
   2. Weakens the bone, allowing pathologic fractures.
   3. Avascular necrosis.
   4. Radiation causes early cell death and conversion of red marrow to fatty marrow (begins 8 days posttherapy). See Chapter 6, Section II, Marrow.
C. Neoplasm:
   1. Exostosis.
   2. Leukemia.
   3. Degeneration to osteosarcoma, chondrosarcoma, or malignant fibrous histiocytoma.
D. More prone to infection than normal bone.

VI. ACRO-OSTEOLYSIS

A. Definition: Lysis of the distal aspects of the phalanges, with a wide range of etiologies.

---

* See also radiation therapy section in Introduction to Chapter 1.

B. Gamut.
  1. Thermal injury.
    a. Burn: May have associated soft tissue contracture.
    b. Frostbite: Characteristically, the thumb is spared. In children, the distal epiphyses are most at risk and may either resorb or become sclerotic.
  2. Environmental: Polyvinylchloride (PVC) exposure causes acro-osteolysis. The most characteristic pattern is a lucent transverse zone across the proximal to middle aspect of the distal phalanges.
  3. Metabolic:
    a. Hyperparathyroidism: Tuft resorption, often accompanied by other signs such as subperiosteal resorption, vascular calcification, or Brown tumors.
    b. Lesch-Nyhan disease.
  4. Arthritis:
    a. Psoriatic: There should be associated DIP and carpal erosive disease.
    b. Neuroarthropathy, especially diabetic.
  5. Connective tissue disease:
    a. Scleroderma: Often associated soft tissue calcification.
    b. Other causes of vasculitis.
  6. Infection: Leprosy: May see associated linear calcification of a digital nerve.
  7. Congenital:
    a. Pyknodysostosis: Associated dense bones with transverse fractures.
    b. Hajdu-Cheney: Familial disorder with acro-osteolysis pattern identical to that of PVC, associated with osteoporosis and multiple facial and cranial abnormalities.

VII. PERIOSTEAL REACTION IN INFANTS

Key Concepts

Age at onset may be useful in diagnosis; must remember to consider nonaccidental trauma (battered child syndrome) as a common cause.

A. *Onset prior to age 6 months:*
  1. *Infantile cortical hyperostosis* (Caffey's disease):
    a. Onset early, occasionally at birth.
    b. Clinical findings: Fever, *hyperirritability,* and soft tissue swelling (reflects the periosteal reaction of underlying bone).

    c. Usually self-limited but may persist, leading to a delay in musculoskeletal development.

    d. X-ray findings:

        (1) *Involves mandible, clavicles,* ribs, scapulae, cranium, and tubular bones, often sequentially.

        (2) The mandibular and clavicular involvement are important findings since they are generally not present in infant periosteal reaction of other etiologies.

        (3) Cortical hyperostosis may be marked, sometimes with osseous bridging.

        (4) No metaphyseal abnormalities.

  2. *Physiologic periosteal new bone:*

    a. Occurs in 35% of infants after 1 month of age.

    b. Bilateral, in long tubular bones.

    c. Incorporated into cortex by age 6 months.

    d. Diagnosis of exclusion.

  3. Extracorporeal membrane oxygenation in neonates may result in significant soft tissue swelling at the ribs and subsequent periosteal reaction.[16]

B. *Onset after age 6 months:*

  1. *Hypervitaminosis A.*

    a. Cortical thickening of tubular bones, most commonly the ulna; wavy or undulating pattern.

    b. Metaphyseal cupping, most commonly distal femurs, may result in coned epiphyses.

    c. Findings of increased intracranial pressure.

    d. Child may be extremely irritable.

  2. *Scurvy or rickets* may show periosteal reaction secondary to a metaphyseal corner fracture and subperiosteal bleed. Prior to 6 months they occur only in the severely stressed premature infant.

C. *Onset at any time during infancy:*

  1. Trauma: *Nonaccidental trauma* is a common occurrence and may be radiographically manifest solely by periosteal reaction (for a more complete description of this entity, see the section of the handbook on trauma).

  2. *Infection:* Many pathogens may be involved, but congenital syphilis should especially be considered.

    a. Osteochondritis with widened zone of provisional calcification and metaphyseal irregularity in tubular bones and costochondral junctions seen in fetus and neonate.

    b. Diaphyseal osteomyelitis: A later change, seen with inadequate therapy.

    c. Periostitis: Widespread and symmetric.

3. Periosteal response to *tumor*.
   a. Neuroblastoma metastasis: Generally metaphyseal permeative change, but periosteal reaction may be the first manifestation.
   b. Periostitis in acute childhood *leukemia*.
      (1) Leukemia may have a paucity of clinical signs.
      (2) Arthralgias and arthritis are common (12% to 65%) and may be the presenting symptom.
      (3) Periostitis seen in 10% to 35%, due to invasion of subperiosteum by tumor, elevating the periosteum.
      (4) Especially prominent in the terminal phalanges.
4. Prostaglandin administration may cause periosteal reaction.
5. Sickle cell dactylitis (infarcts, generally in the phalanges, with associated periosteal reaction).
6. In patients past infancy JRA should be considered since periostitis, especially of the phalanges, is a common feature of that disease process.
7. "Wavy" radius is a normal variant that simulates periosteal reaction.

VIII. LOCALIZED GIANTISM

A. Definition: Overgrowth of both osseous and soft tissues localized to a few digits.
B. *Neurofibromatosis* may have an associated dysplasia causing localized giantism.
C. *Hypervascularity* (as from an arteriovenous malformation) is a second common cause of localized giantism; another is lymphangiomatosis.
D. *Macrodystrophia lipomatosa* is a rare cause of localized giantism of unknown etiology; it is identified pathologically by a disproportionate increase in adipose tissue and osteoblasts lining the periosteum. Second and third digits of the lower extremity are the most common sites.
E. *Klippel-Trenaunay-Weber syndrome* is another rare etiology of localized giantism. It is associated with cutaneous capillary hemangioma and varicose veins. Giantism is attributed to the abnormal vascular supply. Phleboliths may be present.

IX. SOFT TISSUE CALCIFICATION GAMUT

Key Concepts

Presumes normal underlying bone. Excludes vascular calcification and chondrocalcinosis. Details of each entity are discussed in separate chapters.

A. Trauma:
  1. Myositis ossificans: Has a characteristic zoning phenomenon and timing of appearance and maturation.
  2. Burns: Contractures often are associated.
  3. Frostbite.
  4. Head injury.
  5. Paraplegia or quadriplegia.
  6. Hydroxyapatite crystal deposition disease, especially calcific bursitis or tendinitis.
B. Tumor: Any soft tissue tumor may have dystrophic calcification but those most commonly considered include:
  1. Synovial cell sarcoma.
  2. Liposarcoma.
  3. Soft tissue osteosarcoma.
  4. Fibrosarcoma or malignant fibrous histiocytoma.
C. Collagen vascular diseases:
  1. Scleroderma: Calcification is usually subcutaneous, may be widespread; usually other changes of scleroderma are present.
  2. Dermatomyositis: Sheetlike calcification in muscle or fascial planes are described, but other calcification patterns are seen as well.
  3. Systemic lupus erythematosus: Calcification is uncommon but certainly may occur, even in the absence of renal disease.
  4. CREST syndrome—calcinosis cutis, Raynaud's, scleroderma, and telangiectasis.
  5. Calcinosis cutis.
D. Congenital:
  1. Tumoral calcinosis: Periarticular.
  2. Myositis ossificans progressiva: Often axial, bridging bones of the thorax.
  3. Pseudohypoparathyroidism and pseudopseudohypoparathyroidism.
  4. Progeria.
  5. Ehlers-Danlos syndrome.
E. Metabolic:
  1. Hyperparathyroidism, primary or secondary.
  2. Hypoparathyroidism.
  3. Gout.
  4. Renal dialysis sequela: Periarticular calcifications may be very extensive.
F. Infections:
  1. Granulomatous: TB, brucellosis, coccidioidomycosis.
  2. Dystrophic calcification in abscesses.
  3. Leprosy: Digital nerve calcification.
  4. Cysticercosis: Small oval bodies in muscle.

5. Echinococcosis: Usually in liver or bone but occasionally in soft tissues.
G. Drugs:
   1. Hypervitaminosis D.
   2. Milk-alkali syndrome.
H. Miscellaneous conditions:
   1. Synovial chondromatosis.
   2. Weber-Christian disease.

X. MUSCLE (MRI extremely useful, but specificity is limited.)

A. Injury[17]:
   1. STIR sequences are particularly sensitive, T2 slightly less so, and T1 insensitive to injury and edema; T1, however, is sensitive to subacute hematoma and fatty infiltration of muscle.
   2. Spectrum of injury includes rupture, acute strain, delayed onset muscle soreness, and chronic repetitive strain (or overuse)
   3. Clinical evaluation of even complete muscle rupture may be difficult since the defect may be masked by edema or hematoma, or the affected muscle may be deep to intact muscles, or other muscles may be recruited to perform the injured muscle's action; conversely, intact muscles may be functionally impaired by spasm, and weakness may be simply due to pain, spasm, or hematoma.
   4. MR shows edema, as well as the structural integrity of the muscle, musculotendinous unit, tendon, and tendo-osseous junction.
   5. Perifascial fluid collections are common.
   6. The muscle edema pattern may persist for several months following injury, long after the patient is clinically healed.
   7. Fatty infiltration is not common.
   8. Fascial herniation: muscle herniation through fascia may be fixed or intermittent; may present with pain and/or mass; dynamic imaging with isometric contraction of the involved muscle may be required for diagnosis.
B. Muscle metabolism abnormalities:
   1. Usually inherited defects of glycolytic enzyme (for example, McArdle's disease).
   2. Muscle develops a contracture, usually with exquisite pain and rhabdomyalysis.
   3. MR shows myonecrosis and/or fatty infiltration.
   4. Rhabdomyalysis need not be associated with a metabolic or neurologic disorder, but may occur postexertion.
C. Compartment syndrome:
   1. Edema and/or hemorrhage around intact fascial planes, obstructing blood flow to the surrounding muscle.

2. Usually diagnosed by pressure analysis rather than MR; treated by surgical decompression.
3. Exertion-induced chronic compartment syndromes may be evaluated by MR with contrast.

D. Inflammatory myopathies:
1. Polymyositis, dermatomyositis, inclusion body myositis.
2. Inflammatory changes of edema, typically bilateral and symmetric, but sometimes within a single or scattered muscles.

E. Neoplasm:
1. Generally more ''round'' than elongated along the muscle; exception to this is lymphoma, which can infiltrate along the entire muscle.
2. Nonspecific low SI on T1, high SI on T2; may have edema surrounding the tumor, with the margins indistinguishable.

F. Pyomyositis[18,19]:
1. Unusual in the absence of chronic disease such as AIDS, sickle cell, chronic lymphocytic leukemia (CLL), chronic steroid usage, IV drug abuse, diabetes, or antecedent trauma.
2. Abscesses are difficult to distinguish from cellulitis (slightly high or isointense T1, mildly inhomogeneous high SI T2) except with gadolinium, where a high SI rim enhancement surrounds a soft tissue fluid collection if the lesion is an abscess.
3. Such rim enhancement may also be seen in a ruptured popliteal cyst, phlegmon, necrotic tumor, diabetic muscle infarction, and seroma, so is not specific for abscess (though abscess is far more common than the above entities).
4. Ninety percent are due to *S. aureus*.

G. Diabetic muscle infarction:
1. Due to vascular occlusive disease.
2. Clinical presentation is of acute pain and swelling, usually of the thigh; in patients with poorly controlled diabetes who usually already have other organ involvement.
3. MR shows muscle edema, as well as perifascial and subcutaneous tissue edema.
4. Gadolinium may show minimal contrast enhancement due to the vascular insufficiency to the muscle, this may help differentiate diabetic muscle infarction from myositis, pyomyositis, hematoma, neoplasm, and muscle rupture.[20]

XI. PERIPHERAL NERVE ENTRAPMENT

A. Etiologies may be mechanical or dynamic; may be due to tumor, cyst, inflammatory process, trauma (hematoma, myositis, callous formation), edema, or repetitive actions where there is a ''tunnel'' or restricted space.

B. Initial diagnosis is usually made by clinical findings or electromyography; if the diagnosis is difficult, plain film and MR may be requested.

C. Upper extremity[21]:

   1. Suprascapular nerve: Enters the supraspinatus fossa through the scapular notch, making a sharp turn around the scapular spine; branches into supraspinatus and infraspinatus nerves, bridged by ligament; direct trauma, tumors, or cysts may irritate the nerve and result in muscle atrophy (infraspinatus or supraspinatus).

   2. Quadrilateral space syndrome: Compression of axillary nerve in the space formed by the long head of the triceps, teres minor, teres major, and humerus; fracture, mass, extreme abduction of the arm, or hypertrophy of muscle in paraplegics may cause the syndrome, resulting in atrophy of the deltoid and teres minor.

   3. Pronator teres syndrome: Entrapment of the median nerve between the pronator teres and two heads of flexor digitorum superficialis; compression may be due to hematoma, mass, repetitive pronation-supination, Volkmann's contracture, or prolonged external compression (''honeymoon paralysis''); clinically have a motor disturbance of the first three fingers and sensory abnormality of the palm of the hand.

   4. Supinator muscle syndrome: Posterior interosseous nerve (the deep branch of the radial nerve) is compressed as it passes under the tendinous arch of the supinator muscle.

   5. Cubital tunnel syndrome: Compression of the ulnar nerve as it passes through the fibro-osseous tunnel at the posteromedial part of the elbow, or one centimeter distally where it crosses beneath the arcuate ligament.

   6. Carpal tunnel: Median nerve compression within the tunnel formed by the carpal bones and flexor retinaculum, which also contains multiple tendons.

   7. Guyon's canal syndrome: The ulnar nerve passes outside the carpal tunnel, but through Guyon's canal (bordered by the pisiform, flexor retinaculum, and palmar carpal ligament); may have sensory or motor loss or combination, involving the fourth and fifth fingers.

D. Lower extremity:

   1. Be sure to distinguish between radiculopathy and peripheral neuropathy and to exclude systemic causes such as vasculitis or diabetes (the most common cause of lumbosacral plexus neuropathy).

   2. Sensory deficit may be subtle, and motor deficits occur late.

   3. Femoral nerve: Usually proximal to the inguinal ligament.

   4. Obturator neuropathy: Usually either intrapelvic or at the pubis.

5. Sciatic: Most commonly at sciatic notch.
6. Pyriformis syndrome: Pain and paresthesias in buttocks from sciatic nerve compression as it courses under the pyriformis (or through it in the event of anatomic variation).
7. Common peroneal nerve: Usually due to cysts or trauma, with entrapment between the two heads of the peroneal muscle.
8. Tarsal tunnel: Posterior tibial nerve as it courses between the flexor retinaculum and calcaneus, causes paresthesias along the plantar aspect of the foot and toes.
9. Morton's neuroma: Not a true neuroma, but a fibrous degeneration surrounding an interdigital nerve, usually on the plantar aspect of the foot between the second and third metatarsal heads; the nerve is compressed under the deep transverse metatarsal ligament; high-heeled shoes predispose. Gadolinium contrast injection is often required for MR diagnosis.

REFERENCES

1. Wilson D, Prince J: MR imaging of hemophilic pseudotumors. *AJR* 1988; 150:349–350.
2. Deutsch A, Mink J, Rosenfelt F, Waxman A: Incidental detection of hematopoietic hyperplasia on routine knee MR imaging. *AJR* 1989;152:333–336.
3. Mirowitz S: Hematopoietic bone marrow within the proximal humeral epiphysis in normal adults. Investigation with MR imaging. *Radiology* 1993; 188:689–693.
4. Richardson M, Palten R: Age-related changes in marrow distribution in the shoulder: MR imaging findings. *Radiology* 1994;192:209–215.
5. Poulton T, Murphy W, Dvark J, Chapek C, Feiglin D: Bone marrow reconversion in adults who are smokers: MR imaging findings. *AJR* 1993;161: 1217–1221.
6. Shellock F, Morris E, Deutsch A, Mink J, Kerr R, Boden S: Hematopoietic bone marrow hyperplasia: high prevalence on MR images of the knee in asymptomatic marathon runners. *AJR* 1992;158:335–338.
7. Stevens S, Moore S, Amylon M: Repopulation of marrow after transplantation: MR imaging with pathologic correlation. *Radiology* 1990;175:213–218.
8. Blomlie V, Rofstad E, Skjonsberg A, Tvera K, Lien H: Female pelvic bone marrow: serial MR imaging before, during, and after radiation therapy. *Radiology* 1995;194:537–543.
9. Al-Sheikh W, Sfakionalis, G, Mnaymneh W, et al: Subacute and chronic bone infections: diagnosis using In-111, Ga-67, and Tc-99m bone scintigraphy, and radiography. *Radiology* 1985;155:501–506.
10. Alazraki N, Fierer J, Resnick D: Chronic osteomyelitis monitoring by Tc-99m phosphate and Ga-67 citrate imaging. *Am J Roentgenol* 1985;145: 767–771.
11. Hopkins K, Li K, Bergman G: Gadolinium DTPA enhanced magnetic reso-

nance imaging of musculoskeletal infectious processes. *Skeletal Radiol* 1995;24:324–330.

12. Traughber P, Manaster B, Murphy K, et al: Negative bone scans of joints after aspiration and/or contrast arthrography: experimental studies. *Am J Roentgenol* 1986;146:87–92.

13. Steinbach L, Tehranzadeh J, Fleckenstein J, Vanarthos W, Pais M: Human immunodeficiency virus infection: musculoskeletal manifestations. *Radiology* 1993;186:833–838.

14. Sartoris D, Resnick D, Resnick C, et al: Musculoskeletal manifestations of sarcoidosis. *Semin Roentgenol* 1985;20:376–386.

15. Matsuo M, Ehara S, Tomakawa Y, Chida E, Nischida J, Sugai T: Muscular sarcoidosis. *Skeletal Radiol* 1995;24:535–537.

16. Feinstein K, Fernbach S: Periosteal reaction of the ribs in neonates treated with extracorporeal membrane oxygenation: prevalence and association with soft tissue swelling. *AJR* 1993;160:587–589.

17. Fleckenstein J: Role of MRI in clinical evaluation of muscle injuries. *The Radiologist* 1995;2(6):343–353.

18. Hopkins K, King C, Bergman G: Gadolinium DTPA enhanced magnetic resonance imaging of musculoskeletal infective processes. *Skeletal Radiol* 1995;24:325–330.

19. Gordon B, Martinez S, Collins A: Pyomyositis: characteristics at CT and MR imaging. *Radiology* 1995;197:279–286.

20. Chason D, Fleckenstein J, Burns D, Rojas G: Diabetic muscle infarction: radiologic evaluation. *Skeletal Radiol* 1996;25:127–132.

21. Beltran J, Rosenberg Z: Diagnosis of compressive and entrapment neuropathies of the upper extremity: value of MR imaging. *AJR* 1994;163: 525–531.

Index